BIRTH ~~CARE~~ ABUSE

Beverley Chalmers (DSc (Med); PhD)
and
Dana Solomon (PhD)

Grosvenor House
Publishing Limited

This book is published by
Grosvenor House Publishing Ltd
Link House
140 The Broadway, Tolworth, Surrey, KT6 7HT.
www.grosvenorhousepublishing.co.uk

A CIP record for this book
is available from the British Library

Paperback ISBN 978-1-83615-634-5

Dedication

For Bernie

With love, respect and admiration. Thank you for over fifty-five wonderful years. And for three amazing daughters.

For Carmen, Dana, and Tandy

Thank you for giving us a lifetime of pleasure and pride.

For Pearce, Addison, Sadie, Alex, and Aston

May your lives be filled with love, and with respectful care.

For my late father, Dr. "Punny" Wolfowitz

Who provided a professional model that inspired me.

Acknowledgements

Dr. Chalmers

This book is an amalgamation and culmination of over fifty years of work dedicated to mothers, newborns, families, and care providers. It highlights the extent and nature of the many failings of obstetric care, that do not live up to the ideal of respectful care, and may also perpetrate significant harm and abuse against women, parents, babies, and families.

Some of the ideas in this book were initially included in, *Family-Centred Perinatal Care: Improving Pregnancy, Birth and Postpartum Care* (2017)[1] published by Cambridge University Press and presented as a formal academic/educational text for health care providers. I appreciate Cambridge University Press's permission to reformulate the text with a focus on obstetric abuse. I am immensely grateful to my daughter, Dr. Dana Solomon, for her astute contributions to the text and for her considerable editing and manuscript preparation skills. She, as the director of D-Editions, has served as an outstanding, knowledgeable, critical, and supportive editor of most of my books.

I am indebted to the multiple academics who have walked these paths before me and who have inspired my work, assisted me in many endeavours, and contributed to my knowledge and writing in this field over many decades. Most have contributed to my thinking through their academic writings, but many have mentored me in-person, by working alongside me over many years, supporting, instructing and encouraging me, or by facilitating my work significantly, including Dr. Marsden Wagner (Denmark), Dr. James McIntyre (South Africa),

Dr. Octavian Bivol (Moldova), Dr. Murray Enkin (Canada), Dr. Iain Chalmers (UK), Dr. Keith Bolton (South Africa), Dr. Adik Levin (Estonia), Dr. Elisabet Helsing (Norway), Dr. Agnes Gereb (Hungary), Dr. Rick Porter (UK), Dr. Mahmoud Fathalla (Egypt), Dr. John Kennell (USA), and Dalia Jeskaite (Lithuania).

I remain, also, forever indebted to my husband and our three daughters who have supported my life-long journey into perinatal care. My husband, Bernie, deserves particular thanks for our shared, fifty-seven years together: without him, this work, and my adventures, developments, creations, and insights would not have been possible.

Dr. Solomon

It is only fitting that in a book on perinatal care, I should start by thanking my mother. She taught me not only about perinatal care and birth – a dubiously useful skill set in my life – but more importantly about being a good parent. She showed me what it meant to be an independent, powerful, strong woman. She is my academic role model and taught me that being a mom is about more than giving birth. Thank you for taking me with you on this journey, through all the books and adventures.

I would also like to acknowledge Dr. Jennifer Gagnon, Kathryn Douglas-Campbell, Corin Parsons, and the UBC Disability Affinity Group. They helped me better understand disability, as an identity, and in its nuances. Their support has enabled me to re-make my worldview in ways for which I am eternally grateful. I hope some of their lessons have made it into this book.

Nothing I do would be possible without my husband, Simon. It feels like our journey is only just beginning, and fifteen years in, I am still as twitterpated as ever. I could not ask for a better partner or a better husband. You are my everything.

Authors' Contributions

This book emerged from Dr. Chalmers' more than fifty years of work in perinatal care. Most of this work was created by Dr. Chalmers. Dr. Solomon has been collaborating with her in various capacities for more than twenty years and has edited most of her books.

Dr. Solomon's background and experience focus on discrimination and prejudice in a variety of global and local contexts. In the past decade her work has addressed inequities in health care, particularly perinatal care. She has worked in a perinatal health research lab at the University of British Columbia and as a private educator and advocate working to reduce health-related discrimination.

In the process of editing and reviewing multiple versions of this book, Dr. Solomon applied her perspectives and expanded the conceptualization of the text to the extent that she earned co-authorship. Her contributions can be seen throughout the book, providing an invaluable perspective to the original material.

This was, admittedly, an unusual authorship collaboration. Any references in the text that use "I" refer to Dr. Chalmers' experiences in the field. If it is a comment that is shared by both of us, then "we" is used.

Authors' Note

People with all gender identities get pregnant and have children, and for some, there is tremendous trepidation about the prospect of discussing perinatal care in a field filled with pronoun landmines. Our approach to this is to be as inclusive as possible. For us, this does not mean being gender neutral, as that excludes people who identify very strongly with a particular gender (whether that means cis-gendered women or trans men or any other variation). Consequently, we use a range of gendered and gender-neutral language throughout this book, predominantly (but not exclusively) using terms like woman and mother, since the majority of the people who get pregnant identify as such. We use terms like women, pregnant people, and parents, and hope that people with all gender identities can find language somewhere in this book that connects to and represents them, and will likewise recognize their own experiences even when a different pronoun is used. As authors who identify as women, we do not pretend to have any extensive experience of the unique challenges faced by, for example, trans men who have babies, or people with any other gender identity. We very much hope that someone with those lived experiences and relevant expertise can add to the conversation that this book starts.

The issue of appropriate language is a complex one, making the choice of acceptable terminology for both those who do identify with these words, as well as for those who do not, challenging. Our sincere apologies if any of the terminology in this book proves to be offensive to any pregnant person or new parent.

We have abbreviated terms commonly used in perinatal care to their customary acronyms.

WHO:	World Health Organization
UNICEF:	United Nations Children's Fund
NICU:	Neonatal Intensive Care Unit
BFHI:	Baby Friendly Hospital Initiative
MES:	Maternity Experiences Survey
NICE:	National Institute for Health and Care Excellence
HNCI:	Humane Neonatal Care Initiative
NIDCAP:	Newborn Individualized Developmental Care and Assessment Program

About the Cover

The painting on the cover, titled *Care*, by Dana Solomon, reflects the experiences of those whose encounters with the medical, legal, and insurance systems have been torturous, abusive, and harmful. The attacks, pain, and trauma come from innumerable sources, some of which are discussed in this book, and others that extend deeper into the systems that disable and harm those ostensibly receiving care.

Preface

In the social sciences full disclosure of one's philosophy of care is regarded as academically honest and necessary. While this is less common in the health sciences, it seems appropriate for this book.

Central to my approach is the reason I chose to revise and expand my earlier publication of *Family-Centred Perinatal Care*:[2] It is too easy for caregivers to believe or pretend they are providing family-centred care, even when they are not. Few caregivers consider their approaches to be disrespectful or abusive, deliberately or unintentionally. However, multiple studies reveal that abuse and disrespect are common in health care, including in perinatal care. This disconnect between how caregivers choose to see themselves, and how their actions are experienced by clients makes it necessary to publish a book that more explicitly states what is harmful and what is good practice.

An early reviewer of *Family Centred Perinatal Care* (FCPC) advised me to add praise for perinatal caregivers as most readers would not like being criticized. While this was done for FCPC, we do not give a great deal of praise in this book. Not because we do not believe there are good caregivers – we know there are many wonderful doctors, midwives, nurses, and other caregivers. But couching every criticism amidst a flurry of praise to soothe the egos of the health care profession creates the inaccurate view that the abuses we are discussing are rare, or the actions of "a few bad apples," when in fact they are pervasive and systemic problems that urgently need to be addressed. Health caregivers are not toddlers that require a spoonful of sugar to take their medicine – they need to recognize that their profession has serious problems that require serious attention.

I have worked with caregivers across all disciplines related to perinatal care for over five decades. I believe I was able to do this because I was never a clinical threat. I am not an Ob-Gyn, a family doctor, a midwife, doula, or nurse, but a social scientist, a perinatal psychologist, an academic researcher in obstetrics, and a public health promotion advocate. Sadly, perinatal care disciplines often work in competition with each other rather than in collaboration. Inter-professional interactions should not be about whether midwives offer better care or whether obstetricians save more lives. That is not the point; it is not about the caregivers at all. It should be about what is best for mothers, babies, and their families.

My Perspectives

When first embarking on studies in perinatal health, I read an obstetrics textbook, a midwifery manual, and books written for prospective or new mothers. The impact was mind-blowing and directed my life's work in this field. It was almost impossible to accept that all three were describing the same experience. Exposing all newcomers to these widely differing accounts of the same experience, whether medical, nursing, midwifery, or social scientist, might provide a valuable entry point to the study of respectful, non-abusive, family-centred childbirth care. Over my lifetime I have contributed to obstetric manuals,[3] midwifery texts[4] and books written for mothers and families.[5] My approach in all of these has been congruent and reflects a humanistic, holistic, and evidence-based approach, regardless of the target audience for these works.

I have been fortunate to be able to collaborate with colleagues from multiple cultures, countries, and religious backgrounds in the course of my career. I have worked on extensive academic research projects with people from numerous cultures, racial and religious identities, those identifying as LGBTQ+, and people living with disabilities. I have co-authored books and articles with Jews, Muslims, and Christians and with those who are strong adherents to religious belief and those who reject such considerations. When ideological differences that were difficult for me to accept emerged, I was faced with the question of whether I felt comfortable assisting women whose value systems were so vastly different from my own. I quickly realised that women giving birth all need, and value, assistance.

I have worked in peaceful countries and in areas torn apart by war. Although I occasionally feared for my safety, I did not hesitate to offer whatever assistance I could. My concern with a respectful, non-abusive, family-centred, holistic, and humanistic approach to childbearing has emerged from these varied experiences. My own birth experiences, both fulfilling and confirming as well as disappointing and surprising, contributed to my approach as well. A broad approach to humanity is needed if cultural respect and collaboration is to be facilitated, just as a broad approach to childbearing is necessary to meet widely differing women's and caregivers' expectations. Respectful and non-abusive family-centred care is not simply an academic construct but is also a series of real-life actions taken to implement a system of care that values not only clinical excellence, but "whole family wellbeing." It is humanistic and holistic in addition to being clinically precise. Over the five decades of my involvement in perinatal care, I have come to accept that not providing family-centred, respectful, humanistic, holistic, and technologically essential care only when needed, is simply abusive.

Table Of Contents

Overview

Exposing ourselves to the darker sides of perinatal care in this book will be painful, at times threatening, and certainly challenging. We like to think of ourselves as offering humane, holistic, and technologically essential care, but we do not always do so. All too often, our perinatal practice is abusive, involving direct physical, verbal, emotional, or sexual assaults, or less directly abusive, through inadequate clinical care that is not evidence-based, psycho-socially sensitive, family-centred, culturally respectful, holistic, and humanistic.

In the 1990s, shortly after publishing an article in Canada outlining the principles involved in becoming a Baby Friendly Hospital (BFH), and pointing out that no hospitals in the country were, at the time, accredited as such, I received an angry letter admonishing me that all hospitals in Canada were baby friendly: after all, every hospital values good care for their babies. In similar vein, today, all maternity hospitals might claim to offer non-abusive, or even family-centred perinatal care, as they no doubt believe that they are not abusing their clients and that they provide good care for families. Being polite to prospective or new parents, or providing adequate, if not evidence-based, clinical care is, however, not enough. Perinatal care can be, and often is, abusive. Shrouded in a cloak of medical necessity, many procedures, interventions, maternity care settings, care provider attitudes, and perinatal care encounters – perhaps unwittingly – are disrespectful, insensitive, hurtful, and often unnecessary. Respectful family-centred care during pregnancy, birth, and the postpartum period that is evidence-based, psycho-socially sensitive, multi-culturally adapted, inter-and multi-disciplinary, and utilizing only essential and appropriate technology can go far to preventing the many abusive experiences that are reported by women and their families. We have yet to demonstrate our understanding that the person giving birth is not only a uterus, vagina, and perineum carrying a fetus, but a person with hopes, wishes, expectations, and feelings.

Many of the issues raised in this book are controversial as they question the ways that perinatal care has been offered for decades. Solutions to the challenges raised may be difficult to implement, especially for those who are not cognisant, and in some cases willfully ignorant of the impact of their actions, resistant to change, or unwilling to confront their own practices. Caution, care, and sensitivity to the needs of both caregivers and families is needed when implementing changes, but failure to do so is not an option if we truly value not only non-abusive, but respectful perinatal care.

Key Concepts

There are two categories of abuse that are most prevalent in our discussion of obstetric abuse. The first recognizes those actions that are traditionally accepted as abusive and that reflect physical, emotional, social, economic, and sexual abuse. The second category exposes how standard clinical care may also be abusive when it does not meet high levels of excellence that incorporate a holistic, humanistic, psycho-socially respectful, and culturally sensitive approach to care, that is also based on high quality evidence. Both categories should be regarded as obstetric abuse. On one level it is easy to say "Of course I follow each of these principles," but when considered in more depth, the extent to which one follows them may be superficial – and consequently potentially abusive.

Abusive treatment occurs and manifests in multiple ways. Underlying many of these are behaviours or treatments that are based on personal or professional biases, outdated research, or biased research that, among other failures, considers only client reactions to clinical interventions and fails to also consider the impact of caregiver attitudes, actions, and practices on outcomes. While many of the actions taken by caregivers are rooted in personality, biases, prejudices, and attitudes, others are rooted in systemic structures that determine how caregivers may look after clients in the institutions in which they work. Abuse for any of these reasons is unacceptable. These aspects of abuse are discussed in the first part of this book, "Perinatal Abuse."

The second part of this book, "Birth as it Should Be," deals with clinical care as it should be, contrasted with abusive clinical treatment. Some core principles underlying these aspects of treatment are highlighted here.

Clinical Issues

The medicalization of perinatal care has led us to a world in which pregnancy is viewed as a health problem, or in some cases, even a temporary disability. In health settings, this results in pregnant people being treated as if they are ill, "at risk," and in danger. It can lead to friends and family members treating pregnant people as fragile, incapable, or otherwise diminished. It also frequently results in professional consequences, whether employers treat pregnant employees differently, deny them access to advancement or pay raises, or otherwise discriminate against people who are, or may become pregnant in the future. The impact of medicalizing pregnancy (among other aspects of life) extends far beyond the health care setting.

There is a prevalent fashion referring to a "normal," "natural," or uncomplicated pregnancy as a "physiological" birth. There is an inherent danger in following this terminology. Pregnancy and birth are not simply physiological functions: this language emphasizes the biological level of pregnancy and birth and ignores the psychological, social, and cultural components of having children. Emotions, cognitions/knowledge, spiritual implications, and physiological processes all form part of the process of giving life to a newborn with or without clinical intervention. I am constantly amazed at how women and their families, as well as academics, are willing to adopt this medicalized ideology and downplay the importance of the experiential, interpersonal, emotional, cognitive, social, and societal components of having a baby.

"Care"

The term "care" is bandied about with frequent disregard for its actual meaning. Care has even been used to describe some of the most egregious abuses committed by the medical profession, with some even using terms like "abusive care," not recognising the inherent contradiction. We use "care" to encompass two broad frameworks: the first is professional, in the sense that it focuses on clinical, professional, caregiver standards and relationships that are necessary to provide good care, including being individualized, evidence-based, inter-and-multi-disciplinary, and de-medicalized. The second is inter-personal, focusing on the ways in which caregivers interact with their clients, and encompasses ideals such as care being respectful, family-centred, holistic, humanistic, and psycho-socially sensitive, as well as inclusive.

Individualized

Each person and every birth is unique and has unique needs. Care should be individualized, and not blindly follow a rule book or a checklist/protocol. At the same time, however, bias among caregivers emerging from long-standing practices, or prejudices, and incorrect assumptions about sub-groups of women or their economic, social, cultural background, or even their appearance, may be so rife that we require guidelines, protocols, and standards to eliminate the undue influence of these prejudices, traditional practices, and incorrect assumptions to whatever extent we can. Bias may be inherent in the systems in place as well as in the individual caregiver, leading to valid questions regarding the level of trust we can place in either caregivers, care facilities, or care protocols.

Evidence-Based

Care practices should be based on the best available, current evidence usually regarded as practices founded on randomized controlled trials. Yet such trials are limited in their application: it is not possible to manipulate people's wishes or preferences for one of the trial arms, when allocating people to experimental or control groups randomly. Trials may also exclude people with complex medical conditions, disabilities, or differing body types as well as people from marginalized communities, resulting in limited generalizability to these categories of clients. It is not always possible to test the impact of some interventions on pregnant women without risk. Nor are researchers always expert at asking the best questions, interpreting research findings, or avoiding bias in their application. Research protocols are only as good as their designers and we, as researchers, are not immune to our own biases in, for example, selecting which clients we study, what observations we make, and which variables or outcomes are best to include in any research project. Randomized controlled trials also do not often examine variations in health system policies, or caregiver behaviour, bias, or attitude.

Regardless of the quality of available evidence to support care, caregivers should remain open-minded, vigilant, and aware of possible pitfalls in the research on which guidelines are based. They should be open to other possible options, listen to what the mother and the family want and need, be cognisant of outliers and their requirements, and recognize that care is not necessarily one-size-fits-all and that there can be variations in care based on situational needs.

Multi-Disciplinary

A variety of caregiver professionals are involved in perinatal care including midwives, family doctors, obstetricians, paediatricians, childbirth educators, perinatal psychologists, doulas, physiotherapists, social workers, kinesiologists, nutritionists, lawyers, and fertility specialists, to name only the major groups. Communication across these disciplinary boundaries is often lacking, to the detriment of the woman, her baby/babies, and the family.

Demedicalized

Care should utilize only essential and appropriate technology. In all perinatal care, only the most appropriate level of intervention should be involved. In general, the least interventionist approach to care that is appropriate should be employed.

Interpersonal Issues

A lack of respectful and sensitive care remains a central issue in women's reports of disrespectful care, with reports frequently identifying their treatment as perhaps technically adequate but lacking consideration for them as people.[6] Recent publications have begun to address the issue of achieving a balance between technology and humanistic care, but clearly indicate that humanistic perinatal care has not yet been achieved.[7]

Respectful

Caregivers expect to be respected but do not always extend their respect to their patients.[8] There is a difference between genuine respect for clients and acknowledging that clients must "feel like" they are respected. Physician ideology has traditionally viewed medical caregivers as superior – as knowing what is best for others. This ideology is facilitated by regulations that leave caregivers in sole control of all medical records and that prioritize caregiver decision making. This creates power dynamics that – perhaps unconsciously, but not always so – keep patients subservient and uncomfortable.

Family-Centred

Care needs to consider not only the mother and her newborn/s, but the needs of her partner and other support companions of her choice. The most important person in perinatal care is the mother. The needs of the caregiver take a secondary place in this hierarchy unless clinical demands require medical or professional expertise to ensure the safety of mother or baby. In a life threatening/damaging situation the needs of the caregiver to provide such care take priority.

Holistic

Pregnancy, birth, and postpartum care must be holistic. It needs to consider all aspects of human functioning simultaneously including physiological, emotional, cognitive, interpersonal, social, cultural, and spiritual levels. Holistic care is crucial in all aspects of medicine and especially in perinatal care.

Inclusive

Given our global village with its variations in culture, societies, religions, and abilities, we need to adopt an inclusive and respectful approach to care. We need to address racism, gender and sexual diversity, age differentials, religious variety, ableism, body inclusion, and cultural variations in care.

The 10:10 Principles

Perinatal care should incorporate the key concepts listed above. These apply to the care of women having either vaginal or caesarean births, and to those experiencing optimal as well as adverse maternal or neonatal outcomes. These principles of perinatal care can be divided into ten that focus on the needs of families and ten that emphasize the caregivers' role – the 10:10 Principles. These form the fundamental principles of optimal perinatal care.[9] This book addresses how these principles have been used, mis-used, or ignored during pregnancy and birth, and how they continue to be neglected.

Family Principles

1. Respectful care addresses the needs of women/parents, their newborn/s and their chosen family support during pregnancy, birth and postpartum, regardless of the type of birth, and for births with both optimal and adverse outcomes.
2. Care is sensitive to the psychological and social needs of women and their families, including their needs for knowledge, emotional support, and spiritual considerations.
3. Care is culturally respectful and informed.
4. Care is individualized to meet each family's needs.
5. Care is respectful of a person's dignity, privacy, and confidentiality.
6. Families are encouraged, prepared, and supported to be actively involved in the care of their newborn, whether a healthy term infant or a sick or preterm baby requiring intensive clinical care.
7. Families lead decision-making about their care, founded on evidence-based information, provided without covert or overt coercion, and with full understanding of the potential adverse effects of any care procedure.
8. Families are offered knowledgeable and appropriate care to support breastfeeding and when needed, alternate feeding methods.
9. Caregivers and health care facilities should collect, monitor, rigorously evaluate, and implement changes based on feedback from families about their care.
10. Information about parents, families, and infants is strictly confidential. Parents should have full and easy access to their clinical notes and those of their child(ren).

Caregiver Principles

1. Care does not discriminate. It is not biased, racist, ableist, or stigmatizing.

2. Care respects the reproductive and sexual rights of all parents and their families.
3. Care is individualized and based on the best available evidence-based information.
4. Pregnancy and birth are regarded as healthy, normal, life events with caregivers remaining vigilant for the development of complications.
5. Interventions are used only when essential and with informed consent.
6. Care is interdisciplinary, requiring integration among whichever caregivers are appropriate.
7. A holistic and humanistic approach to care is expected of all care providers.
8. Professional education of caregivers should include the diverse principles of non-abusive, respectful, holistic, humanistic, and family-centred care.
9. Families are entitled to full, open, and honest communication about all aspects of their care. They should be entitled to apology and compensation in the event of avoidable negative outcomes.
10. Aggregated information about family-centred, psycho-social, and clinical practices and outcomes is made publicly available and accessible, regardless of socio-economic, educational, or demographic background. Privacy concerns should not be used to conceal non-optimal caregiver practices.

There have been many other attempts to develop universal Principles of Perinatal care including those proposed by the WHO.[10] The 10:10 Principles above are inclusive of the various approaches that have been proposed and are cognisant of a global perspective. They are included as a framework within which to view this text.

To date, however, these various admirable principles of care remain unenforceable. No country has a systematic approach to monitoring and evaluating caregivers' practices or policies with a view to implementing the standards they outline. Where any monitoring occurs it is usually evaluated by professional bodies of caregivers who are tasked with evaluating their own colleagues. Arms length, and thereby likely more objective, assessment of clinical care remains an elusive dream.

We have one last word for readers: It can be difficult to see our own mistakes or shortcomings, particularly when those errors were made with a genuine belief that we were doing the right thing. If you give up part way through reading this book in disgust or anger, we hope it will plant some seeds that may grow, that you may recognize areas of concern in your practice, and perhaps return to the book later with a view to strengthening your own provision of respectful perinatal care.

Perinatal Abuse

In recent decades, we have recognized the reality of violence and abuse in our world, to the extent that measures of violence (towards children, women, and men) have been incorporated into United Nations Agencies Healthcare Indicators.[11] The incidence of violence against women and children[12] far exceeds our previous expectations and provides a shocking reminder of the progress that we have yet to make in building a respectful and healthy social environment. This concern is global and obstetric violence is one part of it.

Clinical Abuse

The USA Aid Translating Research into Action project (US-AID-TRAction) conducted by Harvard University School of Public Health identifies seven categories of disrespect and abuse that may and do occur in the perinatal period in many countries worldwide. These are physical abuse, non-consensual procedures, violating confidentiality, undignified treatment, discrimination based on specific patient attributes, abandonment of care, and detention in facilities.[13] More recently, a mixed methods systematic review has led to the establishment of seven categories of abusive or disrespectful care of women during childbirth. These include: physical abuse, sexual abuse, verbal abuse, stigma and discrimination, failure to meet professional standards of care, poor rapport between clients and providers, and health system conditions and constraints.[14] A recent commentary on obstetric trauma due to abuse and preventable events lists violation of women's rights, disrespect and abuse, obstetric mistreatment, abuse in healthcare, dehumanized care, mistreatment of women, detrimental care, and violence in maternal care as terms that are commonly used to describe adverse events due to obstetric care causing trauma.[15] In the discussion that follows we have added emotional abuse, inequitable treatment, political or ideological abuse, and economic abuse.

Monitoring Abuse

Elizabeth Kakura distinguishes between abuse, coercion, and disrespect when defining obstetric violence, although she acknowledges that these are overlapping categories that might, if occurring in isolation, result in differing degrees of severity of abuse.[16] In isolation any one event may not rise to the level of violence or abuse. Occurring together, or when multiple events occur concurrently, they might. Mistreatment or, more severely, violence against women in maternity care settings, happens globally and affects women at all socio-economic levels.[17] The internet has facilitated the sharing of stories of mistreatment in childbirth that, prior to this avenue of communication, remained hidden. Prior to this, women's stories were silenced and many were afraid to speak out because of taboos, fear of stigma, or fears of retaliation from caregivers. Testimonies now reveal that disrespectful treatment of women is widespread and ingrained in health care systems.[18] This abuse disproportionately affects those who identify as Indigenous, Disabled, 2SLGBTQI+, women and gender diverse individuals, Black people, people of colour, people living in bigger bodies or those with a high BMI, people with lower socio-economic status, and those who are younger or older than is "typical" for perinatal care (from this point forward, referred to as equity-owed or equity-denied groups).[19] Although currently receiving increasing global attention, knowledge about obstetric abuse is not yet widespread, is seldom shared openly but is often revealed to close friends and family, and is not monitored by health care systems.[20] One recent definition of violence in obstetric care that offers a potential working guide to this emerging area of research and interest is: "An event, either intentional or unintentional, that occurs during the antenatal, intrapartum or postnatal period. These events can be physical, verbal, psychosocial or negligent in nature and are caused by the actions of the HCP and experienced by the birthing women."[21]

Some have argued that care can be separated into categories of "Obstetric Violence" and "Birth Trauma."[22] Birth Trauma reflects the birthing person's perception of their treatment, whether clinical or non-clinical. Birth Trauma is an umbrella term that includes both negatively perceived clinical care as well as experiences where caregivers have been directly involved in causing harm. In this text, in contrast, both directly asserted violence against women as well as treatment that leads to negative perceptions of their birthing experiences is regarded as Obstetric or Birth Abuse. The fundamental assumption of this book is that treatment of women should not result in negative birth experiences, even when adverse clinical outcomes occur. Whether a caregiver strikes a woman, ignores her requests, speaks disrespectfully to her, or provides inappropriate clinical treatment, it is Obstetric/Birth Abuse.

While it is almost impossible to believe that obstetric caregivers might be responsible for virtually all women's perceptions of their care, including any negative perceptions that women may have in response to their treatment, this is the reality we must now face in obstetric care. A recent editorial in *The Lancet* was written in a way that implied that women, not caregivers, are responsible for their negative birth experiences[23] – an approach which we strongly opposed in our rebuttal of this article.[24] This *Lancet* Editorial uses phrases such as " 'women frequently experiencing suboptimal care [...and] many women enter labour unprepared'[25] rather than stating that caregivers might provide suboptimal care and fail to prepare women for pregnancy, labour and birth."[26] The editorial advocates for "better mental postnatal care"[27] but does not advocate for providing care that avoids trauma requiring postpartum therapy. *The Lancet* editorial reveals a customary ideology that obstetric caregivers know what is best for all women and that women's needs must be considered ("listened to") but not necessarily heeded.[28] In the editorial, the authors discuss reports of "suboptimal care, and trauma, and propose counselling, instead of advocating for better care and preventing caregivers from traumatizing pregnant people."[29] Our seismic inversion of responsibility for negative birth experiences is challenging for today's caregivers to accept, as well as possibly for parents who have long been indoctrinated to regard clinical caregivers as exceptionally knowledgeable, trustworthy, and beyond reproach. Women have also been accustomed to blaming themselves when things go wrong, especially in pregnancy and birth asking such questions as: "What did I do wrong? Did that cigarette I smoked, or drink I had before I knew I was pregnant, cause my negative birth outcomes, or events?" It is long past time for us to rethink responsibility for negative birth experiences and to shift the emphasis from blaming mothers to holding caregivers accountable, as is the thesis of this book. While abusive care is discussed in detail in the first part of this book, care as it should be offered is proposed in the second.

I have frequently observed outdated, and sometimes cruel, obstetric care practices. Women sometimes emerge from their birth experiences wishing to “never have another child again” or to “never go through such an experience again.” Many times, they appear physically battered after birth, with extremely painful perineums resulting from deep and extensive episiotomies which preclude sitting for some days or even weeks, combined with perineal bruising from excessive manual stretching of the perineum during the second stage of labour, and with extensive bruising of their arms from intravenous lines. Pale and sore they lie unmoving for hours after birth, separated from family or friends, with their babies kept apart from them in nurseries. Such treatment happened in dozens of the countries I worked in, both in developed and developing nations. In some cases, this treatment was based on the best available knowledge of caregivers at that time, or because more up-to-date information was not available or accessible. In others, particularly in developed nations, it happened because caregivers chose not to seek continuing education. Such uncaring actions flourish in health care systems in which reports of abuse and standards of care are not monitored, and where demands on caregivers to maintain updated care practices are not enforced. They thrive in care systems in which there are no repercussions for poor outcomes or mistreatment of patients. Inadequate or out-of-date knowledge; a lack of concern for the perspectives, or rights, of women; lack of respect for women’s bodies and their dignity, privacy, and confidentiality; and, often, inadequate financial resources, are characteristics that can readily be associated with disrespectful treatment. Where no access to current knowledge is available, this treatment is, at least, understandable. More egregious, however, is the disrespectful approach that occurs in countries where up-to-date knowledge is readily available and where caregivers choose not to avail themselves of this information or apply it in practice. Failure of health care systems to monitor and evaluate their health care providers’ practices and to sanction those who do not reach satisfactory standards, is abusive, if not criminally negligent.

Abusive Procedures

It typically takes a decade or even longer to translate evidence-based knowledge into accepted care practices. This egregious delay is aggravated when the evidence directly contradicts longstanding obstetric practices. Consequently, while abusive obstetric situations are increasingly recognized and exposed, there are also situations in which disrespectful practices are, or were at one time, considered necessary or beneficial by caregivers.[30] We can classify some aspects of standard obstetric care as practiced in many technologically advanced societies and in parts of the developing world as violence against women. Those procedures are, and have been, usually performed with the best interests of the woman in mind and supported by what was believed to be best practice at the time. Regardless of the best intentions of the caregivers, they are cruelly abusive. These practices include: routine episiotomy; repair of minor perineal lacerations; lack of appropriate anaesthesia or analgesia for such perineal procedures or for some obstetric or gynaecological treatments and tests; exploration of the uterus or exteriorization and visualization of the cervix following vaginal delivery; swabbing of the vagina with antiseptic after birth; anal exploration after delivery; as well as procedures such as routine perineal and pubic shaving, and enemas during labour. Exerting manual fundal pressure to facilitate childbirth during the second stage of labour (the Kristeller manoeuvre) is not recommended but is still widely practiced, sometimes with the elbow, forearm, or whole body, to provoke birth. It is variously applied across countries, with the highest rates in Honduras at between fifty to seventy percent of vaginal births.[31] Episiotomy, including stitching after giving birth, when performed without informed consent and/or without anaesthesia, may have repercussions for a woman's sexual and reproductive life, as well as her mental health, that can leave lasting scars, both physical and psychological. Routine episiotomy is no longer justified as a medical necessity and can be considered a violation of women's rights and gender-based violence.[32] In some countries, women report being stitched up tightly after episiotomies, known as the "husband stitch," that is supposedly done for the husband's pleasure.[33] This practice also occurs following repair of women giving birth after female genital mutilation/cutting when the remaining labia are again juxtaposed and stitched together, ostensibly to increase the husband's sexual pleasure.[34] To compound the problem, many of the above procedures have been done without effective or appropriate pain relief. Such practices are not clinically, or morally, justified.

Caesarean section, while life-saving for some, can also be considered gender-based violence and even torture when performed without medical necessity and informed consent.[35] There is growing evidence of its overuse across the globe and in Latin America and some parts of Europe it is in danger of becoming the preferred way of giving birth.

Even the commonly used and non-evidence-based lithotomy position for birth is abusive. Clinically, it is the least physiologically beneficial position in which to give birth. While this position may be necessary for some medical procedures, and therefore unavoidable in a few instances, it is the least clinically valid position for birth, but is one of the most commonly used.

In Southern Sudan, I was present with a woman entering the second stage of labour in a local rural clinic, being attended by a Sudanese, western-trained, healthcare provider/midwife. The recumbent woman repeatedly struggled to lift herself into a seated position only to be pushed down onto the delivery bed and told to lie flat. This occurred numerous times. Likely ignorant of the benefits of an upright position for birth, and disdainful of traditional upright delivery positions, this aggressive and inappropriate treatment was probably the result of poor training based on "western" education that has traditionally utilized a supine delivery position, combined with a lack of respect for the birthing woman's wishes. A forced supine position for birth is also reported in the USA.[36] Obstetric procedures, such as the routine use of continuous fetal heart monitoring in labour, that require a supine maternal position for lengthy periods, can be doubly abusive: they are not evidence-based practice and force maternal immobility in the least advisable position for both labour and birth.

In addition, not being allowed to have a companion during labour and birth is non-optimal and out-of-date practice. In South Africa, one of the first randomized control trials showing the value of having a companion during labour was conducted in 1991 by one of my doctoral students.[37] Yet, in 2007, sixteen years later, as many as 84.5% of women in South Africa were still not allowed to have a companion in childbirth.[38] In Brazil, in 2008, 41.8% of women were not allowed to have a companion for labour, and 98.6% for delivery.[39] Whereas these were accepted and beneficially regarded obstetrical routines some decades ago, they are now actively contradicted by evidence.[40] In many developed societies many of these hurtful practices have, fortunately, been discontinued although not completely and not everywhere.[41]

The emergence of Covid-19, with its associated need to restrict "unnecessary" contact with clients in hospitals, rapidly led to the exclusion of companions in childbirth. Clients' fears of contagion, as well as a wish to have a companion of their choice with them in labour and at birth led many women to give birth at home, with (or even without) midwifery support. Midwives developed protective measures to prevent the spread of infection for both their clients and themselves when attending home births. A recent large-scale survey across twenty countries in the WHO European Region including over 48,000 women revealed that always having a companion of their choice and having professional assistance at birth were associated with satisfaction with their experiences during this Covid-19 epidemic. Instrumental births, episiotomies, having fundal pressure applied, or having a caesarean section were linked to less positive birth experiences.[42] This study confirms, yet again, the known benefits of having a companion at birth, and having fewer rather than more clinical interventions.

Discrimination

People from all equity-denied groups, including Indigenous women, women with disabilities, and women with differing gender identities all report inequities in access to and quality of health care, including perinatal care. Access to care, affordability of care, and availability of care, are all obstacles to care for people in these groups.

For example, women with obesity or those living in bigger bodies frequently report emotionally traumatic and clinically inferior treatment when their physical and psychological needs are ignored, such as when insensitive, critical, and derogatory comments about their weight are made, when all their clinical symptoms are simply discounted as due to their obesity and little or no alternate explanations are sought, and when inappropriate facilities that do not support their larger size such as too small MRI equipment, blood pressure cuffs, or examination tables, are all that are available. Such women often report being berated about their weight, or being treated as though they are stupid, lazy, noncompliant, obstructive, or even unclean. They may even be turned away from their nearest health care facility because it does not authorize care of larger women (or women based on their race, or mental ability, or disability etc.). Such treatment is not only disrespectful, it is also not evidence-based, it is incompetent, and inadequate.

People with Disabilities also experience discriminatory behaviour around perinatal care. Many if not most caregivers have little training on how best to offer care for women with varying kinds of disabilities. Even the very concept of a woman with a disability having a baby is sometimes anathema for them. Assumptions about their inability to care for and rear children are made and are often denigrating, questions about their sexual activity and right to have sexual enjoyment arise. At a more fundamental level, appropriate clinical facilities are not always available - such as the accessibility of examination tables or chairs for women with achondroplasia or sign language and/or interpreters for deaf or non-verbal clients.[43]

People identifying as LGBTQ+ also face discriminatory treatment. Not only may the biological needs of these birthing persons be complex and variable, but so too are their emotional needs. Caregivers need to familiarize themselves with the needs and wishes of their clients and to collaborate with them to ensure that they receive the appropriate care they desire. Sometimes, this may be as straightforward as accepting and embracing the fact that families come in all forms and compositions, and all should be respected and welcomed in perinatal care. Other times, care needs may be more nuanced or complex. Regardless, it has long been the stated aspiration that "partnering in care" is the goal with all people having babies; it is past time when this should be the expectation, rather than the aspiration. This is vital for any parent, and any family.

Gynaecological Abuse

Many of the women who experience disrespectful birth procedures are still in their reproductive years and continue to require obstetrical care or fertility treatments for future pregnancies, as well as gynaecological care between pregnancies and after their childbearing years. Gynaecological procedures may evoke traumatic memories of abusive medical encounters during earlier fertility treatments, pregnancies, and births. The gynaecologist needs to remain alert and sensitive to such obstetric experiences and provide trauma-informed care. While these issues are not explored in depth here, they are touched on to acknowledge their importance in the obstetric context.

It would be valuable to explore alternate methods of conducting vaginal procedures, thereby reducing the psychological stress and, for some, physical pain of pelvic examinations. It is also necessary to find approaches that avoid inflicting the emotional trauma that can be evoked through memories of personal, or healthcare related, abuse experienced by some women. Whereas obstetric care is moving towards a more sensitive approach, fertility treatments, have generally escaped criticism. In preference to intimate examinations, non-invasive techniques of diagnosis should be explored and developed. When an alternative to an emotionally harmful or physically painful procedure is available and is not used, that is abusive.

Pain relief or management is a neglected component of gynaecological procedures. For many women, even routine gynaecological procedures such as an internal exam or a pap test can be painful. More invasive exams, such as endometrial biopsies, are also routinely done without any anaesthetic, despite being extremely painful for some. The expectation of pain during gynaecological procedures also creates an environment that is highly susceptible to abuse: women expect to be hurt during these procedures so they do not question it when an abuser inflicts more pain than might be unavoidable. They may not even realise that a procedure during which they experienced significant pain should not have been painful at all. Similarly, women and caregivers discount pain as a symptom of a potential problem, since they have been conditioned to expect gynaecological pain as part of being female. This is particularly true for diagnoses such as endometriosis, one of the symptoms of which is severe menstrual pain. Women reporting such pain may be routinely dismissed with the notion that "periods are painful," thereby delaying a diagnosis. The approach to gynaecology that routinely ignores pain management as part of its practice is symptomatic of a broader problem in medicine in which women are less likely to receive appropriate pain management prescriptions or approaches, and in which women's (or female presenting people's) reported symptoms, including pain, are more likely to be ignored or dismissed.[44] This effect is further exacerbated for women with other intersecting marginalized identities, such as those with disabilities, in bigger bodies, with substance use disorders, and people from racialized identity groups.[45]

We sorely need exploration of what would make women's experiences of vaginal procedures easier. Alternatives to the lithotomy position for vaginal examinations are desirable. Simple changes such as conducting routine examinations while standing at the woman's side with her legs bent and feet resting on the bed rather than with the caregiver seated directly opposite her splayed legs in a lithotomy position may offer women more dignity during these exams, and reduce feelings of helplessness, embarrassment, and fear.[46] Approaches to these exams differ from country to country: In South Africa, the less exposed, former position is preferred by clinicians, while in Canada the lithotomy position is commonly used. At the very least, clients should be offered a choice, and caregivers should be comfortable and proficient with either technique.

In South Africa, while working at Chris Hani (formerly Baragwanath) Hospital in Soweto, I co-taught Obstetrics education for both fourth and final (sixth) year medical students at the University of the Witwatersrand, with an obstetrician, Dr. James McIntyre. We routinely expected our students (both male and female) to role-play the part of a pregnant woman or a woman in labour, requiring them to assume a lithotomy position with their legs in stirrups while – in the classroom setting – remaining fully dressed. A second student acted the doctor's role. Student reflections on their emotions during this role-play revealed embarrassment, powerlessness, vulnerability, and fear; a worthwhile exposure for them that led to far greater sensitivity regarding women's experiences during care.[47]

Non-Consensual Procedures

Widespread lack of informed consent for common procedures occurring at the time of birth (non-consensual interventions), such as for episiotomies, augmentation of labour, some caesarean sections, hysterectomies, blood transfusions, and sterilization, have also been reported in many childbirth settings with some women reporting lack of patient-doctor confidentiality.[48] Once again, people from equity-owed groups are less likely to be asked for their consent than others. In many countries, a patient's consent is obtained for all interventions as soon as they enter hospital, when they are required to sign multiple forms. In effect, these are consent waivers leaving all control of care in the hands of caregivers, and forcing patients to surrender their bodily autonomy. Other consent forms, such as for epidural anaesthesia or caesarean section, may be handed to a woman for signature when she is in labour, sometimes even during contractions, which makes it difficult if not impossible for her to focus or ask questions. Consent obtained under such circumstances does not qualify as "free and informed" and as such, procedures performed based on such "consent" are coercive and abusive. Worse still, she may be coerced into agreeing to interventions by threats of withholding treatment, being abandoned by her caregiver, threats to report her to child protective services, or having to chose between two unwanted treatment options.[49] Performing a medical procedure without free and informed consent is assault and is a criminal offense. In the USA at least, women who refuse to consent to procedures such as caesarean section may be referred to either judicial intervention to enforce the surgery, as well as to child welfare organizations. On occasion, even if they are coerced into agreeing to the caesarean section, they may still be referred to child welfare organizations that are entitled to remove the baby on the grounds that the woman is unfit to parent the child because of her unwillingness to have a caesarean section. The personal, social, legal, and psychological impact of such proceedings are horrendous.[50]

In addition, many women report painful and frequent vaginal examinations in labour, sometimes conducted in non-private settings, and with caregivers denying pain relief.[51] In the former Soviet Union, for example, women could labour together with others in large wards, sometimes including as many as fifteen to twenty women. Vaginal examinations to monitor the progress of their labours, were done on a central bed in front of all the other women. Women's consent for this procedure and for their lack of privacy was never a concern for caregivers. Other women report being neglected or ignored in labour (and even at delivery), having long wait times, being "punished" for not booking prior to delivery, having "rushed" care, and feeling that they were "bothering" or "putting the caregiver out." Women often report inadequate explanations about potential complications or impending delivery; explanations are often scanty, if provided at all.[52] "Don't worry, I'll look after you" is not a sufficient or an appropriate response to enquiries about examinations or progress of labour. This response is never acceptable and simply reflects a paternalistic and infantilizing interaction.

Human Rights Abuse

Forced abortion, forced sterilization and symphysiotomy (determined to be a form of torture and a human rights violation), have occurred in the past and in some places continue to be practiced. In Ireland, the Human Rights Committee against Torture determined that between 1944 and 1987, 1,500 girls were subjected to symphysiotomy – a separation of the fibres joining the anterior pubic bones to enlarge the pubic outlet in the event of an obstructed birth.[53] In Canada, forced sterilizations of Indigenous women have occurred in Saskatchewan,

British Columbia, Alberta, and Quebec, even in recent years.[54] This practice has deep historical roots in this country. Coerced tubal ligation occurred in parallel with, and facilitating, the genocide of these Indigenous people. It is estimated that between 1929 and 1972, 2,800 people were sterilized in the province of Alberta alone. Forced abortion and sterilization have been practiced by health care givers across the globe including in Japan, Germany, Sweden, and the USA,[55] based on a conviction that this is

> in the best interest of the women, or based on the belief that certain groups of women from minority groups, such as Roma women, indigenous [*sic*] women, women with disabilities and women living with HIV are not "worthy" of procreation, are incapable of making responsible decisions regarding contraception, are not fit to be "good mothers" or that their offspring are not desirable.[56]

In Japan, for example, forced sterilization was legalized from 1948 until 1996, during which time over 25,000 people were sterilized, about 16,000 of them without consent.[57] In Nazi Germany, between 350,000-400,000 Germans were forcibly sterilized under the eugenics laws.[58] Equity-owed groups are often the most frequently targeted victims.[59] For example, members of the Roma minority have been forcibly sterilized in the Czech Republic, Hungary and Slovakia, usually during a caesarean section and without their prior knowledge or consent. In the USA, more than half the States had a eugenics law lasting until the 1970's.[60] Project Prevention in the USA is a nonprofit organization that pays women who use illicit drugs to accept long-term contraception: As of 2011 more than 1,300 women had been coerced into sterilization. In 2010 the project expanded to the UK and to Kenya.[61] Indian "sterilization camps" have misled poor and illiterate women into enduring sterilization without knowing or understanding what was being done. Some Indian governmental programs pay private sector physicians per sterilization performed, thus incentivizing them to encourage or coerce sterilization.[62] Similar programs encouraging women with HIV to be sterilized have been reported in Chile, the Dominican Republic, Mexico, Namibia, South Africa, and Venezuela.[63] In Greenland, between 1966 and 1970 alone, at least 4,500 women, including teenagers as young as thirteen, were fitted with IUD's to limit the birth rate among Indigenous women. The practice is known to have continued until at least 1975 or even longer.[64]

Women with disabilities are regularly denied their most basic human rights, including facing non-consensual sterilization on the grounds that it is believed that women with disabilities do not have the right to refuse medical procedures, that they should not have children, or because they do not have the capacity to understand the procedures. Such practices occur in both Spain and Egypt but also in the USA where fifteen States have laws that fail to protect women with disabilities from forced sterilization.[65] China is also complicit in forced sterilization: In the Chinese city of Puning, almost 1,400 elderly people were detained until their children agreed to sterilization.[66]

Abuse Under Anaesthesia

Unwelcome to acknowledge, as it may seem almost unbelievable, is the increasing recognition that doctors sometimes "behave badly" in operating theatres.[67] Comments passed, and actions taken when a woman is anaesthetized may be "inappropriate and disrespectful of patients, harmful to students, and derogatory towards colleagues."[68] In 2015 the Annuls of Internal Medicine published an anonymous account of such behaviours, including the attending physician's comment, while swabbing a woman's labia and inner thighs prior to a vaginal hysterectomy, that "I bet she's enjoying this."[69] Other examples of inappropriate and derogatory, and sometimes racist, comments may be made and are often not countered by embarrassed – and often junior – colleagues. Singh and Posner also report hearing openly homophobic, antisemitic, and sexually charged comments in the operating theatres, with little done to stop them.[70] As they advise, "If you wouldn't say it with the patient awake and your mother in the room, don't say it."[71] They note that the patient should be cared for with the utmost respect whether awake or asleep. It is, for example, never acceptable to undertake pelvic examinations in the operating theatre for the purpose of instruction, without the patient's prior knowledge and consent.

Despite this obvious ethical consideration, it is apparently legal in most USA states for doctors and medical students to perform pelvic exams on an unconscious woman who is under anaesthesia for treatment that does not normally require pelvic exams and who has not given explicit consent to such type of examination.[72] Currently, it is up to caregivers themselves to assume responsibility for ending such bad behaviours, although this is clearly not necessarily a sufficient safeguard. Hospitals, health authorities, patient advocacy groups or similar, need to step in to monitor such events and to manage them.

Students at USA medical schools frequently report witnessing unethical behaviour. In one medical school 35% of first year students reported such observations, with this increasing to 90% by their fourth year.[73] In other surveys, 98% of third- and fourth-year students had heard derogatory comments made by physicians when referring to their patients, while 61% had witnessed unethical incidents. Some events were horrific, including sedating a patient in order to intravenously administer medications to her, which she had earlier offered valid reasons for declining. The physician reported she was "of impaired judgement."[74] A recent survey of Canadian medical students revealed that 63% had performed a pelvic examination on a patient who was under anaesthesia, 35% a rectal examination, and 11% another type of sensitive examination, such as breast, scrotal, or penile examinations.[75] Of those performing pelvic examinations, 28% did not know if consent had been obtained, and 26% reported that no specific consent for such examinations had been obtained. Many students (36%) were uncomfortable with how the consent process had been handled while a further 32% were not sure if they were comfortable. As students progress through their medical training, they are more likely to consider unkind comments or actions to be appropriate.

Problems with these reports exist on multiple levels: first and most obviously, the frequency of these reports suggests that unethical and grossly inappropriate behaviour is not simply a case of a few bad role models, but is rather pervasive and even accepted as normal practice. This is in line with patient reports of their experiences, affirming that abusive, unethical, and wholly inappropriate behaviour reported by patients is not simply a case of occasional misunderstandings or disgruntled patients, but is clearly a predominant presence in multiple health systems around the world. Secondly, there is apparently no or little intervention from medical schools to halt such behaviour, indicating that such behaviour is accepted or at least tolerated, or the behaviour is never reported. If the latter is the case, there are additional problems with failures to provide students or colleagues with safe learning/working environments that enable and encourage them to report inappropriate behaviour without fear of reprisals. Third, is the failure of the health systems in question to prevent, halt, or initiate consequences for breaches of ethics in both practice and training. Clearly this aspect of medical school education requires wholesale and systemic reform.

Physical Abuse

Some examples of physical abuse during labour and birth include: hitting or slapping with an open hand or instrument; pinching, particularly on the thighs; kicking, shouting at, or scolding the mother; exerting excessive pressure on her abdomen to get the baby out; performing episiotomies, enemas, or other unnecessary procedures (sometimes for financial gain); repairing episiotomies without pain relief; tying the woman down during labour; or using mouth gags.[76] In some places incarcerated women are restrained on their beds during labour and are gagged. They report mental health challenges, dehumanization, lack of privacy, stigma, trauma, and lack of emotional support.[77] Some are shackled for hours, or even days, despite the continuous presence of guards.[78]

While such overtly aggressive physical actions are easily recognized as abusive, less obvious forms of physical abuse also occur and are less identifiable. These include performing painful examinations without offering pain relief, for example, while taking biopsies, Pap smears, inserting IUDs, or stitching perineal lacerations. Incompetent actions such as using an incorrectly sized speculum, exerting undue pressure while doing ultrasounds in the hope that pushing harder will get a better image, or not being trained on how to optimally perform such procedures on women with varying body types, can all lead to physical abuse.

Sexual Abuse

The American College of Obstetrics and Gynecology has clearly condemned perinatal sexual abuse, providing guidelines for practices that involve all breast, genital, and rectal examinations.[79] Sexual misconduct in care is more prevalent than previously thought and multiple physicians in the USA have been brought to state medical boards facing such accusations by patients. Individual cases reporting sexual abuse have been reported in news articles by hundreds of women. Sexual abuse during labour has emerged in countries ranging from the USA, to Israel, the Netherlands, Kenya, and Nigeria. In Israel a gynaecologist was accused of using a vibrator and his fingers to examine women seeking help for pain during intercourse.[80] In the USA, one gynaecologist has settled with 147 women who accused him of abusive breast and vaginal examinations.[81] In another USA case, over fifty women have accused one Ob-Gyn of inappropriate breast groping, and of one woman, prior to her marriage, experiencing extremely painful simultaneous vaginal and abdominal pressure resulting in an abortion.[82] Recently, an American army doctor has been accused of secretly recording hundreds of women during intimate vaginal or breast examinations over decades. Investigators have recovered thousands of photos and videos from his cell phone, used to record the examinations.[83] In Kenya a male healthcare provider examined a woman in labour forcefully while touching his own genitals, roughly pulling her legs apart and repeatedly shoving his fingers into her vagina.[84] In Nigeria, sexual abuse of women by a health care worker is reported by 2% of women.[85] Sexual abuse has also recently been reported in the Netherlands as occurring in 0.8% (or approximately 98 women) of their sample of 12,239 women.[86] An emerging reaction to such abuse is the creation of a Birth Monopoly, Obstetric Violence Story and Map which is focussed on exposing obstetric abuse in the USA in particular, but allowing for a global mapping of such incidents.[87]

Abuse of Caregivers

There is also abuse of care providers. Respectful treatment of caregivers is as important as respectful care of clients and their families. In war-torn, Southern Sudan, I asked a large group of traditional birth attendants with whom I was working "if you could have any wish you wanted, what things would you most want to obtain, that would enable you to provide better care for women in childbirth?" They agreed that the most important item was a uniform that others would recognize as a sign of their status so that they would be treated with respect. They also asked for rubber boots for wading through the mud caused by heavy summer rains to reach outlying women in labour and that would keep their uniforms clean, and their appearance dignified. They clearly perceived their lack of status as an obstacle to their providing care for mothers. Years of international pressure to give birth in formal healthcare facilities, rather than with the aid of traditional birth attendants, has led locals to lose respect for traditional birth attendant women, who are frequently the only available healthcare provider in this huge, largely rural country.

Not all challenges to the respectful treatment of caregivers can be solved as easily as with the provision of uniforms and rubber boots for caregivers in South Sudan. In developed countries, inadequate health care systems result in care providers being overworked and over stressed to the point that they experience serious mental and physical health complications.[88] Frustrated clients trying to access care in inadequately staffed care centres may well vent their anger towards their care providers. Caregivers may experience multiple forms of abuse levelled at them by angry, violent, or simply dissatisfied clients. Caregivers from equity-denied groups are particularly at risk of abuse, not just from their colleagues and employers, but from their clients as well. As in all professions, bias influences hiring, promotions, and treatment of these equity-denied caregivers. The global pandemics of Covid-19 as well as the consequent resurgence of excessive flu infections have placed enormous pressures and stressors on care providers, leading to increased abuse experiences. The caregiver abuse pandemic has not yet been named but might well be recognized in the months and years to come. The increasing presence of notices in medical rooms and clinics that state that disrespectful attitudes and actions expressed against medical staff will not be tolerated is evidence of this growing awareness. Caregiver abuse is self-perpetuating. Caregivers who abuse clients, lead to clients who become defensive or hostile when dealing with them, creating a vicious cycle.

Receptionist behaviour can compound the problem. Regarded as the gatekeepers for their clinical employers, they may make contact with a doctor difficult for clients. Receptionists may be less than helpful or sensitive to clients' expressed concerns regarding their painful or worrying symptoms, and may increase client irritation by being unresponsive to their needs. Some – perhaps because of overload, or possibly inefficiency – may forget to send urgent referrals, may leave clients waiting for an appointment that is never made, may ignore or delay paperwork that is needed for government or workplace support programs, leading to clients having to make repeated follow-up calls to trace the documents, and then charging clients for eventually supplying them. Irritation with receptionists can lead to aggression towards caregivers as well.

Physicians sometimes behave in an uncivil manner towards other health care providers. In Canada, more than 75% of health care employees have witnessed uncivil physician behaviour.[89] About a third of physicians (31%) report receiving weekly or daily rude, dismissive, or aggressive communications from other doctors. Trainees younger than thirty years old, shorter than 5'8," junior students, females, non-native language speakers, or those from non-dominant ethnicity groups, all report higher rates of incivility. Disruptive behaviours lead to less patient care, poorer team interactions, and are linked to medication errors, client neglect, surgical complications, or mortality. Health care providers experiencing such incivility have decreased well-being, increased burnout, greater absenteeism, and early departures from the workplace. Students experiencing such behaviour are themselves more likely to exhibit it.[90]

There are also reports of sexual abuse of caregivers by their own colleagues. Registered surgeons of all genders were invited to take part in an anonymous survey and 1,434 did so. Female surgeons in the National Health Service in the UK reported being sexually harassed and, in some cases (n=11), raped by their colleagues. In some instances, this occurred in the operating theatre. Nearly two thirds of women surgeons (63%) who responded to researchers from the Universities of Exeter and Surrey, and the working party on Sexual Misconduct in Surgery, reported that they had been sexually harassed in the past five years: one third (30%) had been sexually assaulted by their colleagues.[91] Almost all women (90%) and 81% of men had witnessed some form of sexual misconduct.[92] A quarter of the male respondents (24%) also reported being sexually harassed. Reaction to the report has been, unsurprisingly, deep shock and embarrassment, coupled with a lack of faith in bodies such as the NHS Trusts, the General Medical Council, and the Royal Colleges, to tackle the problem.[93]

Psychological Abuse

Psychological abuse is reported throughout perinatal care and can be experienced in a variety of ways. Coercion, emotionally and verbally abusive behaviours, disrespectful treatment, gaslighting, and lack of trauma informed care are some of the ways in which perinatal care can become psychologically abusive.

Coercion

Caregivers sometimes manipulate women emotionally – intentionally or unintentionally – to make use of interventions. For example, I have heard anaesthetists asking women in labour: "Would you like your epidural now dear, while I am still around? I may not be here later when you decide you want it." Alternatively, caregivers may try a different approach: "I recommend you have this...you don't want to feel responsible for harming your baby by not doing this do you?" Also, few or no alternatives to pharmacological pain management may be offered. These could include walking in labour, using showers or baths for relaxation, remaining mobile up to the moment of giving birth, adopting differing positions for pain relief, using breathing, relaxation and stress reducing techniques.[94] The result may be that women's use of pharmacological pain management, in contradiction to their original "natural birth" hopes, is understandable. Giving birth is painful and supporting a woman to manage this pain by using time-consuming supportive processes may not be every caregiver's preference, or hospital's policy.

It is striking that, in some Canadian research,[95] 70% of women expressed a need to give birth naturally, without intervention, while the same number actually had considerable intervention in the process. What can explain this discrepancy? Is it that women cannot cope with the reality of birth despite their high hopes? Alternatively, is it that caregivers do not provide the type of support and care that women need to assist them to find the best way possible to experience their births regardless of what happens? Or, is it that we use interventions inappropriately, causing medically induced aberrations?[96]

Emotional Abuse

On a more individualized level, while clinical procedures may inflict painful experiences on women during pregnancy and birth, other actions may be psychologically hurtful. Lack of respect for a woman's dignity, privacy and confidentiality may result in emotional neglect and non-dignified care and is a commonly reported theme from many women around the world.[97] Women from equity-owed groups are more likely to encounter abusive care in general, including disrespectful treatment and interactions.

Non-confidential care related to sensitive patient information such as HIV/AIDS status, age, marital status, or medical history, increases the woman's likelihood of discriminatory care and may deter her from attending a healthcare facility in future.[98] Failure of a physician to provide a follow-up visit for a woman after assisting with her delivery (leaving this to midwives or nurses), reflects disinterest by her caregiver, and may engender a woman's lack of respect for her doctor. Avoiding women or minimizing contact with them following adverse pregnancy outcomes (again leaving this to midwives or nurses) is simply unacceptable, reflects caregiver ignorance, and is cowardly. In some cases, new parents are not only ignored or neglected after birth but may even be left to labour and give birth alone, such as has been reported to occur in South Africa, Ghana, Sierra Leone, Kenya, Brazil, and India, amongst others.[99]

Ignoring women's experiences can, and has, led to major scandals in maternity care services, such as in the UK. At the Shrewsbury and Telford National Health Service Trust, 201 babies and nine mothers died leading to an investigation into how so many avoidable deaths and injuries could have occurred. A toxic mix of factors including staffing pressures, training gaps, and overstretched rotas contributed, but so did staff not listening to clients' experiences, blaming women for their poor outcomes – and even their own deaths – combined with a lack of compassionate care. Added to this was inadequate leadership and a bullying culture among staff.[100]

The UK is not alone in reporting disrespectful care. A Dutch, online survey recently completed by 12,239 women who had given birth in the past five years, revealed that 20-40% of women reported disrespect and abuse regarding their lack of choice, lack of communication, lack of support, and harsh or rough treatment, or physical violence. A third of women (36.3%) experienced at least one disrespectful situation as upsetting: experiencing more categories of upsetting disrespectful care/abuse was associated with more negative birth experiences.[101]

Verbal Abuse

Verbal statements can compound and contribute to emotional abuse. This includes the use of harsh or rude language, judgemental statements, threats of poor outcomes or withholding treatment if women are noncompliant. People from lower socio-economic groups, migrants, those from ethnic minorities, Disabled parents, people with a high BMI, adolescents, and older mothers of high parity, report discriminatory care.[102] The words most commonly used by women to describe the verbal disrespect they experience include "rude, harsh language, sarcasm, swear, snap at, mock, threaten, scold, scream/yell/shout/raise voice, degrade, belittle, dehumanize, intimidate, ridicule, name-calling, humiliate, and insult"[103] reflecting the wide array of disrespectful attitudes held towards these women. Emotional manipulation such as "You don't want to harm your baby, do you?" is an almost irresistible manipulation used to coerce women to comply with (unwanted) procedures. Further, women in Honduras reported being told "you didn't cry when you did it, open your legs or your baby will die and it will be your fault," or "you didn't shout when the penis was inside you, why do you shout now?"[104] Verbal abuse and sexist remarks made to women during birth are made behind the closed doors of health facilities with few caregivers being willing to report their co-workers' comments. Being a whistleblower is risky: even if this is a supposedly protected activity, work insecurity, or retaliation, is feared, usually with good reason.

Disrespectful Treatment

Even the most basic, and often innocent interactions between client and caregiver can perpetuate this power imbalance and appear to be disrespectful. For example, doctors frequently introduce themselves as "Hello Beverley, I'm Dr. Doe." While it is an improvement for caregivers to introduce themselves at all (a sadly low bar to clear), this form of greeting ignores the client's own status and endorses the power imbalance between doctor and client. My response to this type of greeting is almost always "Hello, Dr. Doe, I'm Dr. Chalmers," usually leading to a more balanced discussion. Not all clients are able to assert themselves in similar fashion, and those seeking help from a doctor that is difficult to obtain, feel unable to do so, for fear of retaliation. Regarding all clients as equally unable to comprehend medical terminology and reducing the level of communication to a Grade Five level for all is disrespectful for those who do have a higher level of comprehension. Caregivers need to take a few moments to learn about their clients and to adjust their communication approaches accordingly.

This problem often emerges in medical systems that incentivize shorter appointment times. A family doctor may have ten minutes to spend with a patient. If they do not finish their appointments fast enough, they lose out financially. This type of reimbursement system forces doctors into shorter appointments, eliminating the possibility of becoming familiar with the patient's life-style, or even the possibility of understanding a complex problem.

Gaslighting

One common example of emotional abuse is the practice of gaslighting, with its attempt to deny reality, or convince someone that their perception of reality is false.[105] Gaslighting is designed to make mothers question their sanity and become reliant on their caregiver's advice or opinions, and to doubt the veracity and legitimacy of their own experiences, perspectives, and feelings. This is an under-examined aspect of obstetric violence, but is a commonly reported experience. Denial of mothers' humanity, their knowledge as valid, their judgements as rational, or their feelings as legitimate are all methods of gaslighting mothers. All four types of denial leave mothers feeling non-credible and destabilized.[106] Gaslighting can take varied forms, a few of which could be: caregivers dismiss women's symptoms as being caused by a chronic health condition, their weight, or a disability, rather than investigating alternate possible causes; caregivers dismiss reports of pain as "normal pregnancy pain" and do not explore any further diagnostic or treatment routes; alternatively, caregivers dismiss reports of pain because they believe a procedure should not be painful, regardless of the mother's experiences. Caregivers may also attempt to convince women that an adverse outcome or negative experience is "not that bad," or is the fault of the woman; both narratives being particularly common in situations related to pregnancy loss or infertility. Caregivers may also report procedures performed by other colleagues, apparently without client consent, were likely a misunderstanding by the client of what was to be expected, or "that's just normal procedure." Both responses cover up their colleague's actions by denying the client's experience of what happened. Overemphasising the risks involved in procedures they do not wish to perform, or underplaying the risks of actions they would prefer to take are also forms of emotional manipulation.

As so well depicted in the 1944 movie *Gaslight*, from where the name is derived, gaslighting is increasingly recognized as a form of emotional manipulation that is insidious, and designed to create self doubt to the point of disturbance, distress, and disorientation. It increases client's dependence on the caregiver and decreases their ability to question or challenge the treatment they receive. In addition to being emotionally abusive, gaslighting also results in poor medical outcomes. When caregivers dismiss a woman's symptoms or reports of pain, they can miss important diagnoses or warning signs, which can result in serious negative clinical outcomes. Gaslighting may well be rooted in the stereotypical, and no longer accepted, role of the doctor as superior and patient as subordinate. For example, requiring a client to undress and be placed in a lithotomy position prior to the doctor first meeting the client immediately places the client in a subservient and vulnerable position and is disrespectful and manipulative. Power based relationships where "Dr. Doe" treats patient "Mary" rather than "Mrs./Miss./Ms./Dr. Jones" facilitate authoritarian dismissal of presenting symptoms with diagnoses that are assumed to fit prejudicial assumptions. Such mistreatment leads to humiliation, frustration, and self-doubt in recipients: the standard after-effects of gaslighting.

Trauma Informed Care

The absence of effective, trauma-informed care can be re-traumatizing for survivors of both physical and emotional abuse. The choice to ignore readily available expertise on how to avoid re-traumatizing survivors of abuse in healthcare settings is, in itself, abusive.[107]

According to a 2013 United Nations global review of available data, 35% of women worldwide have experienced either physical and/or sexual violence and about one in ten children under eighteen have been sexually abused.[108] In some individual countries, the estimates of women who have experienced abuse rise to 70%.[109] The implications of previous experience of violence, whether sexual, physical, or interpersonal, for obstetric and gynaecological care can be more significant than for other areas of healthcare.[110] Sexual violence has obvious ramifications given that the same bodily parts are involved. Memories of physical violence may be aroused through the intimacy of gynaecological or obstetric examinations and procedures. Feelings of being restrained for example, with continuous fetal monitoring, or having one's feet in stirrups, can trigger flashbacks of rape or abuse. Not all trauma is physical: Psychological experiences that reflect feelings of betrayal, neglect, fear, coercion, control, and manipulation can all trigger emotional reactions to birth and /or the newborn. Some of these may be complex emotions that are strengthened by repetition or are cumulative or sustained events. Caregivers need to be sensitive to actions, words, or events during the perinatal period that trigger such emotional memories and to work with the client to recognize and cope with these.

At the same time, we need to be aware that clinical perinatal care can also be traumatic for caregivers. Exposure to stillbirths, the birth of babies with anomalies, difficult client's birth experiences or events, and constantly caring for others who might be having traumatic emotional reactions, take a toll on caregivers as well. Providing supports for caregivers is also a crucial component of optimal care.[111]

We should respect requests from patients, including those related to caregiver preferences (whether a preference for an individual caregiver, or those of a specific gender). Trauma informed care mandates that caregivers be sensitive to the possibility that someone under their care may have experienced past abuse, regardless of whether that person has disclosed that history. All care should be trauma informed and sensitive. Caregivers should be trained to recognize the indicators of trauma in individuals and families and take steps to actively avoid re-traumatising people under their care. They should actively work to increase safety and collaboration, reducing power differences between caregiver and patient, and emphasize collaboration, and informed choices for families. Caregivers should earn the trust of those under their care, and work to remain trustworthy throughout their careers.[112]

In situations in which a caregiver knows of a history of abuse, knowledge of the woman's past experience should temper how we touch women, what procedures or interventions we use (when we have multiple options), what preparation we offer for obstetric examinations, what supports they might need to cope with such contacts, and what explanations and advice we give and, particularly, to be aware of the words or language that we, as caregivers, use, or that clients use, that might provide or reflect emotional triggers for the woman.[113] A caregiver's ability to sensitively discuss past traumas and to provide appropriate support for women with these experiences may be facilitated by the use of such instruments as the *Antenatal Psycho-social Health Assessment Tool* (ALPHA)[114] that explores psychological, and social issues that give rise to stress in pregnancy as well as their associated negative obstetric outcomes. While this does not provide tools for caring for clients it does provide some indications of whether clients have, or might have, experienced trauma in their past. It can help to raise a "red flag" as to the need for especially sensitive and trauma informed care.

Discussing and disclosing sexual, physical, or interpersonal abuse is difficult for any woman, despite many societies' (but not all) increasing recognition and condemnation of such acts.[115] When such information is disclosed, we need to protect the confidentiality of that information. This results in difficulties regarding the sharing of information with additional caregivers who need to be aware of the woman's past experiences, and the importance of not simply recording this information on charts where it is available for indiscriminate inspection. It is necessary to discuss this concern with women and to agree on what information we can share, with whom, and whether verbally or through written documentation. Her preferences regarding how such information is disclosed should be honoured, regardless of caregiver preferences or opinions. Many cultures and countries are reluctant to address the issue of family violence and abuse directly. Few have implemented effective training programs for medical and allied healthcare workers to assist them to deal with the abusive experiences of their clients, such as the various Family Violence Prevention Programs supported by the Public Health Agency of Canada[116] or the multidisciplinary, perinatal, trauma-informed health care clinic developed in Portland, Oregon, USA.[117] Even fewer have considered that their own practices may add to that abuse.[118]

Societal Abuse

While physical and psychological abuse are familiar concepts, the idea of societal abuse is less readily understood. In this context, we discuss societal abuse as abusive systems and policies that are imposed at societal levels. These may include health systems, economically exploitative practices, or political interventions or policies that lead to perinatal abuse. This chapter also briefly discusses some historical examples of societal abuse.

Systemic Abuse

Health care institutions may have systems in place that are abusive. Denying equitable care is one example. Some hospitals refuse to treat clients with certain characteristics, such as those with high BMI, Disabilities, lower income levels, without access to medical insurance, or in some countries, clients of colour. For examples, there are reports of health care providers in some hospitals being required to call social services when Indigenous mothers in Canada give birth, often resulting in their newborns being taken from them and placed in foster care.

Religious convictions, and particularly those surrounding the emergence of life, also influence policies and practices in hospitals, as well as in the States/Regions and Countries in which they are situated, leading to controversies regarding the provision of some contraceptives, abortions, and the provision of gender affirming treatment. In the USA, the impact of these anti-choice convictions is leading to national disagreement, conflict, and political upheaval in addition to further imbalances in the care of equity-owed groups. Banning abortion in many USA States has also resulted in more newborns in these States dying shortly after birth: clearly the consequence of allowing a fetus with terminal conditions to proceed to term rather than allowing the mother to terminate an unviable pregnancy early on. For example, in Texas the infant mortality rate increased by 13%, largely driven by the death of babies born with congenital anomalies.[119] Maternal mortality was also impacted with sepsis rates following hospitalization for pregnancy loss in the second trimester of pregnancy increasing by more than 50%.[120] The emotional trauma inflicted by this on the women, their partners and additional family members is inconceivable.

Economic Abuse

A further abusive practice that I observed in multiple countries of the former Soviet Union, involves the payment of bribes to doctors, nurses, midwives, receptionists, cleaners, and guards. These bribes take the form of money, food or drinks, jewelry, or other gifts and are expected in many countries around the world. In many cases these payments ensured such "luxuries" as private rooms, access to water births, and care from more senior members of the health care facility. But they were also expected for the provision of basic clinical care such as for pain-relieving medications for labour and birth and even for the repair of episiotomies or more extensive perineal tears. In some cases, such payments ensured essential services such as cleaning the women's rooms. In former Soviet countries, being paid "under the table" was the norm and may have explained how some heads of departments or senior doctors lived exceedingly well – with mansions and expensive cars – while being officially paid only a few hundred dollars a month. Private hospitals have emerged that offer services – often basic clinical care practices – for (large) fees, thus, in a sense, formalizing the informal bribery system and favouring more affluent clients. "Luxury" care (such as more comfortable rooms, better food or a choice of meals, or private TV's), can perhaps be viewed as justifying private payment systems. In contrast, the provision of standard evidence-based care that is essential, good, clinical practice (such as pain relief) should never warrant special bribes, as frequently occurs.

In some countries including in Asia, sub-Saharan Africa, Latin America, and the Middle East, women have been detained in hospitals after giving birth because of their inability to pay hospital fees. Some women have been detained for weeks, or even years while being forced to sleep on the floor, denied adequate food, and watched over by guards.[121] Detaining women or their newborns in a care facility until they pay for their care is egregiously discriminatory.[122]

In technologically advanced countries, economic abuse takes different forms. Obstetricians and midwives, for example, are paid at vastly differing rates even for the care of pregnancies at similar (low) levels of risk. In countries where both private health care systems exist together with state-funded services, some women pay (usually through their insurance coverage) far more for maternity care than those without access to private medical care. Ironically, in such countries (as in South Africa), the care offered in private health care services is frequently far more interventionist with far higher caesarean section rates (almost double the number) for instance, than the essential care offered in state-funded services.[123] State-funded services that pay caregivers salaries rather than fee-for-service charges attract the most qualified doctors as they are usually larger, serving greater numbers of clients that result in opportunities to treat rare and interesting clinical challenges. Such hospitals, such as Chris Hani Hospital in Soweto, South Africa care for 25,000 or more birthing people each year with responsibility for a further 10,000 giving birth in midwife run clinics affiliated with the hospital. In such large facilities there is little time, and few resources available, to provide excessive rather than essential clinical care, resulting in the most optimal obstetric care for all women.[124] Although Apartheid ended about thirty years ago, there is still deep-rooted systemic racism in South Africa, as Black people to this day, particularly in rural areas, do not have access to adequate health care as it remains inaccessible, unaffordable, and unavailable for this majority of the population.[125]

The question must be asked as to whether remuneration packages influence the use of technology and present a barrier to equitable care. There is clear evidence to indicate that where fee-for-service remuneration packages are in place for caregivers, the rates of technological interventions increase. In countries where both fee-for-service and salaried medical service structures co-exist, the technological intervention rate can be almost twice as high in fee-for-service systems. This occurs most frequently when there is private health insurance available to higher socio-economic groups, compared with salaried care services that care for families at lower socio-economic levels.[126] While this was in evidence in Apartheid South Africa, it is likely still in evidence in South Africa today.[127] Similarly, in the USA, women giving birth in "for profit" hospitals are twice as likely to have caesarean births as women delivering their babies in not-for-profit facilities.[128] It is obvious that where we financially reward caregivers for interventions, they, not surprisingly, intervene more.

Another form of economic abuse is the grossly inequitable treatment that poorer families experience.[129] So too do people from other equity-owed groups such as those with Disabilities, Indigenous people, disparaged racial groups, and those with higher weight. The cost of care for poorer women is also discriminatory, especially in countries that do not have national medical insurance supports in place. In a country like the USA, without universal health coverage, the cost of having a baby can be prohibitively expensive ranging from approximately $19,000 without health insurance or almost $3,000, even with health care cover.[130] If the mother or child requires anything beyond the most basic care, costs can rapidly become financially devastating reaching into the hundreds of thousands.[131] Even in countries like Canada that do have a universal health insurance policy, care for poorer women is influenced by the costs of being poor. Housing further away from health care centres is usually less expensive for lower income families, but this incurs increased travel costs. Not having flexible work conditions, as is more common in lower income jobs, also makes attendance at health care clinics more difficult to arrange. For people working multiple jobs, the obstacles only increase.

The absence of universal coverage for medications, psychological care, or paramedical services like physiotherapy further aggravates health inequities, even in countries with "universal" health care.

Politics and Reproduction

Political systems play a significant role in determining whether childbirth is supportive or abusive of mothers and their families. There are a myriad of examples of how political systems have manipulated childbearing women including: among Black women in South Africa under Apartheid; women giving birth in the former Soviet Union under communist rule; women growing up in societies that practice Female Genital Mutilation, often believed to be religiously required; and women in genocidal situations including the Holocaust, Cambodia, Rwanda, Sudan and other current African conflict zones where rape is increasingly used as a weapon of war with its cruel consequences for childbearing and rearing.[132]

We need look no further than the recent and current outcries in the United States of America regarding the overturning of Roe v. Wade for a further example of political interference in reproduction. Terminating pregnancies on psychological, social or emotional grounds, (for example following rape, incest, newborn anomalies, maternal health considerations, or even desperate social situations of the mother) have been an integral part of respectful obstetric care and women's human rights for decades in America and elsewhere. But concerns for rights and freedoms, as well as religious, political, societal, economic, personal and interpersonal, familial, and emotional reactions to either banning or promoting abortion have split American people, politics and political parties across the nation. Birth, or its prevention, is clearly not simply a physiological process but a multifaceted, multi-layered issue involving religious and political implications that have far reaching and often fatal outcomes for both mothers, fetuses, and newborns.

Historical Abuse

Considerable evidence indicates that disrespectful and non-consensual treatment of women in childbirth is widespread.[133] Such treatment, along with abusive care, is also associated with increased maternal mortality.[134] Disrespectful treatment and obstetric violence have a long history extending back centuries.[135] It often reflects social and political discrimination, oppression, and exclusion, usually manifesting in some form of forced control or legalized abuse of women's reproductive lives and their bodies. In 16th century Rome, for instance, Catholic authorities removed Jewish women's babies from their mothers unless they consented to Christianisation through baptism. In the late 18th century in the Spanish colonies of America, priests performed forced caesarean sections on women having difficult births. The priority was to save the souls of the fetuses and not their mothers. Slavery also incurred obstetric violence in the Americas, through exploitation of women's reproduction to enrich their oppressors. In addition to being forced to bear children for their "owners," they were subject to medical experimentation by physicians seeking caregiving developments in obstetrics.[136]

In the Nazi era Jewish women were forced to abort pregnancies while so-called "Aryan" women were denied termination of pregnancies.[137] Jewish and other "undesirable" non-Jewish women were also subjected to forced sterilization and ultimately murder to prevent them from reproducing under Hitler's eugenics and euthanasia programs. Horrific medical experimentation on reproduction, childbearing and sexuality was a distinct policy under Nazi rule in its efforts to both eliminate the Jewish people and others deemed to be "undesirable," and to promote reproduction among so-called "Aryans" that met Nazi approved racial standards.[138] Sexuality, pregnancy, childbearing, and newborn care were systematically abused during the Holocaust as well.[139]

Sterilization of women deemed to be under-valued has been extensively conducted among some groups and continues in some places even today.[140] In China until very recently, women have, for decades, been forbidden to have more than one child.[141] Muslim Uyghurs in China are still being forced to suppress their birth rate with pregnancy checks, forced insertion of intrauterine devices, injectable contraception, and abortions.[142] The result has been a drop in the birth rate in mostly Uyghur regions by 60% between 2015 and 2018. Even in Canada, where healthcare is purported to be excellent, recent reports have revealed that forced or coerced sterilizations of Indigenous women – a group discriminated against since European contact – have continued to occur in some places.[143] The recent widespread legislation condemning abortion in much of America is only the latest in a long line of politically or religiously inspired interference in women's reproductive freedoms.

The medicalization of birth in the 19th and 20th centuries also separated women from their traditional birth attendants and forced them to move from giving birth at home into institutions with physician-managed hospital deliveries and an interventionist approach. Such medicalized care has also been disproportionally directed towards women in equity-owed groups. For example, pharmacological pain management was increasingly offered to white, middle- and upper-class women and not those of other racial groups or economic status, based on the belief that pain was differentially experienced by these groups: an attitude that sometimes persists to this day. Wilfully ignoring or discriminating against "undesirable" women is commonly reported. Coercive sterilization based on eugenic theories has disproportionally impacted Disabled, impoverished, and racially marginalized groups – a practice that recurs, at times, today.[144] Political motivations in Latin America underpinned the late 20th century repression of women from opposition political affiliations, removing their children and sending them to be raised by families who supported the regimes in power. Even today, many women who give birth while incarcerated may be shackled in childbirth and be separated from their newborns while experiencing coerced sterilization.[145]

Ideological and religious fanaticism directed against abortion also results in medical harm from unsafe abortions, as well as economic harms, in addition to the removal of women's rights to control their own bodies. The results of banning abortion are well known: The example set by Ceaușescu in Romania provides clear warnings of what can ensue.[146] In Romania, illegal abortion related maternal mortality soared to ten times that of any other European country at the time even though, theoretically at least, although likely not in reality, the law allowed for exceptions such as for rape, incest or fetal anomalies.[147] Few caregivers in Romania – and today, some in the USA – were willing to risk performing abortions that were likely legal, for fear of challenging the interpretation of this law – a fear expressed by caregivers in some USA states today. The average annual maternal mortality rate in Romania following the ban and its associated implementation procedures, rose to 170/100,000 births per year between 1980-1989. More than 10,000 women died following ill-performed attempts at pregnancy termination. Thousands of Romanian children were institutionalized following their births because their mothers could not find the financial means or emotional motivation to care for them as they feared the punishment that would follow if their child died while under their care. It was preferable to hand the child over to their doctor, who in turn, and for similar reasons, would send the child to a specialist for treatment, who in turn would send the child to an institution – the last referral possibility – to avoid the draconian government punishments that ensued after child death. When Ceaușescu was overthrown and murdered on 25 December 1989, approximately 150,000 to 200,000 children were in institutionalized care. When I visited a number of these institutions in 1991, the condition of these children was abhorrent, revealing both physical and psychological neglect. One of the very first acts of the provisional government that succeeded Ceaușescu was to abrogate the laws banning abortion as well as oral contraception or condoms – as a public health measure aimed at reducing the rate of unsafe abortions and consequent maternal deaths.[148]

Ethics and Rights

Respectful perinatal care is not just a valued addition to clinical care but a fundamental human right.[149] It is a necessary component of ethical and competent care. This is not an aspirational ideal, but is the bare minimum requirement for adequate health care in any field of medicine. Care that is founded on both good evidence and with a rights-based approach is not only going to prevent abusive practices, but will also provide effective care for clients. Evidence- and rights-based approaches to perinatal care mean that people having babies, whether by vaginal birth or caesarean section, and regardless of their financial means, will:

Generally

- Be viewed as having a normal experience unless evidence to the contrary emerges.
- Be cared for with a family-centred approach.
- Receive up-to-date, evidence-based care.
- Receive psycho-socially sensitive care.
- Have care that is culturally appropriate and respectful.
- Be provided with up-to-date, evidence-based information regarding all available care options, risks, and benefits, available in accessible formats. Be given time to assess and consider this information before consenting to procedures.
- Have access to care that is suitable for their physical, psychological, and cultural needs, including accessible to all people regardless of disability, body type, or health status. This includes access to care in a language they understand and in which they can effectively communicate.

- Have care that is respectful of the woman's, and her family's, dignity, confidentiality, and privacy.
- Be cared for in a facility that conforms to the WHO / United Nations Children's Fund (UNICEF) Baby Friendly Hospital Initiative (BFHI).
- Have equitable access to multiple caregivers capable of caring for both medical and psycho-social needs.
- Be able to discuss their birth experiences with their birth caregivers and be entitled to full, honest, and transparent information about all aspects of their care.
- Be offered an apology and equitable compensation if avoidable negative outcomes occur.
- Have care that is free from prejudice, stigma, racism, ableism, sexism, homophobia, and any other form of discrimination.
- Have care that is free from abusive, disrespectful, insulting and otherwise harmful practices, attitudes, and behaviours.
- Have access to publicly available, aggregated, and understandable information regarding the facility's and care provider's maternity care practices and outcomes.
- Have free and unimpeded access to their medical records, test results, and communications between care providers, in a format of their choosing (digital or hard copies).
- Have equitable access to all appropriate medical care, including termination/abortion procedures.

Prenatally

- Have the option to attend prenatal classes, together with their chosen companion/s, designed to assist families with the physical, psychological, and social changes occurring during pregnancy, birth and the first months of parenthood.
- Lead decisions about their or their baby's care, together with their chosen support companion/s, based on comprehensive evidence-based information, without coercion.
- Have the companion/s of their choice present at all prenatal testing or appointments, if that is their choice.

In Labour and Birth

- Be attended at labour and birth by the companion/s of their choice.
- Be given the option to consent to or decline procedures, with sufficient time to consider and discuss options and alternatives, preferably before being in labour (except in a time-sensitive emergency context).
- Be encouraged to avoid a supine position and the use of stirrups in labour and birth, except when instrumental or surgical delivery is required.
- Be cared for using only essential, unbiased, evidence-based interventions, without discrimination.
- Be offered a variety of both pharmacological and non-pharmacological pain management methods (such as walking, use of birthing balls, alternate positions) as alternatives to pharmacological options. Caesarean section will preferably be conducted with regional rather than general anaesthetic.
- Hold their newborn skin-to-skin from the moment of birth onwards (unless medically unsafe to do so) and breastfeed when the baby shows signs of readiness for a feed – usually within the first hour or so after birth. This includes immediate skin-to-skin contact after a caesarean birth. Caesarean section does not preclude immediate skin-to-skin care.
- Be encouraged to breastfeed their newborn/s. Regardless of a parent's choice to breastfeed or not, all parents should be provided with knowledgeable, unbiased, and respectful care and support regarding the advisability of feeding with breastmilk or breastmilk substitutes.
- Give birth in an atmosphere that is caring and gentle, and remains so after birth.
- Be able to attend the birth of a baby born by a surrogate mother in whatever way is agreed upon by the surrogate mother and the biological parent/s.

After Birth

- Room-in for 24 hours a day after birth, with their newborn and chosen family member/s companion/s.
- Lead the care decisions and care for their newborns.
- Room-in with their baby and a family member/companion in the Neonatal Intensive Care Unit (NICU) if the baby needs NICU care, and share, to the greatest extent possible, in the baby's care, including feeding their child, either by breastfeeding or with breastmilk substitutes.
- Access to community parenting support services and activities on discharge. Ensure that appropriate systems are in place to transfer families in need of further medical care back to the healthcare services/team.
- Be provided with a means of offering feedback to the facility on their maternity care experiences, which are then rigorously monitored, evaluated, and incorporated into future care by the facility.

Reproductive Rights

Reproductive rights have become an increasingly important focus in recent decades. Since the 1990s, the United Nations (UN) Health Agencies have spearheaded reproductive rights in obstetric and neonatal care as universal developments.[150] Most of the member countries of the United Nations, at least in theory, support these principles, although it will take some time to implement these mandates in practice and through national legislation.

A series of global Consensus Conferences in the 1990's led to UN declarations of action agendas for socially equitable and sustainable development in the 21st century.[151] These conferences, including the Fourth World Conference on Women (Beijing 1995) the World Summit for Social Development (Copenhagen 1995), the International Conference on Population and Development (Cairo

1994) and the World Conference on Human Rights (Vienna 1993) resulted in a progressive agenda for development. Arising from these conferences have been the Convention on the Rights of the Child, the Convention on the Elimination of all forms of Discrimination against Women, and the Declaration on the Elimination of Violence against Women. In essence, these declarations reflect a policy of people-centred development based on the following key principles:[152]

- All individuals should be able to enjoy all human rights and fundamental freedoms. Achieving social equality and justice is a priority objective of the global community, in particular for girls and women, Indigenous, and other equity-denied groups.
- Empowering people and eradicating poverty, especially through access to information, resources, and democratic institutions, is the key to unleashing human potential and securing peace and development for all.
- Reproductive rights are human rights. National development cannot be achieved without the full and equal participation of women, and people of all genders, in public and private decision-making, and their access to equal opportunities in all aspects of social and economic activity.
- Men, women, and people of all genders share responsibility and participate in all aspects of family and household roles, including child rearing and child support, sexual and reproductive behaviour, and family planning practice. Gender equity is essential in developing families based on equality and mutual respect.
- Health and education for all are core factors of developments that must be dealt with as a part of inter-related social, economic, and poverty eradication efforts.

These principles form the basis of numerous international initiatives designed to monitor and safeguard sexual and reproductive rights. Although these principles were not specifically stated in gender inclusive terms when developed in the 1990's, they are equally applicable to all people that are LGBTQ2S+ as endorsed by the UN in both 2015 and 2024.[153]

The initial priority of many of these agendas was the development of rights regarding reproduction, and specifically focussing on the right to bear only as many children as wanted and when wanted. In consequence, many of these recommendations, such as the 1968 Tehran Human Rights Conference, the 1994 International Conference on Population and Development held in Cairo, the 1995 Fourth World Conference on Women held in Beijing, and the 2008 Sexual Rights Declaration of the International Planned Parenthood Federation, focus primarily on family planning and freedom of choice. While the United Nations Sustainable Development Goals endorsed in 2015 include some reproductive and sexual health targets, these only cover family planning, adolescent fertility, and sexual education (targets 5.6 and 3.7).[154] Issues such as safe abortion, non-discrimination based on sexual orientation or gender identity, sexual satisfaction, gender-based violence, and the importance of high quality, confidential, and timely sexual and reproductive services, are inadequately endorsed by these goals, due to opposition from some member states and their conservative allies to abortion, adolescent sexual and reproductive health services, and sexual rights. In consequence, *The Lancet*, together with the Guttmacher Institute established a Commission aiming to develop broad-ranging, evidence-based priorities for sexual and reproductive health and rights for the coming decades.[155]

Because the United Nations Health Organizations focus their attention more on developing nations, where there is greatest need for assistance, than on the technologically sophisticated world, which should have the resources to help themselves, their charters and recommendations are often discounted by these more developed nations as not applicable to them. This can lead to better healthcare systems being introduced in developing countries than exist in those that are wealthier. The earlier and more extensive implementation of the BFHI in developing countries compared to more affluent parts of the world is a case in point – much to the potential detriment of babies born in wealthier countries.

Rights of Families

More recently, initiatives have developed that are expanding the concern for reproductive health rights to include that of the mother during pregnancy and childbirth. The White Ribbon Alliance for Safe Motherhood, with support from USA Aid (USAID), is leading the campaign to promote respectful maternity care. The White Ribbon Alliance has developed *The Respectful Maternity Care Charter: The Universal Rights of Childbearing Women.*[156] It identifies that in addition to bringing vital, potentially lifesaving health services, women's experiences with maternity caregivers have the potential to empower and comfort, or to inflict lasting damage and emotional trauma. Women's memories of their childbearing experiences stay with them for a lifetime. The White Ribbon Alliance is attempting to build national, regional, and global awareness, which envisions a world in which the right to Respectful Maternity Care is embedded at all levels of all perinatal health systems around the globe, and that women are aware of them. The Charter addresses the issue of disrespect and abuse among those seeking maternity care. It asserts that all childbearing people need and deserve respectful care and protection. This includes care to protect the mother-baby pair as well as marginalized or vulnerable people (e.g., adolescents, ethnic minorities, 2SLGBTQI+ individuals, those living with physical or mental disabilities, people with obesity, people of colour, those living in poverty, incarcerated people, or those with HIV or other chronic illnesses).

Other national organizations have emphasized the rights of women during childbearing, for example, Childbirth Connection in the USA in 2012 proposed *The Rights of Childbearing Women.*[157] The rights listed reflect practices that occur during pregnancy, birth, and the postpartum period. Childbirth Connection asserts that we must ensure that all childbearing people have access to information and care based on the best scientific evidence available, and have opportunities to exercise their right to make healthcare decisions. Access to legal or other recourse to address their grievances is needed by women whose rights are violated.

The Breastfeeding Mothers' Bill of Rights, promoted by the Department of Health, State of New York.[158] and *The United States Centre for Reproductive Rights* declarations[159] are two further examples of locally developed, rights-based documents that support women during this period. The Canadian Society for Obstetricians and Gynaecologists has also developed a charter of sexual and reproductive rights and health that focuses on sexual issues and includes reproductive health issues.[160]

The above rights-based reproductive health programs, and other similar initiatives, have been predominantly directed towards women in keeping with the "woman-centred" approach to care that has superseded previous "physician-centred" or "baby-centred" attitudes. There is still a dearth of attention being paid to a rights-based approach to "family-centred" perinatal care. Even with this wealth of advocacy for rights-based care, abusive and disrespectful treatment remains a consistent and frequent part of perinatal health practices. Perinatal care practices that are not founded in human rights and equity are not only disrespectful, but also constitute incompetent, inadequate, and abusive health care.

Rights of Newborns

The *United Nations Convention on the Rights of the Child*[161] extended reproductive rights concerns towards the child. These do not, however, specifically address the Rights of the Newborn or the rights of the sick or preterm baby cared for in a NICU. An Italian group has developed the *Parma Charter of The Rights of the Newborn*[162] which incorporates many of the ideals outlined in this book. This charter incorporates the following:

1. Every newborn is entitled to life at the best levels of health.
2. Every live newborn is entitled to appropriate assistance during delivery.
3. Every newborn, be they healthy or ill, is entitled to the best care, social protection, and safety available.

4. Every newborn has the right to be born in the most suitable place.
5. The newborn must be guaranteed vicinity to their parents.
6. No medical procedure, including those for research purposes, may be performed on the newborn without the informed consent of the parents or legal guardian.
7. Every newborn is entitled to be adequately fed.
8. In the case of the birth of a severely ill newborn, appropriate treatment must be guaranteed.
9. Every newborn is entitled to be registered after birth, to be given a name and to acquire a nationality.
10. The newborn is a person.[163]

Clause 3 of this charter specifies that special attention must be granted to the medical, social, and psychological care of the unborn child and the mother, during pregnancy and delivery, as these have direct implications for the newborn's health. Clause 5 requires that all healthy newborns room-in with their mother. Babies cared for in NICUs must have family-centred care providing support for parents who should be involved as far as possible in caring for the baby and in related decision-making processes. Breastfeeding is to be facilitated and encouraged as the optimal feeding method addressed in Clause 7.

(In)Appropriate Treatment

Some clinical practices have decades of evidence behind their benefits, but are still not being implemented. In most cases, implementation adds little or no financial costs (and in some situations may be more cost effective), less requirements for advanced technology, and would reduce the burden on health care systems both in the short-term and through long-term benefits of improved outcomes and better psychological results. With usually several decades of evidence available to support these practices, and without an economic or resource-based justification to avoid implementation, the choice to neglect these evidence-based practices is inappropriate and unacceptable.

This chapter outlines these best practices in a variety of perinatal contexts, including during both normal and complicated births, with normal and adverse infant outcomes, and in relation to psycho-social, inter-disciplinary, and family-centred care. It also highlights the evidence for the superiority of following a profoundly integrated clinical, psychological, and social approach over current practices that routinely neglect the psychological and social aspects of care. In each case, the argument will be made that neglecting these advances in care is harmful and constitutes systemic abuses of mothers and families.

It is impossible to provide competent clinical care without also providing family-centred, respectful care. The two are indivisible and failing to provide both is abusive.

Family-Centred Care

Family-centred care during pregnancy, birth, and the postpartum period can be defined as care offered to the pregnant person and their chosen supportive companions that utilizes only essential and appropriate technology and is respectful, evidence-based, psycho-socially sensitive, inclusive, and inter-and multi-disciplinary. Family-centred care has the family as the central priority. It is devoted to meeting each family's needs above all others. It centres their preferences and respects the family as the primary decision-makers. It places families, not as equal partners (which would still be a step up from what currently exists), but as superiors, with the healthcare team serving their needs. Treatment that does not meet these criteria, in a context in which it could have been possible to do so, is unacceptable.

Alternate definitions have been attempted although most, if not all, omit reference to the centrality of the family. The Canadian National *Family-Centred Maternal and Newborn Care Guidelines* approximate this focus and defines family-centred care as "A complex, multidimensional, dynamic process of providing safe, skilled, and individualized care. It responds to the physical, emotional, psycho-social, and spiritual needs of the woman, the newborn, and the family."[164] It does not, however, prioritize the needs of the family. The *Transforming Maternity Care Vision Team* in the USA, emphasized the mother rather than the family, and provides an alternate definition:

> ...the goals for maternity care are best met by implementing a holistic, relationship-based model of care that is woman-centred, inclusive, and collaborative. Caregivers are included as dictated by the health needs, values, and preferences of each woman, taking into account her social and cultural context as she defines it, and given consideration for evidence of effectiveness, value, and efficiency.[165]

Common to most definitions of family-centred care is the understanding that, for most people, pregnancy and birth are normal, healthy, life events. It should, however, be recognized that family-centred care is applicable to not only healthy mothers and babies, but also to the care of mothers and newborns requiring specialized care such as surgical delivery or intensive care.[166] It is also applicable to all people regardless of their health status, age, ability or disability, body type or size, racial or ethnic background, religion, gender identity or sexual orientation, country of origin, educational level, or socio-economic standing. All too often, the normal process of pregnancy and birth is unnecessarily medicalized resulting in abusive treatment compounded by a lack of sensitivity to the wishes, hopes, and needs of prospective parents. When a highly medicalized approach to birth is necessary and appropriate, all considerations for respectful, inclusive, and psycho-socially sensitive care are often ignored, resulting in abuse masquerading as medical care.

Most caregivers do not intervene in birth to deliberately cause hurt. Many genuinely believe that they want to do what is best for the mother, her baby, and family. Despite these beliefs, many caregivers fail to stay up-to-date on relevant literature. When they do not keep up-to-date, they choose to not do what is best for their clients because it is more convenient for themselves. Those who accept common practices, such as continuous, electronic, fetal heart monitoring, choose this because it is convenient for caregivers rather then because this is best practice for all: it is not. Those who choose to maintain nursery-based newborn care, neglect to fully understand how breastfeeding can be supported, or who avoid skin-to-skin care following caesarean sections, do so because it is more convenient for caregivers and not because it is best practice. The same is true for imposing birth in a supine position, with or without stirrups. These are not best practices in the light of available knowledge.

Similarly, some caregivers fail to challenge and address their personal and societal biases, such as against poorer women or families, and bring those biases into their practice. They work in practices that do not have inclusive equipment, suitable for people of all abilities, or body types, and choose not to learn how to care for people with diverse body types, abilities, sexual or gender orientations, or those from different cultural or religious backgrounds. They may have no desire to abuse or hurt their clients, but their neglect, their acceptance of poor practice that may be built into health systems, and their willful ignorance of innovation and diversity of care requirements, because this is more convenient, makes their practices abusive.

Implementing respectful, family-centred treatment occurs at many levels of the care environment ranging from the individual to the departmental and organizational. It is not a specific set of procedures or practices, but an approach that guides policy and program development, facility design, decision making, and daily activities throughout the healthcare environment.[167]

Emergencies

Some may argue that when emergencies occur there is no time for "niceties" such as sensitive care: clinical needs take priority. It is true that clinical needs take priority, but even within that context, it is still the caregiver's responsibility to be respectful and kind to the birthing person and to the family during the crisis, and to debrief after the emergency is over. People who get the interventions they need are usually grateful for them. For instance, women who hope for a so-called non-interventionist, "normal" or vaginal birth but who actually have multiple interventions are satisfied with these interventions if they were applied in order to try to achieve a vaginal birth, even if this was unsuccessful.[168] It is women who are forced or pressured into unnecessary interventions, or those who think they did not get the interventions that they should have received (for example, those who are given a caesarean section before trying alternate interventions designed to help achieve a vaginal birth), that object to their treatment.

During an emergency, family-centred care requires the doctor to be as kind and gentle as possible, considering things like pain management or minimizing future scarring. It may mean a gentle reassuring touch or word, or even simply saying "I'm sorry this is going to hurt." Simply to acknowledge that the person they are dealing with is a human being. The smallest gesture, such as a reassuring touch, can mean a huge amount.

Standards

The lack of a clear definition of respectful, family-centred care has resulted in many, if not most hospitals and care facilities claiming to be "family-centred" even though there is no standard set for such accreditation. The absence of such an accreditation standard is indicative of how far we have to go to achieve a genuinely family-centred approach.

If academics and health professionals have yet to agree on a definition of family-centred care, families are likely to have even greater difficulties assessing which of the care facilities they could utilize are truly "family-centred," and none would have any real means of establishing whether the care procedures they might receive are respectful or abusive. Even without the complications of assessing care options in advance, it can be difficult for a client to judge whether the treatment they received was abusive. We think of abuse as violence, cruelty, yelling, shouting, hitting, causing pain, etc. In medicine, abuse may be more insidious and invisible. Abusive caregivers may speak in gentle tones, talk to their client about how much they understand how difficult it may be for them, and promise that they want to help. They then proceed to offer substandard or harmful treatment, all with the most "caring" demeanor. When that treatment fails, they may again, with immense "empathy," blame the client for its failure, saying, for example, "your pushing wasn't quite strong enough so we had to…" Conversely, some procedures that are both necessary and appropriate cause pain, such as vaginal examinations during labour, particularly during an inherently painful process like giving birth. Women are conditioned to accept that obstetric or gynaecological procedures are painful, and to simply tolerate that pain, even when pain management options exist, or when the frequency of vaginal examinations is excessive. Consequently, when a procedure causes pain unnecessarily, in a way that is objectively abusive (such as too frequent vaginal examinations in labour), many women may not recognize it as such, telling themselves that they just need to tolerate it, the same way they have tolerated pain in gynaecological procedures throughout their adult lives. When that abuse is inflicted by a health provider presenting as kind, caring, and ostensibly thinking only of their best interests, it can become incredibly difficult for anybody to separate the truth from the medical gaslighting.

This highlights the need for externally validated accreditation criteria and processes to determine if a care provider/facility is "Family-Centred." Such an accreditation process should be externally monitored and regularly renewed. A system of accreditation of family-centredness does not yet exist.

Centering Families

Since childbirth became a medicalized, and usually hospitalized event, a century ago,[169] women, their babies, and their partners, have been relegated to a peripheral role within the clinically focused hierarchy of medical care. Much of this has been done for the convenience of caregivers or health systems, with little regard for whether such practices are supported by evidence of what is best for families.

In the medicalized model of perinatal care, there is a fundamental tension between a medical and a psycho-social approach to childbearing: the perception of pregnancy and birth as a normal process (a "well role") or as an illness requiring close medical management (an "ill role").[170] There is also a (slowly) increasing awareness of psycho-social issues in the care of women during pregnancy, birth and the postpartum period, and a family's transition to parenthood, in addition to their physiological basis. This, alongside a general push for patient-centred medicine, has resulted in a gradual change from physician-centred to baby-and/or mother-centred, then to woman-centred, and more recently to family-centred care.

> Family-centred care reinstates women, babies, and partners from the secondary role to which they are

> assigned, to a central role within perinatal care services. We need to remember that: The mother, her partner, and her newborn are the sole reason for the establishment of the whole structure of perinatal and reproductive healthcare services. Consequently, such services should be totally directed towards best meeting their cognitive, emotional, social, cultural or spiritual needs, as well as their biological needs, during the transition to parenthood. This primary reason for the existence of obstetrics, midwifery, and related services is frequently forgotten, underplayed or neglected. Women, their partners, and their babies, are the most important people in this experience. Their families, available and appropriate technology or facilities, and the caregivers that are best able to give them supportive care, surround them, and serve them.[171]

High Risk

Which pregnancies or births are complicated and which are not? Defining "normal" pregnancy, labour, and birth, in contrast to complicated birth, is complex, and confused by the extensive medicalization of all births in our modern, high technology, world. Yet treatment given to women declared to be at "high risk" likely differs considerably, and might involve far more assessments and interventions, from the care offered to women who escape this classification. Making sure that definitions of "high risk" are accurate and useful is therefore important if such definitions lead to inappropriate, and therefore, abusive treatment.

Attempts to define normal pregnancy and birth have led, over decades, to various scales designed to attribute a "risk score" to a woman with the intention of classifying those who are most likely to develop complications and need specialized care. Nevertheless, as the WHO rightly notes, "accurately predicting which women will develop complications is not possible."[172] In theory, defining and predicting risk may be desirable for the allocation of resources, as well as to ensure that women have appropriate levels of care available to them or their newborn at birth. In practice, such "risk scores" have proved unreliable, and according to the UK's National Institute for Care Excellence (NICE) Antenatal Care guidelines,[173] there is no evidence to suggest that the use of antenatal risk assessment tools improves maternal and neonatal outcomes.[174] Labelling women as "high risk" probably has both psychological and clinical negative effects – just as being classed as "low risk" might lead to missed complications. Current approaches to women with obesity that tend to regard them as "at risk" provide a case in point because this appears to lead to unnecessary interventions in labour – such as caesarean section, augmentation of labour, and episiotomy – that are not justified, simply on the grounds of a high BMI.[175] This chapter examines significant attempts to define normal pregnancy and birth and the pitfalls associated with these attempts.

My own large sample (doctoral) research, published as early as 1983, on predicting obstetric complications on the basis of multiple obstetric indicators, a modified version of the Littman and Parmelee "risk score," biological and biographical characteristics, as well as psychological and social factors, accurately predicted complications of birth in fewer than 7% of women.[176] These findings challenged the concept that adverse obstetric outcomes could be predicted based on classical obstetric risk indicators. I was curious as to the roles that psycho-social factors played in predicting these outcomes in addition to the traditionally used "risk scores" based on obstetric variables. My large sample research revealed that neither a standard risk score, nor most of the multiple psychological or social factors, including life event stressors, that I assessed were reliable predictors of pregnancy complications.[177] My attempts to publish these findings were rejected by obstetric journals, but not by journals publishing on medical/health psychology, as this finding was in stark contradiction to obstetric policy and practice at that time. Ten years later I was thrilled to listen to a presentation given by Professor Mahmoud Fathalla,[178] a globally recognized and respected authority, as a keynote address at the thirteenth FIGO conference in Singapore in 1991. He clearly rejected the notion that risk scoring tools could predict obstetric complications. I felt vindicated! More importantly, the obstetric world began to re-think the value of risk scoring systems as predictors of obstetric complications, but not totally or everywhere.

Risk scoring systems may also be misleading as most women may be at risk for specific problems, or at various times during pregnancy, labour, or birth, but not at all times or for all complications. In addition, the question of the effect on women of being labeled "high risk"' remains. Classification of a woman as "at risk" may well lead to caregiver bias resulting in more routine intervention than is appropriate or effective. It can result in stigmatizing a woman (such as the prejudiced view that women with obesity must be lazy, non-compliant, unhealthy, inactive, and stupid), imposing a stereotypical adverse set of expectations which are unlikely to be true, and clinical practices that might or, more likely, might not be necessary or appropriate in her individual case.

Additionally, the classification of "high risk" has psychological implications for the pregnant person. In cases where there are legitimate reasons for increased monitoring or interventions, understanding what those concerns may be and their possible implications is essential for effective clinical care. Without that understanding, women and families are left with fear, and the unknown, both of which are likely to increase anxiety, which in itself can have repercussions for perinatal health. Alternatively, there are many situations in which a pregnancy is labelled "high risk" based on criteria that are too vague to be predictive. For example, a single high blood glucose level early in pregnancy, with no prior or subsequent glucose problems, can still leave a woman classified as high risk and pressured into interventions. People with disabilities are routinely considered "high risk," regardless of the nature of their disability or whether it has any chance of having an impact on pregnancy. Recent studies have noted an increased likelihood of interventions or complications for people with disabilities, but have also noted that the prejudice/discrimination that Disabled People face, both in life and during perinatal care, are likely significant contributors to those outcomes.[179] These are only a few examples of possible situations in which a classification of "high risk" and the associated increase in interventions may not be appropriate. In such cases, women and their families may find themselves feeling stigmatized or pressured into treatment options they do not consider necessary, and may even be harmful. In many cases, such as for Disabled People or people with a high BMI, they may have extensive experience of mistreatment and prejudice from the medical profession, and consequently, may avoid accessing perinatal care until it is absolutely essential. When health care professionals pressure them into interventions, lecture or berate them for conditions outside their control, or pressure them to terminate pregnancies (as can happen when either the mother or unborn baby has a disability), women are naturally reticent to trust health care professionals, or seek their help, even when complications arise. This can have devastating effects when these reasonable fears result in delays seeking care for genuine complications.

The "high risk" classification also has a psychological impact on the health providers. Health providers who see a pregnant person with a supposedly "high risk" characteristic (disability, higher or lower age, higher or lower BMI, etc.), have a tendency to blame any symptoms, concerns, or complications arising during pregnancy/birth on that characteristic, often without seeking other possible explanations. This leads to missed or misdiagnoses, inappropriate treatments offered, and often serious negative outcomes. This, in turn, reinforces the perception of clients that they will not receive adequate care, even when they seek it out. All these experiences lead to increased stress for the pregnant person, which in itself, can lead to complications.

From the woman's perspective, being classified as "high risk" may have various psychological implications. Anxiety may be increased, fear of unnecessary intervention, or, in contrast, a wish for greater monitoring and intervention to ensure that she and her baby are safe, may occur. Women may believe they are "abnormal." They may anticipate their prenatal care appointments fearing that they will be treated as somehow "less than normal" people, that they may be lectured on their supposedly "high risk" characteristics, and as a result, may even delay prenatal visits or avoid clinical appointments unless it proves essential. When complications arise, people may dismiss their symptoms as an expected part of their "abnormal" pregnancy rather than seeking needed assessment. Caregivers frequently dismiss their symptoms as readily, as being the result of their "high risk"" classification, or to their identity in an equity-owed group (such as a person of colour, poor, or living with a disability), rather than investigating them appropriately to be certain that the symptoms exhibited are indeed related to the obvious "risk factor" and are not arising from a different cause that requires careful diagnosis and treatment. People facing stigma on a regular basis (in any equity-denied group) also live with the stress of these medical encounters, that compounds over a lifetime and can have serious repercussions for health, and specifically for pregnancy.

Clearly, also, complications occur in women who are not identified as "high risk" whereas others, who are so classified, may well go on to have normal births. Every effort should therefore be made to ensure that all women have essential services available and accessible. All women should be regarded as having normal pregnancies until proved otherwise, with caregivers remaining vigilant at all times for possible complications.

"Normal" Birth

Definitions of what is a "normal" or a complicated birth have significant influence on clinical care practices. When a procedure is considered normal, it is used with greater frequency, regardless of whether it is necessary or appropriate. Most available definitions of birth attempt to classify normal birth by means of specific interventions used, or not used, in labour and delivery. This approach leads to confusing, and at times, nonsensical definitions.

In clinical practice, defining a given pregnancy/birth as normal should be a dynamic, rather than a static process. All births should be considered normal, and treated as such, until a complication arises that requires intervention. In a dynamic process, this can also mean that a potential complication may arise in early pregnancy that later resolves, after which point the definition of and treatment of that person should return to considering their pregnancy "normal." For example, if a complication arises in early pregnancy that increases the risk for preterm birth, then once the pregnancy reaches term, that risk is no longer relevant and the pregnancy/birth can be treated as normal.

There are a number of definitions of normal birth: a few are discussed here – those of the WHO, the WHO-Euro Bologna Score, Canada, and the UK. Only the WHO and the WHO-Euro Bologna Score approach the definition of normal birth as a dynamic process with the remaining attempts being based on static classifications of interventions used or not used.

Perhaps the simplest remains that of the WHO that defines normal birth as "spontaneous in onset, low-risk at the start of labour and remaining so throughout labour and delivery. The infant is born spontaneously in the vertex position between 37 and 42 completed weeks of pregnancy. After birth the mother and baby are in good condition."[180] The WHO-Bologna Score develops this approach further, providing perhaps the most useful definition available today. Other definitions by professional organizations in both Canada and the UK, for example, are more complex and less helpful.

WHO-Euro Bologna Score

The WHO-Euro Bologna Score is based on the assumption that no single indicator, or set of indicators, can assess whether labour is managed as "normal birth." The "Bologna Score"[181] attempts to quantify, both in an individual labour, as well as in a wider population, the extent to which labours in a hospital or a region, are managed as normal, as opposed to complicated. It incorporates the WHO definition of normal birth as a pregnancy of more than thirty-seven and less than forty-two completed weeks gestation, with a singleton fetus, vertex presentation, and spontaneous onset, and requires that there is a skilled attendant at birth. This rating excludes women from classification as having normal births if they have induced labours or a caesarean birth (either planned or emergency). In addition, the more normal the management of labour, the more likely it is that women would have (1) a companion at birth, (2) be monitored by means of a partogram or, preferably, its newer version, the Labour Care Guide,[182] (3) not have their labour augmented either pharmacologically or mechanically (including practices such as external pressure on the fundus), (4) use a non-supine position for birth, and (5) have skin-to-skin contact of mother and baby for at least thirty minutes within the first hour after birth. The rationale for these inclusions and exclusions is as follows: having a companion at birth reflects evidence-based care, as well as the attitudes of professionals and the involvement of women (and their chosen partner/s) in birth. It incorporates a family-centred approach to care, recognizing psycho-social needs at birth. It is also indicative of flexibility in the delivery care system and may serve to indicate prenatal preparation of women for birth. The use of an appropriate partogram/ Labour Care Guide for the population being cared for (such as the one adapted for women with high BMI or another being developed in a paperless version[183]) is an indicator of effective monitoring of progress of labour, providing guidance on when intervention is required. Absence of augmentation is indicative of persisting normal progress in labour as judged by professionals using evidence-based measures. Use of a non-supine position for delivery, as opposed to supine or lithotomy positions, reflects evidence-based care, and the attitude of caregivers, and will exclude almost all forceps or vacuum extractions. Use of a non-supine position for delivery will also exclude epidural or spinal analgesia, particularly if this creates an adverse effect on labour. Skin-to-skin care for at least thirty minutes within the first hour after birth is evidence-based practice and can serve as an indirect measure of both maternal and infant well-being and early initiation of breastfeeding. It is also indicative of caregiver attitude. The Bologna Score makes it possible to assess both attitudes and practices within a maternity service towards the dynamic management of normal labour.

Canadian Approach

In 2008, a joint statement of the Society of Obstetricians and Gynaecologists of Canada and other Canadian professional organizations including the College of Family Physicians Canada, the Canadian Association of Midwives, the Association of Women's Health, Obstetric and Neonatal Nurses, Canada, and the Society of Rural Physicians of Canada, distinguished between "normal" and "natural" childbirth. "Natural childbirth," according to this definition, involved little or no human intervention.[184] "Normal birth" was defined as excluding elective induction before forty-one weeks, spinal analgesia, general anesthetic, forceps or vacuum, caesarean section, routine episiotomy, continuous electronic fetal monitoring for "low-risk" birth, and fetal malpresentation. "Normal delivery" however, might include interventions such as induction, augmentation, electronic fetal monitoring, artificial rupture of membranes, and pharmacological pain relief like nitrous oxide, opioids, and/or epidural. "Normal" pregnancy and labour could also include complications including hypertension, antepartum or postpartum haemorrhage, perineal trauma and repair, and NICU admission. This complicated and confusing definition attempted to accept commonly used, current practices such as epidurals and inductions (i.e., the "norm") as "normal" in an attempt not to stigmatise the many women who experience these and other procedures or interventions, as "abnormal."

There are so many things wrong with both this definition and this approach to creating it, that it is difficult to know where to start. Defining normal birth based on what commonly happens is, for want of a better term, backwards. We cannot think of any other medical context in which the definition for appropriate treatment is done based on a survey of what treatments are most commonly used. Clinical care should not be defined based on a show of hands.

While it is laudable that these organizations wish to avoid stigmatizing women, perhaps they should begin by addressing the extensive stigmatization that we know is influencing outcomes, such as stigmatizing Indigenous women, people of colour, those with disabilities, or those in bigger bodies, to name only a few. This attempt to mislead women into believing that their experiences of, for example, induction (after forty-one weeks), or augmentation, epidural, haemorrhage, and NICU admission of their baby, were "normal" is both extremely implausible and dangerous, in that it does not provide anything resembling evidence-based guidelines. Parents are not gullible enough to think that neonatal admission to a NICU or maternal haemorrhage are normal events. The most likely consequence of such an approach is to create mistrust in caregivers.

UK Definition

At about the same time as the Canadian definition was proposed, the Royal College of Obstetricians and Gynaecologists of the UK, in its joint statement on making normal birth a reality, did not distinguish between "natural" and "normal" delivery. It defined "normal delivery" as "without induction, without the use of instruments, not by caesarean section and without general, spinal or epidural anaesthetic before or during delivery,"[185] and would potentially also have excluded augmentation of labour, use of opioid drugs, artificial rupture of membranes and managed third stage of labour from definitions of "normal" birth if data had been routinely available to monitor their usage.[186] This definition comes closest to the WHO-Bologna Score, but omits the dynamic assessment of labour progress in favour of attempting to classify some interventions as normal and others not – a potential quagmire. Fewer than half of all women in both Canada and the UK experience "normal birth" as defined in their countries.

The development of definitions of normal birth based on types of interventions used or not used, as has occurred in the UK and Canada, has emerged from the increasing use of technology in birth over past decades and the need to regard some of them as normal and others as not normal. While we might all agree that any surgical intervention is not normal, we might be in less agreement when we challenge other practices that are traditionally thought of as normal but are, today, changing their status. For example, are interventions such as supine deliveries (as opposed to upright) normal or abnormal, or is skin-to-skin mother-infant contact, or perhaps, father-infant contact at birth, normal or abnormal? Challenging birth to become demedicalized, and as minimally interventionist as possible, while remaining safe, requires us to rethink our preconceptions.[187]

Breastfeeding Support

Most women in the developed and technologically sophisticated world do not get the most appropriate support for maternal and child contact after birth or for the promotion of breastfeeding.[188] The western world's low breastfeeding rates within a week or two after birth are clear evidence of a lack of knowledge, skills, and appropriate healthcare services regarding breastfeeding promotion among caregivers and those who wish to breastfeed and who chose to initiate breastfeeding. In some countries, or in segments of societies, this may be accompanied by a belief that substitute technology, infant formula, is just as good, despite the abundant academic evidence supporting the value of breastfeeding, and particularly exclusive breastfeeding for the first six months of life.[189] Hidden – emotional – losses may also occur: for some people the sense of achievement in their ability to give birth or to breastfeed their baby is lost by their over-reliance on a technologically managed birth or postpartum experience. Nor is it facilitated by widespread lack of knowledge among caregivers about how to support breastfeeding or by an interventionist/medicalized approach to birth including the increasing rate of caesarean sections and their resulting reduction in infant-mother contact and breastfeeding.[190] Separating mothers and their babies at the moment of birth, or in the hours or days after birth, is not helpful either. Studies of the value of skin-to-skin contact for normal term infants have revealed the considerable benefits of this approach.[191] Babies interact more with their mothers and cry less if held skin-to-skin. Mothers are also more likely to breastfeed in the first one to four months, and tend to breastfeed for longer, if they have early skin-to-skin contact with their babies.[192] Findings revealing the benefits of skin-to-skin care for newborns admitted to NICUs, have revolutionized this bastion of high-tech care.[193] The growing re-birth of breastfeeding, driven by the WHO/UNICEF BFHI,[194] is restructuring maternity hospitals worldwide as well as reminding us that technology has not always been in the best interests of either mothers or their babies.

When clinical procedures inhibit practices that are known and proven to be beneficial for long term outcomes, those procedures are, by definition, harmful. In contexts in which those harms are known and possible to prevent (for example, by ensuring caregivers assisting mothers to feed their newborn are knowledgeable and skilled in offering breastfeeding support for all mothers who choose to breastfeed), failing to provide those services is abusive.

Reductionist Approach

The time has come to revise our understanding of birth. It is not simply a biological process. "Normal birth" should not simply be called "physiological birth" as is a current fashion: there is far more to birth than just physiology. Reducing the birthing woman to a physiology, a reductionist approach, instead of accepting a holistic and humanistic view of the person in childbirth is demeaning, dehumanizing, and abusive. Perhaps the term "optimal births" might best encompass the definition of family-centred and respectful care promoted in this book as meeting the best evidence-based use of technology appropriate for each individual person (even if this includes caesarean section or NICU admission), accompanied by the most supportive, sensitive, and respectful care, and caregivers, that are required by that person and their chosen family members.

We need to experience birth in as emotionally and intellectually fulfilling a way as possible, as well as in a biologically safe way that uses only minimal, and essential, technology. These are not incompatible dreams. They simply require a change of approach on the part of caregivers and health systems, and a change of heart among women. Both are achievable. Accepting that unnecessarily medicalized and interventionist birth is abusive, and inappropriate care, would be a good start.

Demedicalizing Care

Demedicalizing all stages of the pregnancy, birth, and postpartum periods is required and integrating the traditional medical model together with a psycho-social approach is necessary to provide respectful family-centred care and reduce the frequency of inappropriate and consequently abusive treatment. Over the past two decades, there has been a significant increase in numerous labour practices to initiate, accelerate, terminate, regulate, or monitor the physiological process of labour, aimed at improving outcomes for women and babies while at the same time often improving convenience for caregivers. Scheduled caesarean births, continuous electronic fetal monitoring, scheduled formula feeds for infants, and hospital-based births rather than home births all make the caregiver's life more convenient. As WHO reports, this increasing medicalization of childbirth processes undermines the woman's own capability to give birth and negatively impacts her childbirth experience.[195] For some, family-centred care, and with that the idea of a humanistic and holistic approach to childbearing, is thought to apply only to normal pregnancy and birth. There is also the misconception that clinical care, psycho-socially sensitive care, and family-centred care are separate priorities. In this view, once complications set in, it is commonly accepted that clinical care becomes the only priority, at the expense of family-centred and emotionally supportive care. With this approach, it becomes more acceptable to implement practices in which the needs of the clinician overtly outweigh that of the person/family giving birth. In difficult situations, however, sensitive, family-centred care is even more important.

Since the late 1980's we have known that many technologies used in perinatal care confer no clinical benefit, and that some are harmful. Two seismic resources reached similar conclusions regarding the effectiveness of perinatal technology: WHO debate, deliberation and published recommendations,[196] as well as meta-analyses of randomized controlled trials resulting in evidence-based guidelines.[197] Although over three decades have passed since this knowledge has been available, and although evidence-based perinatal care has become readily accepted in principle, inappropriate technology and interventions are still used. The choice to continue to practice in ways that are outdated and known to be either harmful, or at least less beneficial than other available practices, is abusive.

WHO Activities

Moves towards demedicalizing birth emerged from concerns regarding the increased use of technology in perinatal care. As early as the 1980's WHO-Euro undertook a survey of birth practices in the European region. In 1985, Dr. Marsden Wagner published the WHO-Euro book *Having a Baby in Europe*[198] as well as what became a classic publication in *The Lancet* entitled "Appropriate Technology for Birth."[199] These publications were controversial as they challenged the existing emphasis on technological management of birth. Questions were raised regarding their scientific basis, implying that these were simply the conclusions of left-wing, radical, or extremist "natural birth" advocates.

It soon became possible to address the question of whether the WHO recommendations that emerged from discussion and debate at consensus conferences were supported by scientific evidence-based research, with the publication of *Effective Care in Pregnancy and Childbirth* in 1989.[200] Virtually identical recommendations for a reduction in the use of many interventions in pregnancy and childbirth emerged in both the WHO recommendations for birth and the outcomes of randomized controlled trials, leading me to conclude at that time, when comparing the two documents, that:

> The WHO recommendations for appropriate technology for birth, as developed through survey research, discussion and debate, are strongly endorsed by the findings of carefully controlled, and critically evaluated, randomized controlled trials.[201]

Since this time, numerous systematic reviews included in the Cochrane Database of Systematic Reviews,[202] as well as multiple national guidelines, including the respected NICE guidelines from the UK,[203] have confirmed these conclusions regarding using only appropriate and essential interventions in care during pregnancy and birth.

Impact

Over forty years later, most countries could still benefit from an examination of their perinatal services in the light of evidence-based knowledge and the WHO recommendations for perinatal care. In 1998, this process of reassessment commenced in Europe with a Perinatal Care Workshop convened by the WHO Regional Office for Europe (WHO-Euro) which led to the development of principles that should underlie perinatal care in future.[204]

Ten principles of perinatal care were listed by WHO.[205] These are:

1. Care for normal pregnancy and birth should be de-medicalized meaning that essential care should be provided with the minimum set of interventions necessary and that less rather than more technology be applied whenever possible.
2. Care should be based on the use of appropriate technology, which is defined as a complex of actions that includes methods, procedures, techniques, equipment, and other tools, all applied to solve a specific problem.[206] This point is directed towards reducing the overuse of technology or the application of sophisticated or complex technology when simpler procedures may suffice or indeed be superior.

3. Care should be evidence based, meaning supported by the best available research, and by randomized controlled trials where possible and appropriate.
4. Care should be regionalized and based on an efficient system of referral from primary care centres to tertiary levels of care.
5. Care should be multidisciplinary, involving contributions from such professionals as midwives, obstetricians, neonatologists, nurses, childbirth, and parenthood educators as well as social scientists.
6. Care should be holistic and should be concerned with intellectual, emotional, social, and cultural needs of women, their babies, and families and not only with their biological care.
7. Care should be family-centred and should be directed towards meeting the needs of not only the woman and her newborn but also her partner and significant family or friends.
8. Care should be culturally appropriate and should consider and allow for cultural variations in meeting these expectations.
9. Care should involve women in decision-making.
10. Care should respect the privacy, dignity, and confidentiality of women.

I was integrally involved in the development of the WHO's ten principles of perinatal care. At the time, I was serving a short-term contract at WHO-Euro and was asked to assist with the planning and implementing of two Perinatal Care Workshops. At the first workshop held in Venice in 1998, nine of the above ten principles were developed and formally approved. At the conclusion of this first workshop, but after the formal endorsement of the nine principles by the attending group, I suggested that the tenth principle be added. It was, but it was only formally endorsed by the group attending the second workshop, held in Bologna in 2000. This final principle added the importance of providing respectful treatment and care for women decades before this concept was highlighted in current research.

These principles strongly endorse the protection, promotion, and support for effective and demedicalized, family-centred, respectful, and non-abusive perinatal care and were incorporated into the technical materials as well as the monitoring and evaluation tools of the European regional office of WHO. Principles five to ten clearly emphasize these aspects of pregnancy and birthing care although evidence-based care remains a cornerstone of all ten. If today's perinatal health care institutions look no further than these ten principles, and commit to implementing them, we will have achieved a great deal.

Evidence-Based

In 1989, the publications of *Effective Care in Pregnancy and Childbirth*, and its summary *Guide* gave a major boost to the move to demedicalize perinatal care. In particular, the *Guide's* strongly worded Appendix 4 identified "Forms of care that should be abandoned in the light of available evidence."[207] Subsequent editions have used less strident wording: "Forms of care likely to be ineffective or harmful."[208] Nevertheless, its primary message was that evidence-based care required less routine use of interventions in perinatal care. Family-centred care acknowledges that optimal care during pregnancy and birth uses the minimum set of interventions regarded as essential, based on the best available evidence, and that when a choice is possible, the more natural, and less invasive, option should be preferred.[209] Not only is the minimum use of interventions optimal, but care needs to be individualized so that interventions are never routinely provided but only used on indication for each individual woman. Despite these recommendations, which, if followed, should result in relatively similar levels of intervention both between countries and within countries, based on actual clinical need, rates of interventions in pregnancy, birth and the postpartum period vary widely.

Increasing Caesarean Sections

Technology in medical care is being used more today than ever before. Because many of these technologies may be lifesaving and beneficial in the right circumstances, there has been a willingness to think that if they are good for some, they might be good for all. Fuelled by the (often legitimate) fear of litigation, in the USA at least, these technologies are presented as the lawyers' redeeming feature: "at least everything possible was done to prevent negative outcomes from occurring" and is an easy defense, even if not always justified by evidence. Belief in the infallibility of technology and doctors prevails subconsciously, if not consciously. The result has been an explosion in the routine use of such techniques as continuous electronic fetal monitoring, multiple prenatal ultrasounds, epidural anaesthetic for vaginal delivery, and caesarean section, among others. None of these is supported by evidence for their routine use, yet they are commonplace interventions. Almost every woman in pregnancy (in developed countries at least) has at least one ultrasound, and most have two, three or even more. While selective ultrasound seeking specific desired information is valuable, routine ultrasound in early or particularly in late pregnancy, is not supported by evidence.[210] Continuous electronic fetal monitoring in labour without fetal scalp sampling may be ineffective or even harmful due in some part to ineffective interpretation of readings. Intermittent auscultation during labour offers some advantages.[211] Epidural anaesthesia in labour is also more likely to lead to an increased rate of caesarean births, primarily due to an increase in the length of first and second stage labour resulting in a cascade of interventions.[212]

In many parts of the world caesarean section rates may range between 25%-50% and in some centres or even countries, may exceed this, despite long-held WHO recommendations to maintain this rate to around 10%-15%.[213] More recently, WHO has indicated that population level rates higher than 10% are not associated with reductions in maternal and newborn mortality, although the effects of increased caesarean section rates on other outcomes such as maternal and infant morbidity and psycho-social well-being, are not known.[214] Below a caesarean section rate of 10% maternal and neonatal mortality increases as caesarean sections decrease. As caesarean section rates increase above 10% and up to 30% no reduced effects on mortality are observed.[215] The value of the useful Robson classification system of caesarean sections for determining optimal outcomes for differing indications underlying caesarean section is still being explored.[216] A recent Norwegian study of 1,172,546 deliveries over a twenty year period, that addressed some aspects of this issue, indicated that lower rates of caesarean section were associated with more frequent occurrence of perineal tears, neonatal encephalopathy, cerebral palsy, and stillbirth but also with less frequent maternal haemorrhage. More adverse outcomes were associated with caesarean rates above 15%.[217] In North America, epidural anaesthesia rates for vaginal deliveries may exceed 70%.[218] This might be regarded as absurd in some other parts of the industrialized world. For example, in the UK, epidural rates remain below 30%.[219] We also know that health care providers who use less epidural analgesia have half the number of caesarean births. They also tend to admit women to hospital later in labour and spend more time with them than doctors who admit women earlier.[220] In addition, the frequent use of oxytocin to augment labour is widespread, but has recently been shown to increase rates of uterine hyperstimulation and fetal heart rate abnormalities. Conversely, reducing the rate of oxytocin use in Norway was associated with reduced rates of emergency caesarean delivery.[221]

Two global reports on optimal caesarean section rates have found no reductions in maternal and neonatal mortality and morbidity when frequency of caesarean section was more than 15%.[222] One of these showed that an increased rate of intervention was associated with higher mortality and morbidity in mothers and neonates.[223] Over the past decade or so, many, if not most, technologically advanced societies have rates that have far exceeded this, such as Canada (28%),[224] the USA (33%),[225] and China (50% particularly in cities).[226] Some countries, however, have annual rates that are far too low, such as 1% of births or even less (Ethiopia, Burkina Faso, Niger, and Madagascar).[227] In a WHO survey, fifty-four countries reported caesarean section rates below 10%, and sixty-nine had rates above 15%. These figures indicate that 3.18 million additional caesarean sections are needed in countries where rates were below 10% and 6.2 million unnecessary sections are performed in countries where rates are above 15%. The cost of the global "excess" caesarean sections was estimated by WHO to amount to approximately US $2.32 billion (in 2010), whereas the cost of the global "needed" caesarean sections was approximately US $432 million.[228] Not only are economic issues of relevance, but perhaps even more importantly, overuse and underuse of caesarean section – or other interventions – reflects inappropriate clinical care.

Intervention Rates

As with caesarean section rates, there has been increasing recognition that, despite evidence-based guidelines, childbirth practices, interventions, and policies differ, sometimes widely, both between countries and across regions within countries, confirming that these are not always performed based on clinical need but for other, non-medical reasons. Further data supporting this observation come from a number of national or large-scale regional surveys undertaken between 1997 and 2006 that explored women's perceptions of their maternity care in various countries.[229] These include surveys in the USA such as the Pregnancy Risk Assessment Monitoring System (PRAMS)[230] and the Listening to Mothers Surveys,[231] the Maternity Experiences Survey (MES) in Canada,[232] surveys in the UK,[233] Australia,[234] Sweden,[235] and a number of former Soviet countries including the Russian Federation,[236] Lithuania,[237] the Republic of Moldova[238] and Azerbaijan.[239] These surveys indicate that intrapartum interventions, including caesarean section rates and epidural usage, were less frequent in the UK than in the USA and Canada but more so than in the former Soviet Union countries.[240] One of the most striking differences in the practices identified in these surveys relates to the presence of the partner or husband in labour and/or birth. Whereas this is now almost standard practice in North America and the UK and well supported by evidence, only about half of all women reported having their partner with them in labour in Lithuania and less than 15% in Azerbaijan or Saint Petersburg, Russian Federation. In these countries, at the time of these surveys, no other companion was allowed to be present either.

Epidemiological data have not always confirmed the value of a high technology approach to obstetric and neonatal care, with countries adhering to this model sometimes reporting poorer maternal child health outcomes than others who rely less on the use of technology.[241]

For example, when comparing the USA and Canada, U.S. mothers consistently reported higher levels of intervention.[242] Yet maternal mortality in the USA is over twice as high (17.4/100 000) as in Canada (8.6/100 000) and many other European countries,[243] and infant health outcomes such as perinatal and neonatal mortality, all occur more often in the USA than in Canada.[244] Reasons underlying this discrepancy when making cross-cultural comparisons may vary widely, including differences in state funded, universal healthcare coverage versus private systems, or demographic differences. Interestingly, the use of non-pharmacological methods of pain management in labour and birth appears to play a considerable role in reducing the caesarean section rate. In a 2022 review of over 3,000 births in Brazil, in a population with a 44.2% caesarean section rate, surgical delivery was reduced by 78% in those using non-pharmacological methods of pain relief.[245] Finding the appropriate balance between effective and minimal use of technology as opposed to its routine use, given such variable contributing factors, is therefore one of the challenges facing this century.

Within Country Differences

If evidence-based practices were advocated within a country (for example, by that country's national guidelines) then one would expect rates to be similar across that country. This is not always the case. In Canada, a national survey revealed that rates of caesarean sections, epidural, continuous electronic fetal monitoring, supine position for delivery, episiotomies, and perineal stitching, among others, differ considerably across its ten provinces and three territories.[246] Similarly, an examination of regional variations in caesarean section rates among women in English National Health Service trusts revealed that maternal characteristics and clinical risk factors accounted for little of the variability that occurred across the country.[247] In Delhi, India, rates of interventions fall short of evidence-based guidelines with relative overuse of interventions in private hospitals and deficiency of patient-centred practices such as labour support in public hospitals.[248] In South Africa, under the Apartheid regime, rates of caesarean section were almost twice as high in private (fee-for-service) hospitals than in state supported (salaried staff) hospitals.[249] These wide variations suggest that the usage of interventions is not only based on evidence or on medical need. Rather, a variety of other factors including the types of healthcare providers in different regions, hospital size, availability of resources, maternal access to care, rural or urban residence, long-established ways of providing care, local cultural variations, medico-legal concerns, availability of technology, maternal demographic variables, and caregiver bias or prejudice against equity-owed groups, influence practice. How maternity care is organized or reimbursed, how and where practitioners are trained, and prevailing attitudes toward pregnant women and their families also affect practice.[250]

Discriminatory Interventions

Evidence-based practice should apply to all families regardless of socio-economic status or other discriminatory variables. Of concern are the findings that some procedures for which there are no medical indications continue to be performed, sometimes in a discriminatory pattern.[251] In Canada, for example, socially disadvantaged women are more likely to have had enemas, lie in a supine position for birth, and have their legs in stirrups, all unproven, if not potentially harmful, practices.[252] Among mothers having a vaginal or attempted vaginal birth, 19.1% had their perineal or pubic hair shaved and 15% reported that someone "pushed on the top of their abdomen to help push the baby down" (the Kristeller manoeuvre).[253] These procedures are performed more often in younger (teenage) mothers, poorly educated women, and low-income women than in those who are older, better off, and better educated. Globally, women of lower socio-economic status have described being humiliated by caregivers for their poverty, illiteracy, living in low-income areas, or for being dirty and unkempt regardless of whether they actually are dirty or unkempt[254] Women of colour, Black, and Indigenous women also report significantly increased levels of abusive care.[255] Many healthcare providers hold strong negative attitudes towards people with obesity.[256] They may be stigmatized to the extent that their management in labour – which requires greater patience as labour is often longer in women with higher BMIs – differs from that of thinner women and leads to unnecessarily increased, non-evidence-based, shorter appointment times, missed diagnoses, caesarean section rates due to their BMI rather than to clinical need, and to more abusive treatment.[257]

Newborn Interventions

Reviews indicate that a range of commonly practiced interventions during labour, birth, and the immediate postpartum period also affect the fetal to neonatal transition. For example, evidence does not support many routine practices such as: separation of mother and baby for some hours after delivery or in postpartum wards, supplementation of breastmilk with water or breastmilk substitutes, suctioning of the newborn at birth, suctioning of meconium-stained babies, and intubation and suctioning of vigorous infants to prevent meconium aspiration.[258] As with maternal care in labour and birth, less intervention, and particularly less routine intervention, in newborn care is frequently better.

In their defense, physicians may quote women's choice, saying that women want this type of "excellent, high-technology care." Each birth has to "be perfect" and every available technique possible may be used to achieve this. Sadly, available interventions are not always supported by sound research evidence as beneficial for either mother or baby when used on a routine basis. Intervening in the normal physiological process of labour and birth in the absence of medical necessity increases the risk of complications for both mother and baby.[259]

Prenatal and Postpartum Interventions

Best available evidence does not only apply to labour and birth but to prenatal and postpartum care as well. There is still debate regarding aspects of prenatal care, including the optimal number of prenatal visits needed (ranging from four or six to at least ten or more), the value of routine first trimester ultrasound when menstrual period dates are known, routine weighing of women at each prenatal visit, as well as the recommended weight gain advised for women at various levels of BMI (whether or not such targets can ever be achieved by women anyway), and routine iron supplementation in pregnancy, among others.[260] With regard to postpartum care, the adoption of the BFHI in many western countries is a clear example of the sometimes slow process of implementing evidence-based knowledge into practice: The BFHI was launched by WHO and UNICEF over thirty years ago, yet there are, with few exceptions such as Norway and Sweden, a small proportion of maternity hospitals dedicated to achieving or actually accredited as "BFHs" in most western countries.

Evidence-Based Care and Interventions

Evidence-based medicine is one response to emerge in reaction to the technological explosion in the developed world. The publication of *Effective Care in Pregnancy and Childbirth*[261] and the subsequent development of the Cochrane database have revolutionized perinatal care. Demanding that technology be applied when, and only when, it is necessary, and ensuring that the strictest scientific rigour be applied to judge such effectiveness is leading the WHO[262] as well as individual caregivers worldwide, to question the over-use of technology. Notwithstanding the above remaining challenges to the introduction of evidence-based care in technologically advanced centres, significant progress has been made in some respects. In general, the rates of episiotomy have plummeted in recent decades and midwifery is rapidly gaining more widespread respect and endorsement. Home birth is being acknowledged in some countries, like Canada, as a safe site for childbirth with the UK's NICE review concluding that healthy women with straightforward pregnancies are safer giving birth with an attending midwife at home or in a midwife-led unit than in hospital under obstetric care.[263] Practices such as immersion in water during labour, offering non-pharmacological pain management techniques in labour, and delayed cord clamping are being introduced; skin-to-skin care and breastfeeding are more often being supported as optimal policy and practice; single room NICUs with rooming-in of the mother and/or partner are being created; and better facilities for fathers/ partners to stay with newly delivered mothers in hospitals are being pursued. In Canada, national guidelines for family-centred care have been revised to reflect these innovative developments while in the UK, the NICE guidelines are continually providing updated family-centred and evidence-based challenges to global perinatal care. It is clear, however, that much work, and change, is still needed. While such changes are being considered and introduced in a few places, traditional interventionist management of pregnancy and birth remains the default position.

Internet and Interventions

The development of evidence-based research and thinking, that continues to assist caregivers to decide on effective clinical and technological care, created a seismic revolution in perinatal care. A second revolution in all clinical care, including perinatal care, is also ongoing thanks to the development of the internet, and more recently, the explosion of AI generated knowledge. Knowledge regarding medical care, procedures, treatments, and interventions is being made more accessible and understandable through websites, blogs, and advocacy reports on the web. Clients are asking more questions of their caregivers (and of their search engines), and notably, more educated, and informed questions. While initially a threatening experience for caregivers, they have had to incorporate this now shared knowledge, much of it accurate and some inaccurate. A more respectful interaction that considers clients' concerns, questions, and understanding is emerging: in short, a welcome, more collaborative approach is being added to traditional clinical and technological care.

Over Medicalized Treatment

Over-medicalized birth, when interventions are not medically necessary, is inappropriate and could be reasonably perceived as assault rather than optimal care. Consider a similar action in a different context; a surgeon performing appendectomies, as a matter of routine, without any medical need. Or perhaps routinely performing bypass surgery on any person with some of the risk factors for cardiovascular disease. We do not accept medical intervention on that level in any other context. Why should it be different during pregnancy or birth?

The challenge is determining when interventions are beneficial for all or most women (such as taking folic acid before and in the first three months of pregnancy[264]) and when, or for which women, if any, interventions might be harmful (such as shaving, enemas, pushing on the abdomen to help get the baby down in vaginal births, and many, if not most, episiotomies).

From a clinical perspective, a "perfect birth" in this medicalized context is viewed as a healthy, live mother and baby, with little else mattering. While this is a minimum desired outcome, it is the lowest possible bar to meet, only one step above the worst possible outcome of mortality. Such an attitude justifies literally anything that does not kill or maim the mother or baby. Over-reliance on medical treatment or interventions results in poorer clinical outcomes, not to mention little concern for the emotional fulfillment that should accompany birth or the full experience of love and tenderness that should surround the birthing woman, the new mother and baby, and her partner. In fact, over medicalization is likely to lead to significant harms, including reduced breastfeeding (and consequently reductions in its long-term health benefits for both mother and baby), less optimal attachment between parents and their newborns with implications for childrearing and child development, more chances of injury with its associations with slower recovery, and probably higher stress, blood pressure, sugar levels, and generally less optimal health outcomes, as well as greater likelihood for trauma, infection, poor postpartum adjustments, and increased health service costs.

Birth As It Should Be

Throughout this book, we have argued that providing substandard, non-evidence-based treatment when better practices are possible is a form of abuse. This refers to the use of practices that are known to be harmful, or avoiding practices that are known to improve outcomes. This is, admittedly, a broad view of abuse. In some cases, the connection between non-evidence-based practices and abuse is easy to find; there are consequent physiological and psychological harms that require ongoing treatment to manage. In other cases, the link is more subtle and can be more difficult to conceptualise for people who are accustomed to thinking of abuse as something that leaves scars, marks, or other measurable effects. In medical care, however, when a caregiver can reasonably be expected to know what good evidence-based practice should be, and when such care is possible, then neglecting to provide that care amounts to a choice to provide substandard, harmful, or at least not optimal treatment. That is abusive. The following chapters focus on what care should look like.

Holistic Care

A holistic approach that encompasses both physical health as well as psychological and social health is essential from before pregnancy, through pregnancy and birth, and well into the postpartum period. Numerous studies have demonstrated the benefits of this type of care, showing poorer outcomes when it is neglected.[265] Anything less than fully holistic and psycho-socially sensitive care is potentially harmful. Yet too many health systems and health care providers treat psychological health as secondary to physical, disregarding these necessities for appropriate care as niceties that are readily discarded in favour of their own specialty or as aspects of care that are/should be provided by others, such as social workers, psychologists, doulas, or nurses. Holistic care is not only essential during childbearing: it applies to all aspects of medicine. Holistic approaches to cancer care, for example, that encompass not only the survivor's physical outcome but also the long-term psychological and supportive care needs of both the cancer survivor and their companions/family members are emerging as issues of considerable importance.[266]

Before Pregnancy

Recent trends have moved towards advocating a pre-conception program for all women contemplating pregnancy, if not all women of reproductive age,[267] as about half of all pregnancies are unplanned.[268] Given this incidence, more effective pre-conception family planning is needed. Most pre-conception programs, however, routinely focus on clinical aspects of care in preparation for pregnancy, without serious consideration of their psychological consequences. For example, they advocate living healthy lifestyles and include (inappropriate) advice regarding weight loss (as this often results in increasing weight gain in early pregnancy),[269] exercise programs (which may require financial outlay beyond a family's means, or beyond the ability of, for example, a person with mobility challenges that demand expensive solutions), nutritious diet (that may also be beyond the reach of a family especially with rapidly increasing food costs), and avoidance of all alcohol (especially if pregnancy is potentially possible), smoking, or substance use.[270] They seldom integrate care for the psycho-social implications of this advice on women, especially if women are unable to comply with it. In addition, there is little if any data or evidence available supporting the efficacy of available programs for many pregnancy outcomes and a Cochrane review concludes that there is insufficient evidence to recommend widespread implementation of routine pre-pregnancy health promotion for women of childbearing age, either in the general population or between pregnancies.[271]

If pre-conception care is to become the norm, over and above effective family planning, it should be evidence-based and respectful, considering both physical and psychological health, as well as considering caregiver attitudes and consequent impact on outcomes. It should be individualized, with advice that is specific, meaningful, and attainable for each individual in their circumstances. Care must be taken regarding what medical messages are provided together with an understanding of their psychological or social consequences if successful pre-conceptional programs are to be developed. As yet, such optimal programs have still to be developed. Nor is it clear as to who is responsible for providing such pre-conception programs. Certainly, family practitioners might be held responsible for them, but such education might also be profitably offered at high school level, and through more readily accessible avenues such as social media.

Schools could be expected to do much more with regard to preparation of adolescents for reproductive life. Education about pregnancy, birth, and parenthood, is glossed over or simply not taught in schools. We need to teach people how not to get pregnant, but also, how to get pregnant, or preserve fertility if they plan to delay pregnancy until their 30's or 40's. We need to alleviate fears about pregnancy and birth and teach about different health care options available for perinatal care (midwives, doulas, family doctors, obstetricians). We need to prepare teenagers for general reproductive health like routine pap smears, how to get them, what they feel like, and how to make them less uncomfortable. We need to answer the "afraid to ask" questions like what kind of personal grooming to do prior to a women's health medical appointment that most if not all young women do not know about and are too afraid to ask about. Assuming that all mothers will prepare their teenage children about such events is not necessarily a valid assumption.

Weight Loss

Much of the pre-pregnancy advice given to women focuses on their weight, with many caregivers inaccurately seeing weight/BMI as a measure of health.[272] Advocating weight loss in preparation for pregnancy among overweight women is unlikely to be either clinically or psychologically beneficial. Current approaches to reducing weight in pregnancy (or at any time in life) have proved to be untenable, and unsuccessful in the long run, and virtually all non-pharmacological or surgical weight loss programs will lead to higher gestational weight gain and increased anxiety.[273]

For decades caregivers have blamed women with obesity for their weight, claiming that they overeat, do not exercise, and are responsible for their size. Clinical care has been influenced by this perception leading to disrespectful, abusive, sometimes insulting, and inconsiderate care, missed diagnoses when caregivers attribute all their problems to weight, and unnecessary and inappropriate clinical interventions, including caesarean sections. A recent ground-breaking paper has shattered this stereotype and condemned such attitudes and actions as invalid and ignorant. Obesity is a clinically based illness over which most people with obesity have little if any control. The global tsunami of weight loss drugs based on semaglutide, such as Ozempic, Wegovy, Mounjaro, and Rybelsus, emerging from this new understanding of obesity and its causes, is revolutionizing the medical treatment of obesity. In addition, caesarean sections are not a necessary consequence of obesity and multiple clinical sites are reporting that more patience especially during the first stage of labour (labour often takes longer for women with obesity), respectful and sensitive care, with supportive and adequate clinical facilities, facilitates vaginal birth.[274] Prejudice and discrimination play a major part in the current disrespectful and inappropriate perinatal care of women with obesity. Classifying them as "high risk" compounds the problem but lends a clinically acceptable justification for this offensive treatment. Hopefully this will change soon as better understanding of obesity and its aetiology as medical rather than psychological or social prevails. To begin with, understanding that women in bigger bodies do not automatically have diabetes, high blood pressure, sleep apnea etc. would be a start. These women may not be at any higher risk than women in smaller bodies.

Weight stigma is rampant in society as a whole and in the health care profession in particular. For example, people with a BMI over thirty-five have been reported to be more than 100 times as likely to face employment discrimination[275] and 64% of adults report experiencing weight bias from a health care professional.[276] Women with obesity have usually experienced a myriad of difficult and embarrassing social and medical encounters. They encounter insensitive and judgemental caregivers who are rude, bullying, and who humiliate them. In those encounters, they frequently report that health care providers dismiss their concerns, advising them to lose weight instead of investigating their symptoms. They encounter facilities and equipment that don't accommodate their size, such as too small blood pressure cuffs, narrow chairs with arms, examination tables that are difficult to get onto or simply do not have a sufficient weight capacity, MRI or other diagnostic machines that do not accommodate a larger person, and gowns that do not cover the bare necessities. They embark on pregnancy with trepidation and anxiety, not only as any woman experiencing pregnancy may be concerned about inherent dangers in the process, but anxious about their potentially abusive encounters with the multiple caregivers that they will confront during pregnancy, birth, and postpartum. They may also be fearful – with good reason – that any complications they experience may be dismissed or ignored due to their weight, thereby compromising their care. In addition, research now suggests that women achieve healthier pregnancy outcomes if they are fit and well, and that being overweight *per se* might not be the determining factor of complications in birth when fitness or other health indicators are also considered.[277] Although the serious adverse outcomes correlated with obesity in pregnancy – including increased risk of pre-eclampsia, prenatal stillbirth, caesarean delivery, instrumental delivery, shoulder dystocia, meconium aspiration, fetal distress and early neonatal death – are fully acknowledged, advocating weight loss is not supported by the evidence as an effective preventative measure or intervention.[278]

In addition, new research is starting to reveal that some adverse outcomes thought to be associated with obesity may, in fact, be a function of obesity-stigma and its impact on health care provider behaviours. How often do we include clinical biases in our assessment of outcomes? Do we, for example, examine outcomes of labour and birth in women with high BMI without implementing commonly held views that such women require caesarean births? If we believe that women with a high BMI usually require caesarean sections, do we perform these sooner, rather than giving women enough time to attempt a vaginal birth? Are our biases, in fact, creating a perpetual cycle where we think bigger women need caesarean sections, so we perform them, thereby driving the statistics saying that bigger women require caesarean sections. Are we providing those caesarean sections because the women need them, or because of our own discomfort with bigger bodies and the necessity of engaging with those bodies during a vaginal birth? Such physician bias in research is often ignored. Over-medicalization of birth for women with obesity is common, leading to unnecessary caesareans and other interventions, many of which are being revealed to be inappropriate care.[279] The lack of understanding about the clinical condition of obesity, until recently, has compounded the problem of disrespectful and abusive care these women face and much change is needed to undo the damage already done and the consequent loss of trust in the health care profession.[280]

Other Equity-Denied Groups

Similarly, bias may also enter into care for pregnant people with disabilities.[281] Most studies do not address clinical or humanistic perinatal concerns relating to Disabled people. Some caregivers may even assume that women with disabilities should not have babies. Or do not have relationships, or sex. They do, and they also have distinct, and individualized, needs for humane care during pregnancy and at birth. How often do we include women with disabilities in perinatal research? Or consider their needs when applying commonly followed "best practices?" There are multiple other groups that commonly experience caregiver bias including racialized people, poor families, teenage mothers, unmarried women, LGBTQ+ pregnant people, or, any people who are different from the religious, cultural, or ethnic category of the caregiver.

In Pregnancy

Optimal care, whether perinatal care or non-pregnancy related, should be based on strong evidence from well-designed and replicated studies. Where such evidence is not available, the best possible evidence should be used and families should be informed of the limitations of that evidence. In all cases, care should be individualized and adapted to suit the unique needs of each family, recognising that some people may not respond the way most do; all evidence includes outliers.

Prenatal Care Guidelines

A 2015 WHO review of eighty-five prenatal care clinical guidelines, emanating primarily from the USA, the UK and Canada, revealed a wide disparity in both the number and types of interventions proposed for routine care.[282] Folic acid and iron supplementation, Rh diagnosis, and management of nausea and vomiting, were the only clinical interventions included in over half of the guidelines.

For thirty-three out of the 171 interventions highlighted across the guidelines, there were conflicting recommendations. For example, recommendations for vitamin or mineral supplementation, such as iron, calcium and vitamins A and D, were extremely diverse with half the guidelines recommending supplementing and the remaining half advising against this. This review examined traditional clinical assessments (not including psycho-social concerns during pregnancy), although advice and treatment included behavioural and emotional suggestions, such as offering advice regarding nutrition, exercise, smoking cessation, healthy lifestyles, self-care, and emotional wellbeing. Such haphazard recommendations reflect ill informed care, based on caregiver conviction rather than evidence. They also frequently ignore the realities facing many, if not most pregnant people, who in addition to being pregnant are likely juggling at least one, if not several jobs, perhaps other children, partners, and extended families, and who may not have several extra hours a day, not to mention financial means or physical ability, to devote to the seemingly endless requirements of so-called "self-care."

Medical-Psycho-Social Care

Giving birth is a psychologically profound experience. At hardly any other time in her life is a woman more psychologically sensitive or vulnerable and yet, today, she may rely heavily on technology that claims to regulate her biological functioning, while simultaneously not obtaining optimal care for her psycho-social, emotional, or intellectual needs.[283] Integrated medical and psycho-social models of care during pregnancy will, likely, be superior to a primarily clinically focused approach – although possibly equally diverse across local, regional, national, and international borders. Evidence in favour of a combined psychological and clinical focus is emerging in many areas with a lack of such an integrated approach being viewed as inadequate. For example, a review of women's experiences of prenatal care in the USA found that psychological and social needs were as important, if not more so, than obtaining good clinical care: some people reported respectful, comprehensive, individualized care; others experienced long waits, rushed visits, and prenatal care that was mechanistic or harsh.[284] Women's preferences emphasized a more psychologically supportive approach, including reasonable wait times, unhurried visits, continuity of care and caregiver, flexibility, comprehensive care, meeting with other pregnant people in groups, developing meaningful relationships with professionals, and becoming more active participants in care. Specific needs included preferring a single provider, counseling, and education (which was lacking in the women studied), being involved in decision-making, and information about physiological and emotional changes as well as common discomforts of pregnancy. A similar global review confirmed these USA reports indicating that women want a positive pregnancy experience that includes maintaining a healthy pregnancy, both physical and cultural normality, and effective transition to positive labour, birth, and motherhood. Simply offering routine, clinically focused services was not sufficient: women needed social, cultural and psychological support throughout, the provision of relevant and timely information, the detection and treatment of potential and actual pathology, and the tailored (rather than routine) use of biomedical tests and interventions.[285] A further 2021 survey of 8,400 women giving birth in Norway similarly reported that women emphasized the importance of both socio-cultural and psychological aspects of care in addition to physical and clinical factors to achieve both a safe outcome and a positive birth experience.[286]

Significant steps need to be made to ensure that women and their families are appropriately prepared for all aspects of pregnancy and birth: failing to do so may well contribute to negative experiences. Providing a balanced approach to clinical prenatal care that considers both clinical issues as well as psychological and social concerns is needed. A psycho-social-medical approach recognizes that women and their partners play an active role in their care and should be recognized as partners in care. Involving partners has been shown to be beneficial for encouraging healthy lifestyle choices among pregnant women, greater prenatal care usage, and fewer low birth weight or small for gestational age newborns as well as improved breastfeeding practices.[287] So too has been the approach of midwives, who tend to offer holistic, continuous care of women and their families throughout pregnancy, labour, and the postpartum period. Studies comparing obstetricians' and midwives' attitudes to birth have shown marked differences in approach.[288] The Canadian Maternity Experiences Survey also revealed that care by midwives is regarded far more positively by mothers compared to care provided by all other caregivers including obstetricians, family doctors, and nurses.[289]

Potentially Harmful Practices

There are numerous common practices that are not only divorced from good evidence, but also potentially psychologically harmful. These psychological harms increase stress for new parents and families, and can create stress and anxiety around every encounter with medical professionals. While this can result in hesitance to attend appointments or consult with medical caregivers, even when it does not, the stress itself is harmful and unnecessary.

Monitoring Weight Gain

As with prenatal weight concerns, monitoring weight gain during pregnancy is fraught with difficulties. This practice is a current, popular focus given the global concern regarding obesity, and some countries and individual caregivers still endorse weighing women at every prenatal visit regardless of the anxiety this might provoke and the lack of evidence to support the practice. Others, with more level heads, such as the UK's globally respected NICE guidelines, do not advocate weighing mothers at any prenatal visit other than the first.[290] The WHO has also long advocated this.[291]

No Alcohol Policy

Advocating a "no alcohol during pregnancy" recommendation, as is the case in Canada, on the basis that we have not yet determined the optimal limit of alcohol intake that is safe in pregnancy, also leads to considerable anxiety among women – especially the many (about half of all women) with unintended pregnancies – who may have imbibed alcohol before learning of their pregnancy. It is also not evidence-based.[292] Reduced alcohol intake and avoidance of binge drinking in pregnancy have known benefits, but careful thought is needed before continuing with such "no risk" policies.[293] Such extreme policies, although intending to be biologically helpful, are not always evidence-based, may cause undue psychological concern, and are unlikely to be beneficial.[294]

A similar caution may be applied to advice not to take any non-prescribed medication during pregnancy or to not use any "recreational drugs." We need to be particularly sensitive to how we care for women who have taken over-the counter medicines or used non-prescription substances during the early days, weeks, or months of pregnancy, either without knowing they were pregnant at the time, or even if aware of this. Balancing the importance of advocating against drug use, and contributing to client anxiety about past actions, is a difficult, but necessary, path to follow, requiring careful understanding of the risks involved based on type of drug use and quantity/frequency of use.

Dismissing Pain

Women need information regarding not only the "common discomforts" of pregnancy, but about "warning signs" indicating when caregiver advice should be sought. Knowing that, for example, nausea and vomiting in pregnancy is a normal "discomfort," or that many women experience pelvic pain, is not sufficient: knowing when these symptoms become pathological, requiring referral to a caregiver for in-depth assessment, is of far more importance and more likely to assuage anxiety. For example, pelvic girdle pain is common in pregnancy but is by no means "normal" and, according to physiotherapy guidelines, requires thorough investigation if reported by mothers.[295] There is a need to develop and implement evidence-based, women- or family-centred guidelines regarding when their pregnancy might be becoming problematic so that anxiety can be reduced, and essential care obtained.[296] Such guidelines are respectful of the significant role that mothers and families can play in monitoring their own healthcare and emphasize that care must be taken to "listen carefully to mothers" as they are not professionals, will not use the terminology that is familiar to professionals, but are often very much in touch with their bodies and their experiences. Such guidelines are particularly important for people who may not fit into the "typical" models for pregnancy; someone with a pre-existing medical condition, a disability, or a trans man, for example, may need far more individualized information about what they should expect or monitor in their own unique circumstances.

Women's reports of pain in any medical setting, and particularly during pregnancy, may often be discounted. For example, one woman, in her second trimester of pregnancy, called her caregiver, between routine visits, to report that she had pelvic pain lasting for a week, resulting in her struggling to walk. She was reassured by telephone that pelvic pain is a "normal discomfort of pregnancy." Not wishing to be a "complaining mother" she did not report this to her caregiver when it recurred closer to her due date, although she did frequently report ongoing difficulties in turning over in bed throughout the pregnancy – a classic sign of symphysis pubis dysfunction. Her case notes did not include this information and at her birth, attended by different caregivers, this information was not known. A prolonged second stage labour of 2-3 hours with virtually no progress, predominantly in a supine position with widely abducted legs, pressed against her caregivers' hips, followed by an epidural and forceps delivery, with abducted legs in stirrups, of a 9lb 13 oz baby (with birth weight accurately confirmed before birth at a 39-week ultrasound), left her with a clear symphysis pubis diastasis and displaced lower segments of her coccyx, as later revealed by X-ray. This, and her long struggle to return to "normal" in the years following her childbirth, with the assistance of weekly physiotherapy, might have been avoided if either she, or her caregivers, had been aware of the clear warning sign of pubic pain in pregnancy causing inability to walk, coupled with the baby's (known) size and her prolonged second stage labour. Almost every position, or procedure used during her second stage of labour is contraindicated in the event of such prenatal pelvic girdle pain/ symphysis pubis diastasis. Listening to the words that this mother used to describe her pelvic girdle pain (difficulty walking for a week, and inability to turn over in bed), should have led to a physiotherapy referral in pregnancy, and avoidance of harmful labour and birth positions (supine, with widely abducted legs and forceps delivery) to help prevent her later complications. Not listening to mothers, or discounting their symptoms, is neglectful and incompetent care that, in this case, led to serious, long-term, adverse, mobility consequences. While it is appropriate to regard most pregnancies as normal, it is always essential to remain alert to potential problems. Discounting a non-routine report of difficulties walking for a week as a "normal discomfort of pregnancy" is an example of how easily this can go wrong, and an example of abusive disregard of women's reports.

Psychological Screening

There is increasing recognition of the importance of psychological health, both prenatally and postpartum. Screening tests have been developed that help identify women who have psycho-social family concerns (such as relationship difficulties, previous experience of abuse, or emotional problems), allowing caregivers to highlight them for increased attention and support. Two that can be used with some validity are the Canadian Antenatal Psycho-Social Health Assessment Scale (ALPHA) and the Australian Antenatal Risk Questionnaire (ANRQ).[297] Life Event scales that identify women with heightened stress levels in their lives are also useful in identifying which women are at increased risk of potential healthcare problems because of the increased life stresses they have experienced, particularly when these are undesirable (as opposed to desirable) events that have a greater impact on outcome.[298] While well intentioned, however, these scales or assessments of women with psychological or social concerns may also be used to stigmatise them further. In combination with existing prejudices against equity-owed groups, such assessments may compound the discriminatory care offered to them. Caregivers need education about the impact of prejudice on care and the potential of such prejudice to lead them to biased treatment. Bais against equity-owed groups such as Indigenous women, larger women, poor women, women of colour, women with disability, or some religious affiliations, are all common influences on care.

Case Study

A case study provides an example of this type of event: A mother of two normal children was diagnosed with an anencephalic pregnancy. A dating ultrasound was conducted at ten weeks showing a normal heartbeat and appropriate growth. At eleven weeks, a scan detected some potential skull anomalies. A third scan two weeks later confirmed anencephaly and termination of pregnancy was immediately undertaken. The emotional trauma experienced by this mother and her family extended far beyond the clinical condition. Shock at the concept of creating a baby with severe brain damage, fear of a repetition of the anomaly in any future pregnancy, or future pregnancies of her own children, finding that regular intake of standard levels of folic acid prior to and during the first trimester of pregnancy had not protected her from this outcome, learning through internet searches that increased doses of folic acid might have provided better protection, and that other current research is exploring additional preventive treatments for the avoidance of neural tube defects (adding inositol – Vitamin B8 – to folic acid prophylaxis although with insufficient evidence to date to require this to be standard care[299]), all contributed to immense emotional stress. Compounding this were the partner's interpretation of the caregiver's words that "I think your baby is OK but we need to do further tests" following the eleven-week ultrasound, that led the partner to be reassured while the mother was not. In cases like these, the caregiver's attempt to avoid alarming the family may have reassured the father, but only caused significantly heightened anxiety for the mother. Waiting for two weeks between ultrasounds was, emotionally, excruciatingly painful. Confirmation of the severity of the anomaly led to acceptance of the suspected problem, and relief that there was no real decision to be taken, for the mother, but shock for the father who had anticipated that all was probably all right. Close emotional support for this family – like any family facing this type of event – was clearly important and is rarely available.

Even though the offer to talk further to caregivers in the period between the two ultrasounds was made, emotional distress, anxiety, tension, and the belief that there was nothing they could do or say until the diagnosis was finalized, resulted in this family not following up on this offer. Especially in situations of such severity and rarity, a follow-up call to this mother/family both in the intervening ultrasound period and following diagnosis, would have enabled this family (and others in similar situations) to avail themselves of helpful counselling or, at least, an opportunity to ask the many unanswered questions that they had, and to confirm or discount the decidedly differing perceptions of each parent as to whether their baby was likely to have a problem. Ideally, parents would be warned about the possibility of a problem when initial indications are discovered, with some information being given to them about what their options might be going forward. A follow-up telephone call could be scheduled so that, after giving parents time to think about their concerns, they can be given a chance to ask further questions. Not calling them to check on their reactions to, and questions about, their diagnosis, or leaving them guessing about what might be wrong, is emotionally neglectful care. Such calls, however, are difficult to manage well and might be best undertaken by a perinatal psychologist.

In this case, it is the absence of psychologically sensitive care that is a central obstacle to holistic, respectful care. This neglect is likely compounded by the limited time that is afforded in medical practice to provide such supportive care for clients. The problem is confounded further by the lack of integration of psychological support into all aspects of care. Should referral to a psychologist have been routine in this case? Is such care covered by health insurance? Are there sufficient perinatal psychologists appointed to maternity care centres? Should caregivers have indicated to the parents precisely what they were noticing and what it might mean at the eleven-week scan? Should the parents have been left with vague, ambiguous information? Should a routine follow-up call have been scheduled between the eleven- and thirteen- weeks scans to check on any questions that the couple might have in response to the alarming briefing they received? Health care systems in place need to be reworked to focus on supportive and client centred care approaches that avoid the psychological cruelty experienced by families facing such traumas.

This incident occurred in a society and culture where termination of an anencephalic pregnancy was fully endorsed. The emotional and clinical challenges being faced by mothers experiencing similar challenges in parts of the USA and in other countries where abortion/termination, even for reasons such as this, is often outlawed, are compounded exponentially. In such cases in particular, the lack of services to assist these mothers and their families is abhorrent.

In Labour and Birth

The clinical birth environment is stressful for many women and their families. Research has confirmed the beneficial outcomes of midwifery care that takes a more holistic, psycho-socially supportive approach.[300]

Companionship

Explorations of the value of supportive companions in labour have shown, with remarkable consistency and cross-cultural validity, the power of this psycho-social intervention to modify any negative impact of the clinical birth environment.[301] Such care is not a bonus or pleasant addition: it is evidence-based clinical care. Care that does not include such support is both clinically and psychologically incompetent.

In 1991, Wendy-Lynne Wolman, a doctoral candidate working under my supervision at the University of the Witwatersrand in South Africa, completed a randomized trial showing the incredibly beneficial impact of providing companionship during labour on maternal-infant birth outcomes. This study, conducted in a hospital that traditionally did not allow partners to attend birth (Coronation Hospital), was the second trial – following Klaus and Kennell's pioneering research into support in labour – to show that social support in labour was the optimal route to follow. A Masters student under my supervision, Sylvia Csosz, in the following year, 1992, also successfully completed a similar randomized control study at Baragwanath Hospital in Soweto (now Chris Hani Hospital), South Africa, yielding similar findings but taking this one step further.[302] Her study showed that it was not simply a Hawthorne effect that was in operation (of knowing that one is in a research study and benefiting from the added attention this brings). Even women who did not know they were in the study until after the data had been collected, and who were then debriefed and retrospectively requested to grant permission for the data collected about them to be included in the analyses, showed similar optimal outcomes. A number of additional studies across the globe followed, changing the birth environment for families forever.[303] While including companions of the birthing person in labour and delivery is now standard practice in many countries, it is still not included everywhere, and is often one of the first sacrifices to be made to the perinatal care environment when it is under pressure, as happened during the Covid-19 pandemic when support people were banned from labour and delivery rooms. Perinatal care that omits these valuable sources of support is still evident and is inappropriate. It is equivalent to banning hand washing, or wearing gloves or masks during procedures; it is banning an intervention that is known to reduce harmful complications.

Companionship and Covid-19

Fears of infectious diseases such as the Severe Acute Respiratory Syndrome (SARS), that shocked the world in the past decade, and Covid-19 which has had far greater societal and economic consequences globally, led to the, thankfully temporary, exclusion of all family members from hospital births. The result was an increasing movement towards home births, not only because of the fear of infection in hospital settings, and reduced access to hospital facilities that were converted to serve Covid patients, but also because of the fear of birth in the absence of support people. In some cases, not only were partners excluded from birth, but some care facilities implemented directives to enforce induction of labour and even caesarean sections in their attempts to manage and control birth under Covid-19. Such injunctions were abusive in addition to being clinically inappropriate.

In this case, the presence of support people in birth was misclassified as a privilege, rather than as a clinically necessary intervention. This is common with benefits that are perceived to be "psychological" rather than physiologically beneficial – they are discounted as unnecessary or frivolous. Such attitudes discount the wealth of evidence that psycho-social interventions have decidedly clinical and physiological benefits and should be adhered to with the same rigour as is used to enforce hygiene standards, for example.

Birth Environment

Maintaining a, gentle, supportive, encouraging environment for birth is a given requirement of good care, in contrast to the common depiction of birth on TV and in film as a frantic, hurried, and traumatic, albeit momentous, event. Caesarean sections can also be performed with psychological sensitivity. Encouraging skin-to-skin care from the moment of delivery, not separating mother and baby, breastfeeding when the baby shows signs of readiness for a feed, in as supportive an environment as is possible in a surgical suite, can make the experience of caesarean section much more psychologically satisfying, for both mother and father/partner, and can facilitate parent-infant attachment and breastfeeding. These are also evidence-based practices.

In the mid 1990's, I was asked by the WHO Regional Office for Europe to develop a course manual and training program to introduce evidence-based, psycho-socially sensitive and culturally respectful perinatal care into the European region and particularly into the countries of the former Soviet Union. I and my co-trainers included an approach to caesareans in the multiple WHO-Euro training programs that we conducted in the 1990s and 2000s: it is now being termed "gentle caesareans" in western countries but it is still, by no means, a routine practice.[304] The approach we advocated was based on the Misgav Ladav (alternatively called the Stark method) approach to surgery that offered a far less debilitating incision and repair procedure that allowed for quicker and less painful recovery from the surgery than had been possible prior to this.[305] A recent review of women's reports of satisfaction with this approach (adapted and re-named as the Charité Caesarean Birth) reveals little difference between satisfaction ratings of women experiencing this gentler approach to surgery compared to women giving birth vaginally. Compared to those with standard caesarean section methods, these women also reported less exhaustion, as is consistent with the Misgav Ladach approach.[306]

The findings of meta-analyses of randomized controlled trials on effective care in pregnancy and childbirth have questioned the routine use of many clinical interventions and are welcome.[307] Even when essential, however, the psychological implications of their use still require attention. The meaning of, for example, caesarean sections, forceps or vacuum extractions, or the more recently introduced Odon method for assisted vaginal births,[308] inductions, augmentations of labour, or a supine lithotomy position, on the psychological experience of giving birth, have yet to be fully understood. Large scale survey research into women's perceptions of their care in North America and in Canada indicate that such interventions are often associated with experiences of extremely disrespectful care.[309] The slow adoption and assessment of such innovative approaches to caesarean section methods such as the Misgav Ladach approach, first reported in 1999, and only now receiving significant research attention in terms of its impact on women's perceptions of their care, is regrettable.

Postpartum Family Care

Providing care for parents and baby together, in the immediate post-birth period, is a central need in humanistic, holistic, family-centred care if we want to avoid abuse. This applies to the care of the family with a normal, term baby and equally, if not even more so, to families whose newborn requires admission to a NICU. Applying the concept of rooming-in to include the father/partner on a routine basis is needed.

Adjustment to Parenthood

The primary focus of most care in the perinatal period is on the pregnancy, birth, and the first few days after giving birth. Far less attention is given to the adjustment to parenthood, either physically, emotionally, or intellectually. Physically the mother has experienced enormous demands on her body during both pregnancy and birth, whether by vaginal or caesarean delivery. She is likely to feel bruised and battered with discomforts – sometimes significant – arising from episiotomies, hemorrhoids, urinary or fecal dysfunction, and painful breasts, combined with considerably disturbed sleep patterns. Hormonally her body is undergoing rapid changes oftentimes leaving her with swirling emotional reactions that are compounded by insecurity regarding mothering abilities contrasting with excitement and pride in new parenthood. Life certainly turns upside down when a new baby arrives, for the entire family. Few of our supportive care services address these changes and their resulting needs, either in terms of providing adequate cognitive or emotional preparation for them or in assisting families to cope with them in the first months after giving birth. Well-baby clinics, postpartum new-mother get-togethers, community health care centres that offer postpartum facilities, or courses, are all options to strengthen going forward. Neglecting to assist mothers and families to prepare for and to cope with this period of adjustment is harmful.

Family Planning

Family planning is also an important consideration. The focus of family planning should be tailored to each family's needs. For some, that may mean discussing contraception options for preventing or spacing out pregnancies. For others, that may mean planning for future fertility treatments and support. And for other families who have experienced a serious adverse neonatal outcome, it may mean support for the loss of a current baby, as well as planning for a future pregnancy to avoid similar outcomes.

Language

The terminology and language used by professionals regarding pregnancy, labour and birth reflects our approach to these events as "normal" or "complicated." They also reflect our respect, or disrespect, for women and their families. A brief comment on this to a member of the Editorial Board of the British Journal of Obstetrics and Gynaecology in 1992, led to an invitation to publish a commentary on the psychological meaning of the language we use when talking about pregnancy loss.[310] Some two decades later, I proposed that we again revisit this question, applied to the language we use regarding childbirth in general, as a "Roundtable Discussion" for the USA based journal *Birth*.[311] On both occasions the issue was warmly welcomed as sorely needed, suggesting that little had changed over the two intervening decades. Two issues emerge from this: the first is that even after twenty years this issue was still supposedly of significance, but had yet to result in any meaningful change, and the second, that we have yet to learn not to use "jargon" when caring for families, and particularly jargon that implies women are to blame for complications.

The "Roundtable Discussion" of this issue in *Birth* acknowledged the increasing importance of the language we use when caring for pregnant people and their families.[312] We frequently substitute technological terminology for simple experiences and a number of papers in this issue drew attention to the "medicalization" of terminology used regarding pregnancy and birth, in addition to practice. For example, we describe breastfeeding as lactation (ignoring that the mother and not only her lactating breasts, as well as her newborn, are involved in the process of breastfeeding) and caregivers who assist with breastfeeding as lactation consultants. The term "lactation" actually applies to the production of milk by the breasts: it does not include the appropriate positioning of the baby on the breast, or the effective transport of this milk to the baby, which is what breastfeeding is about. Lactation consultants can usually do little to directly improve physiological lactation, but they can, and should, encourage effective latching and encouragement to feed often which will increase milk supply. One does not need a degree to breastfeed: every mother and baby can do it, so why do we need to invent technical terms for those who care for this simple process? We use "non-nutritive sucking" for the need of a baby to suckle for comfort. We use "non-clinical touch" to describe the comfort of a kind caress to support a woman in pain. It is as though we seek status and recognition for the importance of our work through official sounding, medicalized titles. Using "non-nutritive" and "non-clinical" also implies a lesser worth to such actions: nutritive or clinical action is valuable; all other actions are not. Medicalizing our language when interacting with parents does little more than reflect our wish to sound important and to reiterate and emphasize the doctor-patient power imbalance. Like many of today's graduate students who are taught to include jargon and complex technological or linguistic terminology when writing academic papers, using complex terminology is simply disrespectful and obfuscating. Being a sesquipedalian is as obnoxious as this word sounds.

Language can also maintain doctor-patient power differentials in the childbirth setting (for example, "I am *just* going to examine you" instead of "Please may I examine you now?" or, "What is she?" (Meaning how far dilated is the woman's cervix?), and are used mindlessly and meaninglessly, without respect for the woman as anything more than a "case" ("the section in room twenty-two").[313] Language may be used imprecisely, such as "trial of labour" (applied to women with previous caesarean sections, carrying implications that labour is likely to fail – or that the woman might fail – when all labours are, in reality, trials of labour), or "failure to progress" (when this might mean "failure of the caregiver to wait" rather than failure of the women to labour effectively).[314] The word "failure" too is denigrating for mothers: after all, other women whose labours progress smoothly are successful, while they are failures despite the fact that the baby/ies, doctors, caregivers, health care systems in hospitals or at a place of birth all contribute to the progress of labour.

The excessive use of acronyms, including those used to reflect differing issues (for example, IUD may be an intrauterine device or an intrauterine death) also plagues our language of birth[315] but bolsters a medicalized/clinically focused role rather than a sensitive, normalized interaction between caregiver and woman/family. Use of technologized words also reinforces the power position of the doctor who supposedly has superior knowledge. Even the word "sensitive" when applied to care (as occurs throughout this book) may be perceived negatively as meaning "touchy-feely," or "hippie" style thinking rather than simply being the optimal and normal approach to care that defines clinical competence as mandating care for an entire person, including their physical needs, cognitions, emotions, and social interactions.

Using acronyms is common in obstetric care but not restricted to this profession. When I first joined the WHO, Regional Office for Europe in Copenhagen, in 1991, I was met with a welcome e-mail sent from a Canadian colleague. The entire message was a series of acronyms that took some time to decipher. In essence, it said welcome to the world of acronyms and the MCH (Maternal Child Health), MPS (Making Pregnancy Safer), and IMCI (Integrated Management of Childhood Illness),[316] programs! I soon learned how apt this message was in the United Nations world. Our medicalized language regarding birth adopts a similarly distanced view of a very common, human, experience.

Terminology

A family-centred approach needs to retain constant consideration for how the terminology we use is perceived by women; it must remain respectful of both clinical and psychological needs. For example, describing an unwanted early pregnancy loss as an "abortion" may be hurtful, as this term is frequently associated with a deliberately induced abortion. Women typically prefer the term "miscarriage" to describe unwanted pregnancy loss.[317] Caregivers often use terms such as "failed pregnancy," "incompetent cervix," "inadequate germ plasm," "abnormal chromosomal material" to explain pregnancy loss, but these may be understood by women as reflecting their personal failure, incompetence, inadequacy, and abnormality.[318] These terms have their roots in a time when women were blamed for not producing male children, or for having problems in pregnancy and birth. They serve to "keep women in their place" as responsible for their pregnancy outcomes. These terms reinforce women's common reactions to miscarriage as shame, feelings of failure, insecurity, and depression. Early pregnancy loss is often referred to as loss of "the products of conception" by caregivers and as a "baby" by mothers or parents. These outcomes are usually "disposed of" by sluicing or incineration, rather than by burial, further denying the "human" aspects of this difficult experience. As Freud would argue, our language sheds light on our true feelings and thoughts and, thereby, our degree of humanistic "family-centredness." Our language can be, and often is, structured to reinforce the power dynamics and psychologically insensitive approaches that facilitate other abusive approaches to care. Medicalized language may also assist caregivers to avoid becoming too emotionally involved in their client's experiences.

In contradiction to this, however, is the thought that such medicalized language can possibly help some women distance themselves psychologically from the idea of losing a baby. Losing a "collection of cells that would never have become a baby" might be an easier mental adjustment for women to make to a miscarriage: caregiver discretion is advised regarding when to use medicalized language in order to make the pregnancy loss easier to adjust to for some women.

Language of Loss

A more sensitive approach to the care of women experiencing the loss of a baby in early pregnancy has recently been advocated in the United Kingdom.[319] An Independent Pregnancy Review has made seventy-three recommendations for improving care for people who experience a baby loss before twenty-four weeks, including more empathetic care that recognizes both emotional and physical care needs, better ways for remains to be collected and stored with dignity, and issuance of a certificate recognizing their loss for parents. Also included are recommendations to provide education in schools regarding symptoms of baby loss, routine offers of mental health support for women and their partners, assistance with understanding why the loss occurred, private spaces in hospitals for those experiencing baby loss, and further research on the occurrence of baby loss among differing, and more vulnerable families. A pilot study examining the value of offering advice following a first baby loss in early pregnancy rather than only after the third miscarriage is also being undertaken.[320]

Challenges

The objective of care should be to protect the woman from stress as much as possible. Incorporating psycho-social concerns into our medicalized perinatal care world is challenging for caregivers who are likely to be inadequately prepared for these aspects of care. The closer (or more approachable) one appears to be to the client, and the greater the trust that is developed, the more likely it is for her to discuss her concerns. Most caregivers are not trained to deal with such intimacies and feel threatened when they occur and incompetent to manage them. They may also regard psycho-social support to be too time-consuming and beyond their scope of practice. In some medical systems, restrictions on how much time a caregiver can spend with a client, or what they can discuss, impose limits that caregivers cannot control. This can be an extremely frustrating experience for caregivers who are trapped between systemic ineptitudes and patient care. Caregivers in training may even be encouraged to dissociate themselves from their patients' emotional states (for example, by wearing white coats with the status-conveying stethoscope dangling around the neck) so as to allow them to provide (sometimes) painful clinical care, or bad news. Revised preparation of caregivers is surely needed to help them adopt a more personal, family-centred model and to feel competent in caring for psychological as well as biological considerations. This likely means that current educators need retraining if the cycle of neglect of psycho-social issues it to be interrupted. Additionally, adding perinatal psychologists to the care team can provide emotional supports for both parents and caregivers at all stages of the family's transition to parenthood.

Loss and Abuse

Loss occurs both in pregnancy and when women are unable to get pregnant. Some couples are unable to conceive without fertility treatments, and failure of these procedures results in the loss of the potential to become a parent. Once pregnant, miscarriage, stillbirth and neonatal loss can occur. Although this varies across the globe, approximately one or two in 100 pregnancies ends in a stillbirth and about the same number are followed by the death of the newborn. Many more, about fourteen in every hundred pregnancies, results in miscarriage or spontaneous abortion. While physiological processes, such as inappropriate placental function can lead to pregnancy loss, these events can be exacerbated by social factors such as domestic violence.[321]

Reactions to Loss

Reactions to these events may be severe, and may have long lasting effects. A whole range of emotions may be felt after the loss of a wanted pregnancy or newborn including hurt, pain, denial, anger, guilt, depression, frustration, sorrow, and loss of self-esteem. Mothers frequently feel that they have failed as women, and desperately need love, support, and comfort. They may also feel used and abused by medical routines and procedures.[322]

Parents

Emotional reactions to the death of a baby are influenced by the events surrounding the birth, or death experience.[323] Many women who experience miscarriage reveal that this loss is downplayed, ignored or regarded as a minimally stressful event, contrary to their own feelings of loss.[324] This loss is not only a loss of a wanted baby but also a loss of self-esteem – and the fear of the loss of the ability to be a mother.[325]

Most couples say that in the event of a stillbirth, being able to see and hold their newborn to accept the baby and its death is helpful. It is important to say hello to the baby before having to say goodbye, even though this is a difficult experience. Caregivers, however, on seeing the emotional pain that being close to a stillborn baby elicits, are often inclined to take the baby away as soon as possible. Removing the baby too soon can lead to later recriminations and regrets by the parents. Parents may appreciate opportunities to see their stillborn baby on a few occasions over the following days before finally parting with the baby. Such contacts must always be supported by professional staff, such as perinatal psychologists, who are trained to handle difficult situations like these. At the least, photographs of the baby should be taken by the hospital and kept on record for the parents' later reference if requested. Ideally these photographs should be set in the same kind of setting that one would use to photograph a live baby. While the parents may not wish to see their baby at the time of the birth, they may want to see the baby photographs later. Parents must be informed that this is possible.

The more the parents can do to care for the baby, even at this time, is important for their adjustment. The baby who lives for a few days may be cared for to some extent by the parents. Whatever little can be done by the parents may allow them to feel that the baby really is theirs and that it had some life of its own outside the womb in which they were involved and in which they shared.

With a stillborn baby, it often helps the parents to actually see the efforts made by caregivers to revive their baby at the time of birth. The more they observe the efforts, care, attention, and skill that is devoted to their baby, the easier it is for them to accept that everything possible was tried to save their baby. For this reason, it is probably better for the mother to be awake and aware for the delivery of her baby even if this is an emotionally difficult experience. These babies should also be named by the parents, and conversations about the baby should refer to the baby by name. Similarly, a formal burial of the baby may make mourning the baby easier.

Caregivers

Caregivers also feel anger, guilt, sorrow, pain, frustration, and discomfort when a pregnancy/birth ends with a loss. Their own feelings of confusion and unhappiness may cause them to avoid the parents after birth. Caregivers are seldom trained to cope with expressions of grief, their own or those of others.

In response, caregivers may focus on providing physical care for the mother rather than attending to her psychological wellbeing. Attending to the mother's physical needs is essential: she has just given birth and may be sore and bruised, be experiencing episiotomy pain, or caesarean section aftereffects, have hemorrhoids, be constipated, and will develop painful milk-laden breasts. These all need nursing care, but so too do her and her family's emotional needs. Caregivers need to stop and listen; they need to provide whatever support they can to the family, even if that is only to listen and provide a shoulder on which to cry.

Some caregivers try to avoid expressing their own emotions for fear of upsetting the family further. There is, however, no harm in letting the mother or parents see the expression of emotion in their caregivers: it might actually do good. Knowing that their own feelings are understood and that they are in a supportive environment can support the mother's or parents' self-confidence.

Communicating with a mother who has just miscarried, had an abortion, given birth to a stillborn baby or lost a newborn, is difficult. Often words are hard to find and behaviours must suffice: a squeeze of her hand or a quick hug can say an enormous amount. Even just saying "I am sorry this happened to you" can be incredibly supportive. Caregivers must avoid telling the mother or parents how they should feel. Words such as "Don't worry, you'll have another one soon" or "At least you can have other children" are not helpful. The baby that is lost is the one that is being mourned: no other baby can replace this loss.

Changing the subject is another way in which caregivers may try to communicate with the parents. Not knowing what to say when parents express strong emotions often leads caregivers, family, and friends, to try to move the conversation to safer, unemotional ground. All that the mother or parents may want (or need) at this time is to express their grief. Smalltalk does not help.

Expressions of anger directed towards the medical staff and especially to nurses who are often left to deal with the brunt of the parents' reactions, can sometimes be necessary and important stages in the parents grieving; the process of coming to terms with their loss. The caregivers on facing these expressions deserve support to manage their own responses and feelings. Likewise, there need to be systems in place to differentiate between expressions of grief and reasonable anger over avoidable harms, the latter of which should be investigated for the appropriate compensation and corrective action to be implemented

While talking to parents at length at the time of the birth or death of their baby is essential, offering an opportunity to revisit these events some time later, such as at a month or two after the loss, can be helpful for parents.[326] There are possibly many questions that they may have at this time regarding the possible causes of the baby's death, or the potential implications of this for their future reproductive health. Discussions regarding fertility treatments may be essential and are not ideally embarked on at the time of the loss. Arranging an appointment to discuss such issues within a few months after the birth/death of their baby, or when the parents are ready to face it, is important. As women are choosing to or face social structures that require delaying reproduction until later in life, their window of opportunity to retrieve eggs for later use diminishes. Discussing the value and importance of such procedures, in case these eggs are needed, can prevent much heartache should pregnancy success prove elusive for some years.

Caring for parents who have lost a pregnancy or baby is difficult. Care that does not include an extremely sensitive and knowledgeable approach is abusive, and egregiously so, given the sad and hurtful experiences involved.

Infertility

Most discussions of perinatal care focus on care for people who are or have been pregnant or given birth. Those whose treatments do not result in a pregnancy or birth are rarely, if ever, included. This silence and exclusion is harmful. The focus of this section will be on the abuses related to fertility treatments in general, but particularly focused on the experiences of those attempting assisted reproductive technologies (ART) without success.

There have been numerous highly publicised reports of clinical abuses as they relate to ART, including reports of doctors using their own sperm in fertility treatments.[327] Beyond these egregious and very public examples, however, abuse has not been clearly defined in the context of ART.[328]

There is very little research available on this subject. What information does exist is often based on non-empirical methodologies such as case studies.[329] The examples of abuse discussed here are not intended to be either comprehensive or representative without significantly more study.

Physical/Sexual Abuse

Opportunities to abuse clients physically or sexually are prevalent in those undergoing fertility treatments. Such procedures can often involve repeated and frequent internal exams, trans-vaginal ultrasounds, and intimate testing. Those with experience of gynecological exams are conditioned to expect these tests to be uncomfortable, and for some, the expectation is that they will be painful and emotionally difficult. Primed in this way, women undergoing fertility treatment are often unaware that their experiences could be anything other than difficult and/or painful. Moreover, the emotional context in which fertility treatments often happen – with intense desire and motivation to start a family – mean that many people are willing to endure or tolerate almost anything to achieve success, and are unwilling to potentially compromise their chances of having a child by questioning or reporting problematic experiences.

Many tests and procedures are described as "uncomfortable" which can be a euphemism for extremely painful. Pain management options are rarely even mentioned. One woman described an experience of a trans-vaginal ultrasound (a procedure that should be, at worst, mildly uncomfortable), as excruciatingly painful after her doctor used the opportunity to exert extreme pressure on her cervix with the ultrasound wand, pressing and shoving against her cervix for several minutes while she desperately tried not to cry or scream. The doctor, in his records, described the difficulty he had visualizing her ovaries during the procedure, in an explanation that appeared customized to justify her pain should she file a complaint. Since more than fifteen subsequent ultrasounds were performed by a different doctor with only minimal discomfort and no difficulty getting clear results, the problem was unquestionably not anything inherent to the patient. This woman believes her doctor intentionally assaulted her.

Painful Procedures

Some procedures are, by their nature, painful to varying degrees, though frequently this pain is underplayed and misrepresented when described to clients. For example, an HSG (hysterosalpingogram) is often downplayed to clients as causing mild to moderate discomfort similar to menstrual cramps, however many women describe the pain as extreme, the worst pain of their lives, and ranking it as a 10/10 on the pain scale. An online search for pain during an HSG reveals numerous posts describing screaming, crying, cursing, and feeling violated or destroyed afterwards. Whether the pain is caused by lack of competence performing the test, individual variations in pain experiences, or any other cause is irrelevant. When meaningful pain management options for a procedure that might be painful are not offered, this is abusive.

Doctors do not get to decide what level of pain is acceptable to inflict on their clients.

Psychological Abuse

There is significant vulnerability involved in seeking help to have a baby. Many people do so because they desperately want to start or add to their family, and that desperation can mean that they are willing to endure significant physical hardship, emotional trauma, and financial cost in order to achieve that goal. With stakes that high, psychological abuse can flourish. In some cases, this can manifest as significant or excessive pressure to use assistive reproductive technology (ART).[330] In others, false hopes and dishonesty about the potential outcomes of treatment may occur.[331] There are also reports of fertility specialists being blatantly cruel: One woman was told by her fertility specialist "The idea of you getting pregnant is morbid."

Systemic/Procedural Abuse

Systemic structures and policies around ART are often discriminatory, which, in itself, is arguably abusive. There are reports of abuse both in people being pressured to use ART, and being excluded from treatment options.[332] People may be excluded from treatment based on characteristics like HIV status[333] or high BMI, to name only two examples. In Canada, different provincial health systems offer differing coverage for ART, meaning that access to this type of health care is inconsistent between provinces and blatantly discriminates against those without significant financial resources. In other cases, exclusion takes place in a more roundabout systemic way. For example, a woman with a high BMI may be a good candidate for IVF in every other way, but regulations may require that the necessary anaesthesia for her BMI only be performed in a hospital and fertility specialists in that system are not given hospital privileges. Consequently, the system excludes high BMI women from IVF, without explicitly stating that they are doing so. Exploitation and abuses in fertility care often intersect with other forms of discrimination, with those from equity denied or marginalised populations being more vulnerable.[334]

Social Abuse

So much of how we define being a woman is centered on having children. Even clumsy attempts at gender neutrality focus on reproduction, with phrases such as "people with ovaries" or "people who menstruate" being used in an attempt to create more gender-neutral categories. Such descriptions vividly exclude women who do not menstruate, or people who have had a hysterectomy. Simultaneously, the emphasis on the relationship between being a woman and having children inherently excludes those who have a pregnancy/birth but do not identify as women just as much as it excludes women who do not have a pregnancy/birth.

Socially, the role of being a "mother" is frequently linked to women's capacity or qualifications. Female political candidates, leaders, and public figures often lead with, or at least lean into, their roles as parents, often citing motherhood as a qualification for other roles. The implication being that a woman without children is less qualified, less valued, and simply less. Sometimes, this implication is stated outright, as was the case with then Vice Presidential Candidate J.D. Vance's denigrating comments about "childless cat ladies."[335] He went further to state that such women are miserable with their life choices, as if there were no way for a woman to live a fulfilled productive life without having reproduced – whether by choice or not.

Even without these explicit social or familial pressures, there is a broader social expectation that, in itself, is coercive and can be harmful. When one of the authors of this book, Dr. Solomon, got married, she remembers the comments from colleagues she barely knew: "last year you got your PhD; this year you're getting married; we all know what is coming next year." These are the stages of life for a young, professional, heterosexual woman: professional qualifications, marriage, children. Failure at any one of those feels like a failure in life. When the absence of children is not a choice, but rather an imposed state, the constant need to explain or justify that is deeply painful.

Infertility as Loss

There is an old guideline given to potential mothers; to not tell people they are pregnant until after the first trimester and the risk of a miscarriage is lower. While this is slowly changing, the impact of it, and the underlying belief, is still widely felt. Loss is not something to discuss; it is not something to share; and it is perhaps something to be ashamed of. In recent years, there has been some movement for people to discuss fertility struggles more publicly. Notably, most of these public discussions are from people who have had success with fertility treatments. Those for whom the treatments do not result in a baby are still, by and large, silent.

For those who have tried ART and not been successful, that in itself can feel like a loss, but is seldom treated as such. People can understand loss after a miscarriage or stillbirth, but the failure of fertility treatments is less readily understood. One woman, who is not cited here at her request, described her experience in this way:

> Every few days, I had another ultrasound. I would watch the screen in the hopes of seeing something, anything that might mean the treatments were working. I didn't care about the hormones or the medications, the daily injections, or constant tests. They were irrelevant compared to the repeated anguish of endless negative pregnancy tests. Then one day, there was something there. The doctor called it a follicle. We watched that follicle every few days for weeks, watching it grow, far more slowly than it should have, but still growing. After weeks of treatments and ultrasounds, it was finally mature, we could trigger ovulation. I watched this tiny follicle grow, I thought about it, and when it was "launched" through ovulation, it was the embodiment

> of all my hopes for a family. And when I got that next negative pregnancy test, it was like I had lost that potential baby; that potential life I had watched grow was now dead. I knew, intellectually, that it was never life, it was never a baby, but emotionally, I mourn it. In all my fertility treatments, I had a total of three follicles that made it as far as ovulation. They are as close as I will ever get to having children.
>
> At times, it can feel like every interaction with the world is designed to torture you. Holidays like Christmas are focused on children, and the joy one once found in these now has a powerful undertow of sorrow. The seasons are marked by child-based calendars of "summer holidays" and "back to school." Halloween is a night filled with everybody else's children visiting. Mother's Day is an annual tribute to the children you imagined, the life you envisioned, and their loss. Social media is a torture chamber of your friends, siblings, and co-workers marking the milestones of their children, or worse, complaining about how difficult parenthood is. It would be a dream to have a child throwing a tantrum, screaming through a flight, refusing to wear shoes, or running me ragged taking them to various classes and events. These are the problems I can only fantasize about. The urge to scream at the world, to tell them how unbelievably lucky they are for not having slept for three months with a screaming newborn, is almost overpowering; but those screams remain silent.

An understanding of the experience of loss – of a follicle, the ability to have a pregnancy, a miscarriage, a stillbirth, or a neonatal death – is essential for caregivers so they can avoid adding to the emotional trauma experienced by women who lose a baby or the ability to bear a child.

Normal Birth

Providing sub-standard treatment of all those giving birth, that falls short of evidence-based best practices, is inappropriate. The optimal practices for care of women having normal births, outlined in this chapter, have been the benchmark standard for care for more than two decades. They have numerous benefits for the health (physiological and psychological) of both mother and child, as well as long-term benefits for child development. The fact that they are not universally practiced in every context in which they are possible is evidence that caregivers and health systems are not committed to providing evidence-based care for all people. This is particularly true for those giving birth by caesarean, where the lack of evidence-based practices to support breastfeeding are particularly egregious.

Parent-infant attachment is facilitated by events occurring at the time of birth and in the ensuing months and is important for long-term development.[336] Uninterrupted, skin-to-skin, mother- and/or parent-infant contact, for the first hour or more after birth, is the goal to strive for in both vaginal and caesarean birth, to facilitate attachment. Most routine maternity and newborn care procedures, such as cord clamping, eye prophylaxis, and clothing of the infant, can and should be delayed for at least an hour or more to allow for parent-infant time together, with both mother and baby covered to ensure warmth. Thereafter, rooming-in 24/7, care by parents, and demand (baby-led or cue-based) breastfeeding is the optimal approach. Providing postpartum family support is desperately needed for all mothers, but is even more important for women who have given birth by caesarean section. Caesarean birth is associated with far less mother-infant contact, less skin-to-skin contact, and less breastfeeding in the first two hours after birth, together with more pacifier use, more distribution of free formula samples, and more schedule feeding than for mothers delivering vaginally, with subsequent poorer breastfeeding outcomes.[337] The only national survey to report on mother-infant contact immediately after birth in Canada reports that this is not always practiced, even in the best of maternity care services. In this survey for example, 86% of women having vaginal births reported holding their babies within five minutes of birth, although only 29% of mothers giving birth by caesarean section did so. Only 39% of women having vaginal births and 8% of those giving birth by caesarean held their babies skin-to-skin at this time. Almost three quarters (71%) of women reported 24-hour rooming-in after vaginal birth, although fewer than half (47%) of mothers giving birth by caesarean section did so. Only half of all mothers (50%) reported baby-led breastfeeding.[338]

Rooming-In

It has long been recognized that healthy mothers and babies should room-in together after birth. Essential for effective breastfeeding, this practice also promotes mother-infant attachment and develops confidence regarding infant care. After nine months of pregnancy, and probably a much longer period planning for and dreaming about having a baby, it is somewhat incomprehensible why mothers would wish to be separated from their newborns as soon as they are born. Yet many long-standing hospital practices enforce this. Some argue that mothers are tired after labour and need rest – or perhaps use this as an excuse to send mothers to their rooms, and babies to the nurseries, so that the caregivers' work is done. Also, hospitals have, for so long, been organized with nursery-based care that physical layouts do not always facilitate rooming-in. In the immediate post-birth hours, however, sleep is likely the last thing that a mother can do. She is hyper-alert at this time: tiredness will set in later. Her infant, too, is primed to be hyper-alert at birth (unless drugged by medications administered to the mother in labour). Such immediate post-birth alertness is probably an instinctive survival mechanism, ensuring the development of a mother-baby connection. Although maternal tiredness does ensue, sleep will be in short supply for a new mother due not only to the after-effects of labour but to the need to breastfeed her infant every two to three hours for many days and weeks, continuing, with longer inter-feed intervals, for many months. This is the price of motherhood.

Healthcare providers need to assist this process, not by separating the mother and baby but by assisting the woman to care for and feed her baby while obtaining as much sleep as possible between feeds. Whether or not she breastfeeds herself, or a feed is given to the baby by someone else, her breasts will fill with milk within a few days, causing discomfort and wakefulness and potentially making latching more difficult if her breasts become too swollen and engorged with milk. Frequent suckling before the mother's milk comes in encourages milk supply and flow and allows the mother to learn to position and latch her baby well, before her breasts fill with milk. Frequent feeding in these first few days will help to avoid excessive engorgement with its consequent difficulties, and, overall, will probably be much less sleep disturbing than coping with breastfeeding difficulties. In the immediate post-birth period, practices such as disturbing mothers during a feed, or even frequently between feeds, to check on blood pressure, vaginal discharge, medication distribution, caregiver check-ups, and meals, need to be clustered and kept to a minimum. Although we have begun to recognize the importance of protecting infant's sleep patterns in NICUs, we have not yet realised that interfering with maternal sleep needs following the birth of a normal term baby, by frequent interruptions, is equally deleterious. While these actions might suit caregivers, they are simply disrespectful of women's needs and interfere with the mother's recovery from birth.

Involving Partners

We have also not yet accepted that in families, involving the father or partner(s) with the newborn and mother is probably just as important as including them at the birth. Encouraging a companion in labour and at birth is strongly endorsed by randomized controlled trials,[339] although encouraging family support in the post-birth period is as, if not more, important. Isolating mothers from their partners or families in hospitals after birth is a product of the medicalization of birth developed in the past century, and is not a physiological need. On the contrary, it is counterproductive. If ever a person needs assistance from others, it is in the hours and days (and weeks/months!) after giving birth. Expecting nurses or midwives in the hospital setting to provide this is unrealistic and inappropriate: rather, the chosen companion(s) – whether it is family members, the partner, or a friend – is the optimal companion. Although nursing care is needed to care for the physical after-effects of birth, practical support with caring for the newborn is also needed. So too is time to share the joys and wonder of new parenthood together, as a family. Providing rooming-in for families is clearly the next, urgent, step to take in providing family-centred care. Although many hospitals do "allow" partners to stay overnight with the new mother, usually if she is in a single room, little is done to accommodate them other than to provide an often extremely uncomfortable, extendable chair or perhaps a rollaway cot. This is, of course, far better than excluding partners altogether, and hospitals that do provide this option should be warmly praised and encouraged to continue working towards offering even greater comfort for partners. Meals are not usually available for partners, requiring alternate arrangements to be made, although, given the notorious quality of hospital food, not providing it may be an act of kindness. Better care/support for partners could and should be introduced into most maternity centres.

I was taught an invaluable lesson regarding family rooming-in in Estonia. The paediatrician in the hospital to which I was consulting, Dr. Adik Levin, had pioneered rooming-in of babies, and especially sick and preterm babies, with their mothers. Learning from this, the hospital had instituted rooming-in for all new parent couples. This occurred at a time when birth rates were lower across the country and many mothers were able to have single rooms even though the rooms had two beds in them. Partners were invited to stay with the mothers for the entire duration of their hospital stay. If they needed to go to work, they did so, leaving the hospital in the morning and returning after work: or they simply stayed in the hospital all day. I walked into such a room and was so impressed that I asked if I could photograph it. To my surprise it was the father who instantly jumped up, picked up his baby from its bassinet, sat next to his partner on the bed while he held the baby, and invited me to photograph them. He was excited, involved with, and proud of his new family, and was delighted to share this joy with me. Much as we think we have all the answers to "best care practices" in North America and other technologically advanced societies, we can learn much from other countries that have developed their humanistic and family-centred care far beyond ours.

Support People

We need innovative thinking to improve the transition to parenthood for all new families, whether birth is by vaginal delivery or caesarean section. As a minimum, chosen support people for the mother should be encouraged to stay with her, to pick up the baby, change the diapers, allow the mother to sleep while calming the baby, and carry the baby to the mother for feeding in addition to helping her to move around. They can also offer emotional support and much needed advice at this time and serve as maternal advocates. We cannot expect nursing staff to do all these tasks for all mothers: they are traditionally provided by family members but could also be provided by professional postpartum supporters or doulas. Yet healthcare facilities do not support this assistance from others, often limiting visiting hours or times as well as the number of visitors allowed. Developing systems that allow for extensive family, or postpartum doula support in the hours and days following birth, while still in the hospital environment, can go a long way towards both helping people recover from birth, and making this a truly family-centred experience. Those facilities that are already changing in this direction are to be praised and encouraged to develop this approach to care as far as possible.

Encouraging supportive family care can lessen the ill effects of a difficult birth or can support postpartum adjustment, and is optimal care. Such supportive companions could be family members such as sisters, brothers, cousins, grandparent. etc. or simply a friend who accompanies the birthing person to prenatal classes, and/or the birth, and helps particularly during postpartum recovery. Traditionally, the birthing person's mother (or mother-in-law) may offer extensive assistance to a new mother if she lives within reasonable distance from the new family. For many this is invaluable: for some this is an uncomfortable experience, depending on the relationship between family members. While the practical help that this can offer the new family is wonderful, the differing experiences of the new grandmother regarding her own birthing and infant feeding and current care practices, can add additional tensions to this period of major change and adjustment. Ideally, grandmothers could be included in prenatal preparation classes to learn about newer approaches to infant and new mother care prior to the birth of a new baby in the family. One of my valued colleagues, Shula Werner, a pre- and postpartum Physiotherapist, from Israel, always taught that grandmothers have to learn a new role: they cannot continue to play the mother role to which they are accustomed.

Breastfeeding

With the introduction of the WHO and UNICEF's BFHI and its associated Code of Marketing of Breastmilk Substitutes, an increasing awareness of the benefits of breastmilk for babies has been generated globally.[340] Initially emphasized in less developed parts of the world, where infant mortality is increased when mothers do not breastfeed, the movement has infiltrated the technologically sophisticated world as well.[341] The WHO/UNICEF BFHI, supported by extensive research evidence,[342] promotes exclusive breastfeeding (with no other liquids or solid food) for the first six months of life and continued breastfeeding, together with complementary foods, for two years or longer.[343] Many benefits – both maternal and infant – accrue from breastfeeding.[344] The Canadian led Promotion of Breastfeeding Intervention Trial (PROBIT), the largest randomized trial ever conducted in the field of breastfeeding, provided strong evidence that the BFHI increases prolonged and exclusive breastfeeding, which in turn improves infant health in the first year of life and results in children's improved cognitive development at school-going age. Other benefits, confirmed by meta-analyses, include protection against child infections, malocclusion, and probably reductions in overweight and diabetes for children and protection against breast cancer, and possibly ovarian cancer and type 2 diabetes in mothers.[346]

Despite the well documented evidence of the benefits of breastfeeding, and established best practices to support mothers to do so, health systems and providers around the world continue to neglect these evidence-based practices. We are willing to, adamantly, advise mothers not to smoke, drink, or use medications during pregnancy, but we hesitate to say that breastfeeding is best for fear of making mothers feel guilty. We do, however, often imply that mothers are to blame for not attempting to breastfeed, or not succeeding in breastfeeding. Many of the people who are brought in to encourage breastfeeding are fanatical and highly judgemental of women who do not breastfeed – for whatever reason. The healthcare system and society at large frequently regard women who do not breastfeed at all, or for long, as bad mothers, erroneously equating breastfeeding with good mothering. In response to the "breast is best" concept, the "fed is best" movement has arisen which aims to destigmatize the choice not to breastfeed. In one of my earliest publications on maternity care, first printed forty years ago, in 1984, I modified the "breast is best" slogan by adding "but not at all costs."[347] I noted that good mothering is not made up of breastfeeding multiple times a day but by caring for a baby at all times of the day (and night), and throughout life. I was criticized for my attitude by the hardline breastfeeding support groups at the time. Although I remain a staunch supporter of breastfeeding, and served as a Master trainer for the WHO/UNICEF BFHI for some decades, I remain firm in this approach: Good mothering is more than just breastfeeding. Mothers who cannot, or do not breastfeed for long, feel guilty, defensive, and angry at being berated, scolded, and judged – rightly so. They are the ones standing up with the "fed is best" campaign, because they do not want other mothers to be abused for choosing to feed their babies in whatever way they could/chose to. While research clearly supports the importance and health benefits of breastfeeding for both mothers and babies, we must be careful to remember that good mothering comes from a multitude of actions taken to care for and provide a loving family for new babies and not only from breastfeeding.

We also need to address the multitude of factors that contribute to mothers being/feeling unable or unwilling to breastfeed. We need to address the failures of caregivers to give the appropriate practical support and assistance regarding breastfeeding skills. We need to make it not only possible but easy for parents to breastfeed comfortably in public, without judgement, staring, or hostility. We need a society that supports paid family leave for new parents to facilitate exclusive breastfeeding without losing one's livelihood or prospects for career advancement. We also need to normalize breastfeeding in the workplace, after parents return to work but continue to feed their children, with workplaces and daycares set up to facilitate these processes as normal, expected events, not exceptional "accommodations." This can be even better managed for some professions by normalizing and valuing remote work and flexible work arrangements, which enable parents in professions that can be done remotely, to manage both their careers and their families in the way that is most productive for them. As with many aspects of pregnancy and parenthood, breastfeeding is not only a simple physiological action, but ties into our social, professional, personal, and emotional lives. Until our entire society supports mothers to breastfeed, from our medical professionals through to our workplaces and social environments, we also need to condemn those who judge mothers for doing the best they can in their circumstances, who publicly or privately berate or admonish parents for not living up to an "ideal" that society and systems actively prevent them from achieving. Our judgement and scolding should be reserved for those who believe they have the right to attack others, and we should protect, advocate for, and support mothers for doing the best they can.

Breastfeeding Rates

Even though substantial randomised control trial evidence supports the BFHI,[348] relatively few hospitals in North America are accredited as Baby Friendly and only some twenty to thirty thousand worldwide. For example, at the time of writing, only about ten of

Canada's maternity hospitals are accredited "Baby Friendly Hospitals." Breastfeeding is becoming the cultural norm in Canada, with 90% of women intending to, and initiating, breastfeeding.[349] Significant challenges exist, however, with regard to exclusivity and duration rates. According to the Public Health Agency of Canada's MES only 14.4% of mothers giving birth in 2005-6 achieved the Canadian and global standard of breastfeeding exclusively for six months. This figure has slowly increased so that in 2017-8, 54% of women exclusively breastfed their babies for four months but only 34% continued to give at least some breastmilk, if not exclusively, for six months.[350] In 2005-6, 21% of breastfeeding mothers added alternate liquids to their baby's diet within one week of birth and by 14 days, 25%. In 2017-8, this figure had not changed much with 15% of all mothers who initiated breastfeeding stopping altogether in the first month after birth. Breastfeeding rates also vary widely across Canada with rates being higher in the west than the east, and among older mothers.[351]

Canada is not alone in their less-than-optimal breastfeeding practices. Many industrialized countries are aware of the BFHI, and endorse its guidelines, although they are unable or unwilling to implement it fully. While UK rates of breastfeeding initiation, as reported in 2015, have risen to 81% only 55% of women were still breastfeeding at six weeks, and just 34% at six months.[352] About 23% were breastfeeding exclusively at six weeks and only 1% at six months. This drop off is not planned, with 80% of women who stopped breastfeeding in the first six months saying that they would have preferred to continue. Reasons for this are many, including the need for mothers to return to work where breastfeeding supports may not be available, and the intention to involve partners in more active care of their newborn including the possibility of infant feeding. Most important, however, is a widespread lack of appropriate training for healthcare providers regarding the skills and techniques involved in effective positioning and latching of newborns to optimize breastmilk flow and to minimize nipple pain or damage.[353] We need a concerted effort to ensure that all caregivers including obstetricians as well as paediatricians, family doctors, nurses and midwives are trained on the basic and simple skills of breastfeeding that, judging from our less than ideal global outcomes, are lacking at present. In addition, contradictory advice is often given to new mothers about breastfeeding concepts or practices. We also downplay the breastfeeding challenges faced by mothers who have caesarean sections and who face more breastfeeding challenges.[354] We need greater awareness in societies of the benefits of breastfeeding for both mothers and babies, and the consequent provision of societal support systems, such as paid parental leave, that endorse and facilitate breastfeeding.

Skills of Caregivers

Breastfeeding is not rocket science: almost any mother and baby can do it. Skills in monitoring effective breastfeeding, however, are lacking. For example, many postpartum caregivers do not know what an effective latch looks like. Even academic journal reviewers, who are supposedly "experts in breastfeeding," are sometimes unable to recognize appropriate latching. When I submitted photographs of an effective newborn latch for publication in a prominent journal, these were rejected with the comment "Why are you trying to change breastfeeding practices?" Even so-called "expert reviewers" are swayed by the repeatedly published drawings of an effective latch showing the newborn baby's nose well clear of (about one cm away from) the mother's breast instead of, correctly, virtually "buried" in breast tissue.

There is still much to do to promote, support and protect breastfeeding. It is not mothers who are failing to breastfeed their newborns but caregivers and society who are failing mothers.[355] This failure comes despite decades of evidence and literature available to caregivers and health systems to provide the necessary support for this health practice.

Fortunately, in Canada and in many other countries globally, awareness of the benefits of breastfeeding for maternal and infant health and cognitive development of offspring is growing and is gaining some momentum. Rates of breastfeeding, and specifically exclusive breastfeeding for longer periods after birth, are increasing – and are welcomed. But it is not only mothers who need encouragement to breastfeed, but training of healthcare providers about the mechanisms of breastfeeding so that they can provide effective and practical assistance and not just encouragement. Not knowing how to assist a mother to attach her baby to her breast, through correct positioning of the baby in the mother's arms, and effective latching of the baby's mouth onto the mother's breast, resulting in the easy transfer of milk from mother to baby is inadequate healthcare. There are many possible positions for breastfeeding, and caregivers should be able to support mothers to find the positions that work best for them and their baby/ies. They need to have the knowledge and flexibility to support breastfeeding for mothers in all contexts, with different body types, abilities, and needs. Blaming mothers for their inability to breastfeed, in consequence, is abusive.

WHO/UNICEF BFHI

The BFHI, endorsing the importance of breastfeeding, developed in response to repeated resolutions of World Health Assemblies, and repeatedly approved by member states, is designed to create a favourable environment for breastfeeding in maternity hospitals and their associated institutions. The principles underlying the WHO/ UNICEF BFHI are summarized in the *Ten Steps to Successful Breastfeeding*[356] which form the essential components for breastfeeding supportive practices in any healthcare facility caring for pregnant, birthing, or new mothers. The recently revised Ten Steps are provided below:

Ten Steps to Successful Breastfeeding

Critical Management Procedures

1. Comply fully with the International Code of Marketing of Breast-milk Substitutes and relevant World Health Assembly resolutions.

   b. Have a written infant feeding policy that is routinely communicated to staff and parents.
   c. Establish ongoing monitoring and data-management systems.
2. Ensure that staff have sufficient knowledge, competence, and skills to support breastfeeding.

Key Clinical Practices

3. Discuss the importance and management of breastfeeding with pregnant women and their families.
4. Facilitate immediate and uninterrupted skin-to-skin contact and support mothers to initiate breastfeeding as soon as possible after birth.
5. Support mothers to initiate and maintain breastfeeding and manage common difficulties.
6. Do not provide breastfed newborns any food or fluids other than breast milk, unless medically indicated.
7. Enable mothers and their infants to remain together and to practise rooming-in 24 hours a day.
8. Support mothers to recognize and respond to their infants' cues for feeding.
9. Counsel mothers on the use and risks of feeding bottles, teats, and pacifiers.
10. Coordinate discharge so that parents and their infants have timely access to ongoing support and care.

Marketing Breastmilk Substitutes

A prerequisite for accreditation as a BFH is adherence to the International Code of Marketing of Breastmilk Substitutes.[357] The United Nations has repeatedly endorsed this Code, initially adopted by the World Health Assembly as long ago as 1981. It aims to "contribute to the provision of safe and adequate nutrition for infants, by the protection and promotion of breastfeeding, and by ensuring the proper use of breastmilk substitutes, when these are necessary, on the basis of adequate information and through appropriate marketing and distribution."[358] Infringements of the "Code" still occur globally. In North America, where the formula industry has a strong hold and is a lucrative enterprise, we disregard many aspects of the Code. The Code, and the BFHI, call for hospitals to desist from accepting free or low-cost supplies of breastmilk substitutes, or any other benefits that accompany the obligation to distribute such supplies to mothers within the facility or through its associated healthcare professionals. A small proportion of babies require breastmilk substitutes but a BFH must purchase these supplies out of their own resources. In a BFH, most babies (at least 80% and usually closer to 95%) will breastfeed from birth until discharge and will never require bottles, teats, or infant formula. A few will, but the associated costs of the formula needed for them will amount to only a few thousand dollars a year even in high-care facilities.[359]

The Code of Marketing of Breastmilk Substitutes

- No advertising of breastmilk substitutes to families.
- No free samples or supplies in the health care system.
- No promotion of products through health care facilities, including no free or low-cost formula.
- No contact between marketing personnel and mothers.
- No gifts or personal samples to health workers.
- No words or pictures idealizing artificial feeding, including pictures of infants on the labels or the product.
- Information to health workers should be scientific and factual only.
- All information on artificial feeding, including labels, should explain the benefits of breastfeeding and the costs and hazards associated with artificial feeding.
- Unsuitable products should not be promoted for babies.
- All products should be of high quality and take account of the climate and storage conditions of the country where they are used.

At first glance, the BFHI's Ten Steps appear to be simplistic, although their implementation is difficult. Almost all of them require extensive revision of traditional maternal and infant healthcare practices that have been in place in modern hospitals for decades. Many also require substantive changes in prenatal, intra-partum and postpartum obstetric and neonatal care practices. As a package, their implementation has an impact on medical, psychological, social, and economic assumptions underlying maternal and infant care. Dedication, commitment, and conviction regarding the importance of breastfeeding are essential ingredients for successful implementation of this health promotional program.[360] The paucity of accredited BFH's throughout North America and in many other technologically advanced societies reflects a lack of serious commitment to the best health options for our mothers and babies.

Breastfeeding NICU Babies

The BFHI firmly established the importance and practice of breastfeeding newborns, particularly normal, term infants. Strongly supported by WHO and UNICEF, this program went far in creating awareness of optimal feeding methods and the importance of maternal-newborn contact and closeness from birth onwards. However, it did not directly address the newborn requiring intensive care. In addition, its focus was on the importance of breastfeeding, rather than on the inherent needs, and rights, of both the mother/family and the newborn to have psychologically sensitive and supportive pregnancy and birth care, evidence-based practice, and well-trained caregivers. I clearly voiced the BFHI's lack of attention to the NICU setting as well as its neglect of the rights of parents and newborns to both clinically and psychologically supportive obstetric and postpartum care in the British Journal of Obstetrics and Gynaecology in 2004.[361] The name "Baby Friendly Hospital Initiative" has, in reality, been largely misleading. It is, in essence and as originally conceived, a Breastfeeding Friendly Hospital Initiative. To be truly "Baby Friendly," – or preferably "Family Friendly" – hospitals need to incorporate breastfeeding support as well as "friendly" or psycho-socially supportive, evidence-based, obstetric and neonatal care, which is respectful of the rights of babies as well as of their parents.

Postpartum Care

Many changes have occurred in maternity care settings in recent decades. Mother-infant contact was, in decades past, limited to regular three-hourly feeding sessions with nursery-based care for newborns between feeds being the norm. Fortunately, this has slowly evolved into encouraging rooming-in and mother/father-infant contact and care for many, but not all. Coming to grips with the concept that a new baby belongs to his or her mother and family and not to the birthing hospital – an old cliché – has yet to be fully assimilated into healthcare provider practice in many parts of the world.

First Weeks

The first few postpartum weeks are the most neglected components of family-centred maternity care. Preparation for parenthood is rare, either in schools or during pregnancy, even though this is the one career that most people will undertake during their lives. For some mothers, their own baby may be the first newborn they hold. Few first-time parents truly conceive of the enormous physical and emotional demands made by a new baby on the family. Early discharge from postpartum wards to home is a welcome recent development. Spurred on by financial issues (postpartum care in hospital is not lucrative for hospitals), it is also welcomed by many families who prefer the comfort of home compared to the sterile and impersonal hospital setting and the ability to minimize the time spent away from any other children. Early discharge has, however, also resulted in mothers having less time with professional assistance close at hand. Sufficient time was available, when hospital stays lasted five to ten days, for healthcare providers to care for the physical health of the mother and newborn, assist mothers to bath and care for the baby, establish breastfeeding, discuss sexual behaviour and contraception/family planning, advise families on immunization programs, consider safe infant sleeping practices, warn against shaken babies, plan maternal nutrition, advise about symptoms of postpartum depression, and to link the mother or family to appropriate peer and community support groups. With early discharge, these tasks are simply too overwhelming for nursing staff to implement adequately. New families are simply left to their own devices with family support (that is not always available) being their primary source of help. Most maternity hospitals today have reduced the length of postpartum stays largely in response to pressure from families to request early discharge but also because it is financially better for the health care service to encourage this. While early discharge may well be ideal for a confident, well-supported, new mother/family it may not be the best option for mothers who require greater support or assistance. Ideally, however, additional professional support at home when early discharge is preferred, (as is usually offered by midwives), is an alternative and probably most optimal service. Offering an optional discharge time to accommodate the needs and facilities available to these differing types of mothers/families may well be a goal to work towards.

Six Week Check-Up

The six-week postpartum clinical care check-up has been offered/ encouraged less frequently in recent years. When this consultation does take place, it too can be abusive. One mother who attended a six-week postpartum check-up, who was struggling to breastfeed her newborn but was desperate to do so (long before the knowledge that became available in the 1990's with the launch of the WHO/UNICEF BFHI) and who was clearly experiencing postpartum depression (diagnosed later by a psychologist) asked her obstetrician for help at this visit. His response was "You have a beautiful baby. You should be happy. I know many who would love to have such a baby. Would you like me to sell her/arrange an adoption for you?" Such heartless and disrespectful gaslighting of a woman's feelings – no doubt stemming from ignorance of how to support a new struggling and unhappy mother – also reflects a disgusting and abusive sense of superiority, and disdain for women. Such memories last a lifetime in mothers and are recalled with anger. While one would hope that care has improved over the decades, similar experiences are all too common, with new mothers being told to be grateful and happy that they have a healthy baby, regardless of the disrespectful treatment they experienced along the way. This attitude also raises the question of whether mothers of disabled newborns or sick or preterm infants are not happy and cannot be expected to be happy. Such stereotypical views of illness and disability require reassessment.

Postpartum Support

New families experience uncertainty about their abilities and their activities. Companionship from family and friends, if not professionals, is welcomed and essential. Seeking alternate models of providing home-based support for new parents is a growing and essential need for family-centred care. Exciting alternate models have been developed in some countries, particularly in Scandinavian settings and the Netherlands, such as maternity hotels where families stay together for a few days in postpartum hotels adjacent to the maternity hospital, or the growing availability of postpartum doulas, called *Kraamverzorgsters* in the Netherlands, who provide mother-baby and home care for days or weeks, or, at least, overnight assistance, after birth.[362] Internet-based support can have mixed value: Some sites are reputable while others offer misinformation. Mothers and families cannot readily judge which are more reliable. An evidence-based rating of pregnancy and birth websites (i.e., a "family-friendly" website rating system) is sorely needed. Telemedicine networks,[363] or emergency nursing pools that mothers could draw on for a day or night's assistance when the going gets tough, might well be valuable models to develop going forward that may complement the network of community clinics and home visiting or telephone contact services that currently exist. No matter which options are made available for mothers, not developing effective support systems for new families is neglectful of an extremely important aspect of healthcare.

Stillbirths

We consider the care needs of the mother who has had a stillbirth or intra-uterine death, and those of her partner and other family, even less. Caregivers, and especially the obstetrician and paediatricians involved, should spend as much time as needed with these families to assist them to deal with their loss. Yet physicians are often not prepared to take on this role, or make the time to undertake it, and health systems and hospital practices may restrict their ability to do so. In 2022, a survey of 3,769 parents of stillborn babies in forty-four countries, revealed that a quarter (25.4%) reported disrespectful care, and 23.5% noted disrespectful care of their baby.[364] Families reported not having their concerns taken seriously, not having enough time with their care providers, and not being able to create memories with their newborn. Care providers reported not being adequately prepared for discussions with parents about the stillbirth, or not having the time to do so. Hospitalizing these families in standard postpartum wards surrounded by healthy newborns and their families is psychologically cruel. Placing them in gynaecology units is probably more acceptable: however, their obstetric needs must still be met. Discharging them from care as soon as possible may well leave them bereft of clinical explanation, as well as psycho-social and emotional discussion and support. Health care provider training and system level support to reform these practices, including for example, the provision of perinatal psychologists, is desperately needed. Respectful stillbirth care of mother, father, and baby is a neglected human right.[365]

Sick or Preterm Newborns

"Why do we put sick babies in jail?" This is a question Dr. Adik Levin, an Estonian neonatologist, poses about current practices for treatment of sick and preterm babies. The need for and value of the exceptional care that we are able to provide for babies in the NICU is not in question. Some elements of our current approach to that care, however, are problematic, particularly the practice of separating newborns from their parents and families. In most centres across the globe, mothers and preterm or sick newborns are separated. Highly specialized clinical care is viewed as a priority with far less attention being paid to parents' or the newborn's psychological needs. This chapter does not question the importance of specialized clinical care, but does question the prevailing approach that isolates babies from their parents which is both abusive and not evidence-based. As with many of the practices identified in this book, they prioritize convenience for the caregivers/hospitals over the needs of the parents/family. This chapter proposes an alternate model that provides for a family-centred approach to NICU care.

NICU

The NICU environment is clinically essential but psychologically isolationist. It is characterized by separation of mother and baby, with minimal contact between them, and especially little skin-to-skin contact, as well as feeding with breastmilk substitutes either totally or in addition to breastmilk. In most of the industrialized world, these practices were accepted, for some decades, as essential means of providing optimal care for the sick or preterm newborn. As a rule, parents do not stay with their baby in a NICU, but are discharged from maternity units to home. During their stay in the maternity unit, mothers are generally encouraged to be with their babies at times during the day, but at night, they are in their own rooms, apart from their babies. After discharge, mothers can spend the day, or at least some hours, with their babies in the NICU, but they usually leave the hospital for the night. In some progressive units, a few days before discharge of the infant, mothers may live-in with their babies in a private room in order to learn how to care for their infants. Other family members can visit the baby in NICU care, although this practice (as with others) varies from country to country and hospital to hospital. In some centres, virtual visiting is facilitated allowing parents to "connect" with their babies in NICUs remotely.[366] These units have one thing in common: the infant is in constant contact with changing medical staff, is exposed to high technology care, and has limited contact with the parents. These conditions impede the mother's ability to attach emotionally to her baby, are detrimental to optimal infant recovery and growth, and increase the risk of infection through exposure to multiple caregivers. Traditionally the experience of having a baby in a NICU or special care baby unit (SCBU) is a traumatic one for parents and probably also for babies.

Re-Visioning NICU Care

NICUs do not have to be organized in ways that separate families.[367] It is possible for NICU care to be both clinically excellent and humane. Mothers (and fathers/partners when feasible) and babies need to be hospitalized together, remaining together 24/7. In that context, mothers become the predominant caregiver for the newborn (shared with professional caregivers), and are supported and encouraged to offer extensive skin-to-skin contact (the latter often called Kangaroo Care).[368] Infants in these circumstances can be breastfed or fed breastmilk with or without technological assistance, as required. The care offered by both the mother and hospital staff needs to be as demedicalized as possible. Introducing this kind of approach challenges the way in which clinical care in NICU's is provided.

Unnecessary Interventions

Traditional western models of NICUs provide stressful care regimens for sick and preterm babies. For example, during a 24-hour period, such infants may be handled, on average, more than 200 times.[369] Not surprisingly, caregiving itself is associated with three-quarters of all hypoxic episodes[370] as well as increased levels of stress hormones.[371] Painful procedures are commonplace in the NICU baby's life. Repeated heel pricks, for example, which may occur hundreds of times in a few weeks of care for the sick newborn, are currently well acknowledged to be perceived by them as painful and at times may even lead to iatrogenic anaemia.[372] We may choose not to heed their cries, but this does not mean that babies do not feel pain, discomfort, or unhappiness. All the evidence points to the reality that they do.[373] We fully acknowledge, respect, and admire the necessity of high technology care, the exceptional knowledge and skill that it takes to provide it, and the life saving procedures that are necessary for severely ill newborns, including accepting their unpleasant and unavoidable side effects. It is the unnecessary interventions, regardless of how carefully administered or even supposedly painless they may be, that when taken together, create a traumatic experience for the new family. All too often care becomes routine, and the evidence supporting continued repetitive tests and interventions becomes less reliable. The approach advocated here is specifically directed towards this aspect of care: do what is essential and take deliberate steps to avoid what is not. In adult care, permission for every test performed must be obtained and questions should be asked regarding the necessity of any intervention. With neonatal care, and particularly in units where mothers are viewed as "occasional guests," questions of this kind are not usually asked. Even when such permission is asked of the new parents, the fear and worry that accompanies having a sick baby may influence parents to give permission for more than what is necessary. Coercion, even if unintended, is possible, if not probable.

For example, being asked to give permission for a series of tests with the caveat that "you wouldn't want to take any risks with your baby" is coercive. As described in the Parma Rights of the Newborn Charter, no medical procedures should be performed on neonates without their parents' informed consent.[374] Informed consent cannot be coerced. The evidence suggests that it is not ethical to continue using our traditional approach. We cannot continue using painful, less effective, and more costly treatment when more effective, less painful, and less costly alternatives are available. Encouraging feeding sick and preterm newborns with breastmilk, and by breast as soon as is possible, in contrast to continuously providing breastmilk substitute feeding is a simple example. Nor can we continue to deprive newborns and their mothers of contact with each other. We can no longer ignore these insensitive aspects of our current models of care.[375]

Loving Preterm Babies

Several decades ago, a young resident in the NICU at (the then called) Baragwanath Hospital in South Africa (now Chris Hani Hospital) recognized the importance of providing love and touch for the babies under his care. At the start of his rounds in the ward, he would lift a stable but tiny preterm newborn to whom he had become attached, and insert the baby into his lab coat pocket where it would nestle, close to his body, for a considerable period of time each day, before being returned to its incubator. The resident's name is unknown, but he is to be credited as a forerunner of thinking about the importance of love, touch and caring for NICU babies. While the outcomes for this particular baby were not specifically documented, preterm and sick newborns cared for in Dr. Adik Levin's unit in Estonia gained weight more rapidly, had reduced duration of infections and less need for antibiotics, when cared for skin-to-skin, and breastfed, by their mothers.[376]

NIDCAP

Heidi Als and colleagues[377] developed a supportive approach for preterm newborn intensive care called the Newborn Individualized

Developmental Care and Assessment Program (NIDCAP). Care is planned to be responsive to the infant's needs while treatment and diagnostic procedures are timed to complement the baby's wakefulness or sleep state. Detailed observations of the baby's behavior are made so that care can be paced based on the infant's cues. It advocates individually appropriate infant positioning using comforting aids, individualized feeding support, opportunities for skin-to-skin holding and collaborative care for all procedures so that the parent can concurrently oversee the infant's comfort and well-being. The emphasis is on a quiet, soothing environment that supports the family's comfort and provides opportunities to feel close to and affectionate with the infant. This approach to care contributes to reduced morbidity, including lowered rates of intraventricular haemorrhage, reduced severity of chronic lung disease, less need for ventilator support and/or oxygen, earlier moving to oral feeds, better weight gain and significant cost savings due to earlier discharge and improved behavioral outcomes.[378]

Humane Neonatal Care Initiative

Even more family-centred, and worthy of emulation globally, the Humane Neonatal Care Initiative (HNCI)[379] was first established in Estonia in 1979, following a special request to the Soviet government, by Dr. Adik Levin, to create an experimental unit, unique in that region and in the world. It involves the mother (and/or her partner) in a rooming-in, neonatal intensive care service, with direct parent-care of the sick or preterm baby and close skin-to-skin parent-baby contact with breastfeeding (or breastmilk feeding) from birth until discharge. Except for technical medical and nursing care, the mothers are taught and expected to provide *all* of the infant's routine care and to stay in the hospital until discharge. Nurses administer drugs and injections, supervise the infant's feeding program, and assist with infant examinations. They also prepare mothers for caregiving and act as consultants. Generally, one nurse supervises ten to twelve newborns and their parents. The leading principles of care in this unit are 24-hour care provided by the mother, with assistance from nurses and hospital staff as necessary; promotion of breastfeeding and skin-to-skin care whenever possible and from as soon as possible after birth; minimal use of technology, and little contact between the baby and medical or nursing staff, who might expose the infant to pathology. This approach emphasizes the value of mother/parent care for NICU babies rather than primarily care by the neonatologist and nurses. Full-time perinatal psychologists, employed in the NICU, provide support for both parents and staff who are not always provided with good preparation for dealing with death, loss, and grief, all of which occur in NICUs.[380] "Second victims," or the healthcare providers who are involved in (usually unexpected) adverse outcomes of childbirth, may also experience loss of self-esteem, grief, fear in future caregiving, anger, and guilt, and also benefit from psychological support.[381] The HNCI is endorsed by WHO-Euro, forms part of their perinatal teaching program, and is being introduced in many countries.

Parent Care

Dr. Levin's initial motivation for initiating this system emerged from a nursing staff shortage that led to involving mothers in the care of their sick or preterm newborn/s in the NICU. Similar overloaded nursing responsibilities exist in many, if not most hospital settings today, recently aggravated by the after-effects of Covid-19 on caregivers. Continuous rooming-in (24/7), and significant primary care of the NICU baby by parents, improves infant growth, facilitates earlier discharge, supports breastfeeding, and creates maternal confidence and competence. In Levin's unit, mothers are encouraged to hold their baby skin-to-skin as much as they can and to "bed-in" in special baby cots designed by Dr. Levin, that attach to the mother's bed (now a commonly available accessory called a co-sleeper or sidecar). Care must, however, be taken to ensure that these cannot allow for entrapment of the newborn between the mother's mattress and the cot. The encouragement of (almost) *continuous* skin-to-skin care is the norm. This practice should be carefully distinguished from the current regimens of relatively brief, *intermittent* skin-to-skin care often advocated in modern NICU settings and with Kangaroo care. Care involving significant physical contact is very different from a few stretches of close contact at fairly regulated times during each day. In Levin's approach, close skin-to-skin contact with the sick or preterm baby is regarded as a normal expectation of caring for a baby. Benefits of continuous skin-to-skin care for babies in NICU's include lower mortality, optimal thermal regulation, improved mother-infant adjustment, improved immunological response, decreased risk of neonatal sepsis and need for antibiotics, reduced hospital readmissions, and increased exclusive breastfeeding.[382]

Mother-Baby Care

Both Levin's and Als' approaches are innovative ways to care for sick and preterm newborns. Distinctive to Levin's approach, and differing from Kangaroo Care's primary focus on skin-to-skin care and breastfeeding, is the concept of predominantly mother/family-centred care in preference to nurse/physician-centred care. In Levin's system, if the infant is the most important person in the NICU, the mother and father are the next most significant. Systems of care prioritize meeting the needs of the family. It is this feature of predominantly parental care, together with its emphasis on predominantly skin-to-skin care and breastmilk feeding, which makes Levin's approach so appealing and effective.

Clinical Benefits

The practice of mother/father-care of NICU babies has multiple physiological benefits. Extensive skin-to-skin care of NICU babies leads to fewer severe infections or sepsis, less hypothermia, earlier discharge, improved breastfeeding initiation and duration, and fewer severe illnesses at six months follow-up.[383] In Levin's unit, babies cared for this way gain weight more rapidly, have enhanced immunological defenses against infection, have infection durations reduced by three to five days, have reduced needs for antibiotics to treat infections, have three to five times fewer respiratory infections during the first year of life, higher rates of physiological interferon, improved neurological development, and a stronger immunology barrier.[384] Levin's findings appear, at first glance, to sound almost magical, although readers who remain skeptical, might recall the remarkable improvements that occurred in behavior with the abolishment of institutionalization as a method of care for children some decades ago, as well as of the classic, and dramatic, Harlow studies conducted on monkeys isolated from their mothers and provided with surrogate caretakers. What is remarkable is not that the babies in Levin's care unit thrive with loving parental care, but that we, in the 21st century, still enforce separation of babies and mothers as well as institutionalization of the neediest of our infants, even in the best of our units.

Not surprisingly, benefits similar to those reported by Levin have been reported by participants in other programs that provide facilities for mothers to stay in the hospital and care for their babies in NICUs such as in: Chris Hani (formerly Baragwanath) Hospital in South Africa, as well as in Ethiopia; Buenos Aires, Argentina; Santiago, Chile; and High Wycombe, UK.[385] Current research also indicates that, at least with regard to the not uncommon practice of mothers abandoning their newborns in maternity hospitals in Thailand, the Philippines, Costa Rica, and Russia, Levin's approach leads to fewer babies being abandoned by their mothers.[386] A large, multicentre, randomized controlled trial conducted in twenty-five Level three NICU's in Canada and Australia, requiring at least eight hours of parent-infant contact a day, has examined the impact of Levin's approach to care for babies in NICUs.[387] Findings indicate that Family Integrated Care, or FiCare, as it is called in this trial, results in greater weight gain over twenty-one days of enrollment in the trial, and a significant decrease in stress and anxiety scores among parents compared to standard care.[388]

Precursor to HNCI

In the 1980's, an innovative neonatologist at Chris Hani (formerly Baragwanath) Hospital in South Africa, Dr. Keith Bolton, independently resolved to give preterm and sick babies back to their mothers and to encourage breastfeeding of these NICU-based babies by their mothers.

His actions were in response to knowledge that many NICU babies were not being breastfed – as their mothers were discharged from hospital shortly after giving birth. These babies died shortly after their return home some days or weeks after birth, due to malnutrition and/or infection in the poor community that the hospital served. He created the ability to have what he called "lodger mothers" – women who stayed in a special ward nearby their babies in the NICU ward and who breastfed them regularly throughout the newborn's hospital stay. Newborn and infant mortality and morbidity were, not surprisingly, reduced.

Global Application

Although the Family-Centred, Humane Neonatal Care Initiative (HNCI)[389] approach has long been advocated, it is yet to be extensively implemented globally. Mothers, fathers, and siblings are now welcomed into many NICUs to observe, touch, hold, and feed small and sick infants. In the FiCare trial, parents in numerous NICU care centres, have, for about eight hours a day, been integrated into the care routinely offered by health care providers. It is time for all neonatologists to encourage the next logical step: of having mothers assume significant responsibility for all, except clinical, aspects of their baby's care, stay with their infants twenty-four hours a day with maximum skin-to-skin contact, provide breastmilk and breastfeeding as well as much of the direct care of the baby (under supervision), and participate in individualized baby appraisal and care programs. Careful attention to the needs of the parents for contact, rest, support, encouragement, counseling, attentive listening, and close collaboration with their baby's caregivers will enhance parents' ability to meet their infant's needs.

Family Limitations

Family-centred NICU care may be difficult for families living far from hospitals, and those having other home commitments. Parental leave restrictions may also limit family-centred care and need legislation designed to support family-centred care of sick or preterm newborns. While first-time parents may be readily able to utilize such facilities, those with older children or other home or work responsibilities may find this more difficult to manage. Some countries are recognizing this need and have established or are moving towards formal provisions for both parents of a baby in a NICU to take parental leave to at least allow for one partner to stay home with older children while the other partner stays with the newborn, or for both parents to stay with their baby in the NICU. Grandparents, other extended family, or close friends, if available, can also contribute to support if needed. No doubt community support services will develop to meet this growing need in much the same way as doula care for women in labour is now extending to doula services for home care of the new mother and baby. Even if the mother of a sick or preterm newborn that requires constant NICU care cannot remain with her baby 24/7, whatever time she can stay with her baby should be unrestricted and encouraged by healthcare facilities.

Designing NICU's for the HNCI

In addition, single-room family care, in contrast to large multi-baby NICU wards, is emerging as one potential model for the design of new NICU units. Benefits of single-family rooms in NICUs include reduced environmental noise, increased parent visiting, improved breastfeeding outcomes, reduced infections, shorter length of stay, and increased staff satisfaction.[390] Further initiatives encouraging twenty-four-hour rooming-in, of either or both parents, with a newborn requiring special care, should be strongly encouraged.

NICU Survival Rates

The survival of very low birth weight (<1500 g) infants has increased from 50% to over 80% since the initiation of NICU care in the early 1970's. A concomitant decrease in morbidity has not taken place.[391] For instance, the incidence of long-term pulmonary morbidity seems to have remained unchanged at 25% to 30%,[392] possibly because of the increasing number of surviving babies of extremely low birth weight (<1000 g). Furthermore, neurodevelopment outcome is associated with disability in 15% to 25% of all very low birth weight infants,[393] figures that have remained relatively unchanged over time. In addition, and as these children reach school age, additional minor conditions, such as difficulties with attention, behavior, visual-motor integration, language performance, and academic skills emerge and seem to occur in about 40% of the children.[394] It will be interesting to see whether Levin's and Als's innovative approaches to NICU care, offering more sensitive, family–centred care, lead to fewer long-term, adverse outcomes as these are monitored more systematically in future. Given the promise offered by such programs, it is unethical not to test them further.

Obstacles

The switch from a hospital/nursery system of care to a rooming-in approach for the sick baby, or the acceptance that neonatal hospitalizations should include the child together with the mother/parent, may prove to be just as difficult to achieve as was the change from a nursery-based system of care to a rooming-in approach for healthy term infants. Nevertheless, it is possible, and more importantly, it is essential; the physiological and psychological benefits have been proven over decades. Staff may see caring for emotionally sensitive mothers as an added burden and may think that it is easier to send the mothers home and care only for the babies. Similar resistance was also initially encountered when caregivers faced increasing demands for fathers/partners to be present at the birth of their babies, despite the enormous value of this emotional support. Concerns about having parents of sick and preterm newborns room-in with their NICU based babies have proved groundless in the Estonian unit and, although while some staff felt, at first, that it was threatening to have parents permanently "observing" them, the care provided jointly by the mothers and staff led to better outcomes. Some staff may also believe that their jobs are at risk if mothers/families are able to take on some or many of their former responsibilities, as occurred when rooming-in became an alternative to nursery-based care for newborns. Having parental collaboration with overworked medical staff may also help to avoid accidental medical mismanagement that is common in NICUs, with particularly life-threatening consequences in this fragile patient population.[395] As much as caregivers may work to provide error-free care, and safeguards are in place to avoid mistakes, it is clear from the number of errors that do take place, that existing precautions could be strengthened. Given that one quarter of medication errors in the NICU are attributed to misidentification of the patient, having an adult present who is able to identify their child, and assist caregivers to avoid such mistakes, may be lifesaving.[396] Having a parent whose sole interest is in caring for their baby may ensure that there is one person for each baby who ensures that their baby's care is consistent across the multiple caregivers who are usually responsible for any one baby in the hospital setting.

Separating Parents and Babies

Health systems often encourage parents to accept that it is the modern hospital equipment and care given by well-trained nurses and doctors that their babies in NICU need most. Parents return home, or stay in hotels near the hospital, hoping that they can maintain some connection to their sick baby. They live in helpless fear and worry, wanting to trust the specialists, but knowing how easily mistakes can happen and wondering, if they were there, could they do something to help? They want to know everything that is happening but are afraid to ask as much as they would like for fear of being "problem parents" and getting even less support. The stress of being away from a sick child, unable to help or know what is happening, is far worse than the reality of learning to care for them. And if the worst happens, and the child dies, parents are left to wonder, for the rest of their lives, if that death could have been prevented if they had only insisted on staying with their baby, or if their baby's short life could have been a little happier if they'd had their mother to hold them. The psychological stress of that "what if" is far, far worse than anything they could have experienced in the hospital with their baby. We have adapted to the challenges of hospitalizing parents/mothers together with sick older children. It is time for the role of caring for a sick baby to return to the parents, while at the same time providing those parents with appropriate psychological support and technological aid.

Costs

A further objection to mother-based NICU care is the fear that caring for mothers/partners together with their babies may add expense for hospitals. The reverse has proved to be the case. Reduced costs of earlier discharge and less need for therapies quickly outweigh the minimally increased cost of lodging a parent with their baby. The NIDCAP system of care, for example, although continuing to incur the expense of highly trained NICU nurses, reduces costs by US $4,000 to US $120,000 per infant, depending on severity of illness and initial birth weight.[397] It is likely that the Levin approach would reduce costs even further.

Changing Mindsets

The greatest obstacle of all, and the most abusive aspect of opposition to change, is overcoming the mindset that imposes barriers to finding creative and innovative solutions to the challenges of facilitating family-centred and psychologically respectful care of sick and preterm newborns. As is common when staff responsibilities are altered, the erroneous perception that their responsibilities are being eroded, their jobs threatened, that parents would observe, judge and interfere with their work, are strong factors leading to resistance to accept the new care regime. When caregivers put their own jobs, egos, or fears above improving patient outcomes, it is abusive. If hospital systems/staff/doctor convenience is more important than caring for the patients, that is abusive. Ultimately, care providers realise that adding parents to the care resources on hand actually makes their tasks easier. Not providing education for all caregivers on the importance of psychosocial needs of all parents and their families during their transition to parenthood, especially with a sick or preterm newborn, remains a further overwhelming barrier to implementing effective and sensitive care.

Psychological Support

Levin notes that the infant's growth may be affected by the mother's psychological adjustment.[398] Growth is slowed for as long as turmoil prevails, and once the emotional struggles subside, the infant benefits. The importance of good psychological counseling and sensitive care from the staff is obvious. Psychological care needs to be individually directed towards each family. Parents who are young, or old, having their first or a later baby, with or without previous experience of NICU care, those considering giving up their baby for adoption, or mothers who have struggled for years to give birth to a baby, all require different psychological supports. There is little data available yet to support or dispute these observations. They are, however, founded on solid psychological counselling theory: they provide rich hypotheses for future investigation.

Care for babies in NICU's requires sensitive care for their parents as well. It is extremely abusive to discount the mother's/parent's fears, concerns, wishes, and needs as well as those of the newborn. Little is known about the psychological reactions of mothers or fathers who care for their sick and/or preterm babies, although Levin's observations on their adjustment are interesting.[399] Adjustment is different in mothers who have full-term but sick babies as compared to those with preterm babies: full-term babies are easier for mothers to accept psychologically. Also, mothers of first-born babies admitted to a NICU find it easier to adapt to the NICU environment compared to those with a second or later child.

First Contact

The most difficult contact time between parents and staff is in the first few days in the wards.[400] Most important is the family's first contact with the NICU. Being met by and introduced to the NICU setting by a very skilled staff member who makes good contact quickly is important. Psychological support for mothers/families may be through individual counseling and/or in groups. Parents have just experienced the birth of a sick or preterm baby – a far cry from the birth of the healthy full-term infant they had envisaged. Individual counseling is particularly important in the first hours and days after arrival in the unit. It is essential that mothers not be abandoned completely at this time but be supported in their adaptation to their new situation and to the events surrounding their birthing experience. If this is not provided, parents may become frustrated, afraid, and unhappy, making close contact between staff and families difficult. The more parenting that the parents can undertake themselves, the quicker these feelings subside. Support for mothers at this early stage includes midwifery care for her, breastfeeding or breastmilk expressing instruction and assistance, nursing support with handling the baby, and psychological support for the family regarding their feelings and fears. It is most important to listen to the parents and to assist them to emerge from their stressful situation and to adapt to their baby. Providing a comfortable space in the NICU unit for parents to meet with their own family members to share both their joys and concerns is important. Teaching the mother/family about their stay in the NICU is crucial.[401]

Abusive Communication

Parents' adaptation and acceptance are facilitated through appropriate and sensitive communication with the mother (and partner) from the moment the baby's challenging situation is recognized, through to explaining her baby's condition and his/her immediate and long-term care. Some mothers of babies with anomalies have reported extremely disconcerting experiences regarding the way they learned about their baby/ies' problems, and the lack of honesty and consistency in the information, support, and care they received for their infants.[402] Some parents' reports of the treatment they received are, on occasion, so offensive and disrespectful as to be scarcely credible. In my research into parents' experiences of giving birth to a baby with Down's syndrome, limb differences, or achondroplasia (dwarfism), parents added extensive qualitative comments to a predominantly quantitative survey.[403] Some of the negative comments were:

> The doctor came to us on the waiting benches not even a waiting room, it was a passage and we had unknown people around us and he told us "Your child is abnormal and will not be able to walk or talk and will not go to a normal school and would need us to do things for him for the rest of his life."[404]

Another participant shared this memory:

> When we asked if there was a possibility of having another achondroplastic [child] he said "What are you worried about, you can always start a circus."[405]

On the more positive side, some comments included: "The most amazing thing about having a child like this is the things he had learned to do that we never dreamed he would be capable of."[406] Another parent said "I had to be fairly accepting of the things I cannot change, and for me this is the only fatherhood that I know – and it's wonderful."[407]

Establishing the importance of the mother and family as a member of the caregiving team right from the start is crucial. Creating a partnership is essential rather than developing a doctor (superior) to mother (inferior) relationship. Unfortunately, health services training does not appear to prepare potential caregivers for this changing role – or at least, judging from the dissatisfaction often expressed by mothers with their care this is not done well enough.

Sensitive Care

Although the importance of psycho-social and cultural issues in obstetric care has been increasingly acknowledged in recent decades, there is still neglect and misunderstanding of what women (and partners and siblings) want and need during pregnancy, birth, and the postpartum period with regard to their care. There is a lack of acknowledgement that optimal biological care must incorporate psycho-social factors as these levels of functioning are integrally related. Excluding psycho-social concerns results in disrespectful perinatal care and can hinder recovery.

In 2011, *The Lancet* published an editorial regarding its then, recently published, series on "Stillbirth."[408] The editorial expressed surprise at the worldwide emotional and heartwarming reaction the journal received in response to the series. What is remarkable about this is not the global response to the stillbirth papers, but the Lancet editorial. When will the medical world realise that behind every stillbirth, miscarriage, birth of a baby with an anomaly, and even difficult birth, unwanted caesarean section, failure to breastfeed successfully, or similar severe or less severe, negative outcome of childbearing, lie real people with hopes, feelings, wishes, expectations, and dreams? If they did, there would be no surprise at readers' emotional reactions to the "Stillbirth"" series.

A woman giving birth is not just a uterus, vagina, and perineum. This phrase has been reiterated for at least the fifty or more years that I have been active in promoting more sensitive care for women and their partners/families during their transition to parenthood. Biological functioning is not the only level of functioning that characterizes a pregnant woman: her cognitions, emotions, interpersonal interactions, social setting, and her spiritual needs all require care. Sadly, our western medical world neglects most additional levels of human functioning to concentrate almost exclusively on the biological when the emphasis should be holistic, including psychological needs encompassing at least emotional, cognitive, and spiritual concerns. We have yet to learn from many of our neighbouring cultures that there is more to having a baby than the functioning of our biological/physiological selves. As noted earlier, our language of birth – denoting "normal" or "optimal" birth as "physiological" only reinforces this reductionism.

Evidence-Based?

An examination of Tables 1-6 of the *Guide to Effective Care in Pregnancy and Childbirth*[409] from a psycho-social and cultural perspective is an interesting indication of the evidence available for the value of psycho-social interventions in pregnancy and birth. At least nine of the forty-one interventions listed in Table 1 as beneficial forms of care address psycho-social concerns. Some examples include:

- Assisting women to stop smoking during pregnancy.
- Providing physical, emotional, and psychological support for women in labour.
- Providing continuous support at this time.
- Providing child care for disadvantaged women and for breastfeeding mothers.
- Encouraging unrestricted breastfeeding.
- Providing consistent support for breastfeeding mothers.
- Trusting women to carry their own case notes in pregnancy.
- Support for socially disadvantaged mothers to improve parenting.

Approximately thirty-four of the 122 beneficial forms of care listed in Table 2 refer to psycho-social issues. Some of these include:

- Prenatal classes.
- Continuity of care.
- Respecting women's choice of place of birth.
- Respecting women's choice of birth companion.
- Presence of a companion on admission to hospital.
- Giving women as much information as they desire.
- Freedom of movement in labour.
- Choice of both labour and birth positions.
- Maternal movement and position changes to relieve pain in labour.
- Touch and massage to relieve pain in labour.
- Attention and distraction to relieve pain in labour.
- Non-pharmacological pain management tools, including music and audio-analgesia.
- Early mother-infant contact after birth.
- Consistent advice to mothers.
- Offering choice of length of stay in hospital.
- Social and financial support.
- Breastfeeding support.
- Telephone service for advice and information after birth.
- Support for bereavement or misfortune, and postpartum depression.
- Self-determination regarding hospitalization and birth experiences.

In contrast, virtually none of the interventions listed in Tables 5 and 6 that include forms of care that are harmful or unlikely to be beneficial are psycho-social interventions. Some psycho-social interventions are however included in this section as lacking evidence supporting them including:

- Routine pubic shaving in preparation for childbirth.
- Routine restriction of mother-infant contact.
- Routine nursery care for babies in hospital.
- Giving samples of formula to breastfeeding mothers.
- Advising mothers to restrict sexual activity in pregnancy.
- Prohibition of all alcohol intake during pregnancy.

- Imposing dietary restrictions during pregnancy.
- Withholding food or drink from women in labour.

Although not a statistically sound or methodologically exact classification (and consequently not truly evidence-based) this evaluation gives rise to much food for future psychological and obstetric thought. It also sheds light on the importance of respectful and psycho-socially sensitive care. Ignoring them is inappropriate, non-evidence-based, and, in consequence, abusive.

Supporting Families

Having a companion during labour is one of the most well documented, beneficial, practices to emerge in perinatal care in recent decades. Remarkably, we think of this as an intervention, even though this was standard care before hospitalization of births about a century ago. In addition to a supportive companion, optimal healthcare includes having one-to-one nursing care for women during labour and birth, although women are often left alone in labour between routine monitoring visits.[410]

Meta-analyses of studies exploring the role of emotional support for women in labour[411] have shown the remarkable strength of this simple intervention in minimizing negative outcomes such as prolonged labour, pain medication during delivery, less effective breastfeeding, and postpartum depression, among others. Outcomes of these meta-analyses conclude that all women should have continuous support throughout labour and birth, as this has clinically meaningful benefits for women and infants and no known harm.[412] The specific details, such as who is best able to offer support, and what support entails, given cultural differences in these preferences, are still being debated, although the message is strikingly clear: women do better when their emotional concerns are cared for. If this intervention could be packed in tablet form, at no or little cost, every woman would be prescribed one.

Caregiver support for women when complications arise is even more challenging. I recall co-teaching a class of fourth year medical students together with an obstetrician and discussing stillbirth. When we asked students what they would say or do when confronted with a woman with an intrapartum fetal death, the immediate response at the time was "call the midwife" (or obstetric nurse) and leave it to her. Such situations are extremely difficult for caregivers to handle, but require increased psychologically sensitive, trauma informed, and family-centred care. Medical (and nursing/midwifery) students need preparation for such situations: leaving the room, as my medical students would have initially preferred to do, is not an option. Moreover, there is no script or prescribed procedure that can be automatically applied in emotionally fraught situations; caregivers need to develop significant empathy and communication skills in order to be able to adapt to the needs of their clients. These requirements apply to any outcome that is not what the family hoped for or expected. These can be shocking, or at least, disappointing outcomes for any family when they occur, no matter how non-life-threatening, or even routine, they may appear to the caregiver. Families are capable of recognizing when things are not going as planned or hoped for: what is most important for them is to be kept informed of what is happening, why actions and choices are being taken, and the implications for them and their family. Reducing the "unknowns" in the situation can help them cope with difficult events.

Psychological needs are paramount during the birthing process. Women are extremely sensitive to the words used around the time of birth and may remember them for decades. Supportive verbalizations are far more appropriate than jokes or "smart-aleck" comments. The popular TV series "*Call the Midwife*" reflecting on midwifery care in the mid 20th century, based on the memoirs of Jennifer Worth,[413] emphasizes the consistently encouraging, respectful and sensitive support that many midwives try to offer women in labour, theoretically at least, no matter what the woman's background, or their personal feelings towards the mother or their family situation. In contrast, is one woman's predominant recollection almost fifty years after her first baby was born (not in the Jennifer Worth books or TV series!) of being told, while being catheterized, that at last "Now you can pee like a man!" As if this was something that a woman giving birth might regard as an achievement!

Support for Partners

Support for those giving birth is essential. In addition, some have highlighted that partners, in addition to their supportive role, have needs of their own during labour and birth that require support during the transition to parenthood: these needs are not usually considered.[414] Research into, and support for, fathers'/partners' experiences is still needed.

Companionship During Procedures

Surprisingly, although for the most part the technologically developed world has agreed to admit partners or companions into the birth setting, they are routinely excluded from other aspects of care. "Wait outside while we do this procedure and then we'll call you in again" is not an unusual instruction for a companion. At the precise moment when the woman needs the support of a known and trusted person, this is removed. There is very little, if any, research on the value of a supportive companion during treatment procedures. Women should be able to choose whether they would like their chosen companion to be with them during procedures for which they are awake and aware. Would this reduce the fearfulness of these procedures and contribute to her acceptance and coping with them? Should companions be encouraged (and prepared) to sit at the mother's head during pelvic examinations, cervical biopsies, or for dilatation and curettage procedures conducted under local anaesthetic? Would providing emotional support for people during these difficult moments reduce anticipatory fear or facilitate acceptance and recovery from the procedure? Such an approach allows lay persons to infringe on the traditionally defined "medical territory" of the operating theatre or the treatment room. However, this is precisely the same situation that prevailed some decades ago when encouraging fathers/partners to be present at vaginal birth was first broached and caused horrified reactions from caregivers such as "He'll faint! He's not sterile! He'll be too shocked! Women don't want him there! He'll never have sex with her again!" Yet now, this is practiced in much of the developed world, with beneficial outcomes. Considering encouraging partners to sit at the head of the woman's bed during a caesarean section under epidural or spinal anaesthetic is equally challenging today. "Humanising" the medical setting has become a clichéd term: yet still, it is needed.

Continuity of Care

A significant variety of caregivers may look after a single woman even for a normal birth experience. Some studies report up to sixteen different caregivers in a six-hour period.[415] Continuity of care hardly exists in this setting and may be even less possible when care extends over a longer period. Team approaches involving case conferences among caregivers are endorsed in theory, but not always successfully implemented in practice. Women, in contrast, want continuity of care and this need appears to be a significant contributory factor to women's positive evaluations of their perinatal experiences. It may also be one contributory factor to why women rate their pregnancy and birth care by midwives more positively than for any other category of healthcare provider.[416]

It is necessary to re-evaluate this component of care in obstetrics and gynaecology today. Obstetrics has recognized the importance of this earlier than gynaecology. There is, for example, significant evidence supporting the value of doulas, either in addition to or instead of partners, for labour and delivery, if not also for prenatal and postpartum care.[417] Such companions provide continuity of care and offer an advocacy link between various caregivers that look after women and their families. On the other hand, women may find themselves referred from one specialist to another with remarkable discontinuity resulting. Concerned with their own areas of specialization, healthcare providers are not always aware of what the woman has been informed or even what examinations have been performed or are planned, before, or following, their input. They may also not be empowered to inform women of their own findings, but need to report these back to the referring caregiver, leaving women wondering what was found for some days or even weeks following assessment. Moreover, communication between caregivers may resemble a game of broken telephone, with critical information being neglected, because its importance for one specialist is not recognized, although it may be crucial for another. For the woman, the extremely frustrating experience is one of falling through the cracks in the system.[418] Such disjointed care is abusive precisely because of the harms it often causes. To achieve continuity of care, the model offered by the doula might be a good one to explore. Providing a "companion" for the woman to escort her through all components of her care will provide a continuous supporter as well as an advocate on her behalf. Companions can be trained health care providers, such as doulas, employed by the woman, family members, or hospital staff, although access to one trained healthcare provider as the primary responsible coordinator of care is needed.[419] Current research into this model of care is revealing positive outcomes, although some types of companions may be more effective than others.[420]

Respectful Care

The lengthy delays often encountered when seeking consultations with specialists, or when requiring diagnostic assessments, obtaining results, or having treatments, is a significant contributor to women's unease about both obstetric and gynaecological care and reflects a lack of respect for her.[421] Once a problem develops, anxiety levels are high, particularly when fear of severe illness (such as cancer), potential surgery (such as a caesarean section), or potential fetal anomaly becomes a possibility. Yet women and their partners frequently have to wait weeks or longer for simple diagnostic procedures such as an ultrasound and even longer for tests that are more sophisticated. Further delays before receiving the outcomes of tests (such as following biopsies, or screening procedures) then add to family's anxiety, and could potentially compound the clinical concern. Such delays are simply disrespectful of clients' concerns and reflect attitudes of not caring. Covid-19 contributed even more to these delays. It is not surprising that frustration and helplessness arise in clients as a result, together with irritation, anger, and suspicion of the healthcare services.

In some industrialized countries, such delays may be due to financial restraints, although better management of resources would likely improve care despite any perceived or actual financial restrictions. If reorganization of systems of care is undertaken, the primary goal should be to re-think the processes in place from the perspective of the woman/family, with the goal of providing prompt care.

Impersonal Treatment

Disrespectful treatment is also evidenced by providing impersonal care, continuing conversations with colleagues while administering routine procedures such as blood collection, glancing at, or talking to passing caregivers while interacting with a client, failing to provide privacy for a client during procedures or while they move from one treatment area to another, and not preserving the dignity of clients while undergoing procedures. Respectful treatment requires avoiding such actions and is an essential and elementary component of care.[422] One example of disrespectful treatment occurred in Canada, where a woman who had undergone a Dilatation and Curettage under local anaesthesia was told that she could personally fetch her husband from the waiting room to join her in her post-surgical recovery room. She learned, much to her dismay, and only after entering the room still dressed in surgical gown and boots, *en route* from the operating theatre to the recovery room, that the waiting room was filled to the brim with family members of all patients receiving care that morning, who all simultaneously turned to see who had entered the room. Embarrassed, and still shocked by her recent clinical experience, she rapidly withdrew from the waiting room, asking her caregivers to call her husband for her. Although probably well intentioned, such advice from caregivers is insensitive to the needs for privacy, dignity, and confidentiality of patients as well as reflecting a lack of concern for her emotional state within minutes of undergoing a painful and disconcerting experience. Not all clients are as comfortable walking around public areas wearing standard, embarrassing, hospital gowns that are designed to allow ready access to all parts of their bodies, as are their hospital-based caregivers who see clients wearing these gowns every day, and see them as "normal." Nor are clients comfortable walking into a room full of strangers, post-surgery, and sharing their medical experiences with them.

Clients as Consumers

We frequently use the term "consumers" to describe healthcare clients. If commercial stores treat shoppers with similar delays in service and impersonal attention, customers will simply shop elsewhere. Within the healthcare service, with its more threatening and intimate experiences for clients, and its lack of real alternatives from which to choose in most instances, there is reluctance to apply a similar model. The fact that clients stay on does not mean that all is well in the state of healthcare. It simply means that getting care elsewhere is difficult, time consuming, and inconvenient, especially when part way through receiving care for a problem. Today, with the shortage of health care providers in many countries, finding an alternate caregiver may be impossible. There is also no guarantee that the next caregiver will be any better; they may be far worse. That dissatisfaction exists is evident in increasing litigation, the high numbers of women who report disrespectful care, and the low ratings of satisfaction with care that are common.[423]

Vast differences in respect for women in childbearing exist across countries. For example, the following story would be shocking to most caregivers in industrialized countries but this type of action is common in countries with less sensitivity to psycho-social concerns. As an international health consultant visiting a hospital in eastern Europe, I recall being taken to meet a mother in the recovery room shortly after she had given birth. I had recently asked my host – the obstetrician in charge – whether the hospital routinely shaved women's pubic hair before vaginal birth. We entered her room, and without any introduction or, in fact, even speaking to her, my host simply pulled her covering sheet off showing me that she was shaved. I apologised profusely and left the room as quickly as I could.

Legal Issues

Litigation, and fear of litigation, strongly influences healthcare, particularly in the USA.[424] The benefits that might be gained from discussing healthcare complications with women and in understanding areas of possible caregiver neglect, however, outweigh the risks. Fear that this might encourage litigation proceedings when care has been unsatisfactory is possibly unfounded. Discussing adverse experiences with clients might do more to prevent litigation than to precipitate it. Litigation may be more likely to occur when there has been minimal or inadequate communication between doctor and client than when the communication channels have remained open and supportive, despite unwanted outcomes of care occurring.[425] The development of "apology law" which is not a legal admission of fault, but is a means of apologizing to patients for errors and non-optimal care, provides a means of clarifying "what went wrong" for patients and offering, hopefully, heartfelt concern.[426] By requiring caregivers to be fully transparent, and to disclose safety breaches and caregiver errors, this law holds promise of a means of meeting clients' overwhelming needs for explanation of adverse outcomes, and psychological "validation" of their experiences. Such emotional validation for a family that has experienced a traumatic birth outcome likely arising from medical error is essential respectful care. Cases like that of Laura MacGregor who gave birth to a son with multiple brain injuries eventually determined to be due to medical malpractice and which remained unresolved for thirteen years of horrifying litigation without ever receiving an apology from her attending doctors or health care service should never occur. Mathew's birth resulted in a diagnosis of spastic quadriplegic cerebral palsy, intellectual disability, gastroesophageal reflux disorder, sleep disorder, and reactive upper airway disease. He had seizures, could not speak, and was dependent on a feeding tube. His mother, Laura, provided virtually all her son's 24-hour care for thirteen years before a malpractice award provided some badly needed relief. The demands on her time to care for Mathew prevented her from sharing in the lives of her other two sons, leaving their father to carry this burden, as well as the overwhelming financial costs of caring for Mathew. He lived for twenty-one years: their legal case continued for thirteen of these before the family was ultimately awarded a multi-million-dollar settlement and a judgement of medical error. In all these years Laura and her family have never received an apology from the medical profession or the caregiving facility in which her son was born. As Laura writes, "Even in the presence of decided culpability and profound injury, no one in medicine has ever said, 'I am sorry that this happened to you.' "[427] As she writes, "No member of the medical community has expressed remorse for my son's injuries, his abbreviated life, my caregiver trauma, or the ongoing impact felt today, almost five years after his death."[428]

It is also abusive that the only recourse when there has been malpractice is an adversarial legal process that, by its design, denies any recognition of fault from the caregiver and forces the victim into years or decades long battles for basic compensation. Alternatives may exist that offer a more respectful way for clients to engage with the medical profession on more equal terms. In some countries, such as Norway, clients may appeal to an independent committee to lodge a disagreement regarding their medical care. That committee judges what compensation might be fair to offer the family and settles the financial payment. The committee, consisting of medical and legal experts, then takes up the case with the caregiver.

The Canadian Medical Association Journal has published an editorial condemning the lack of empathetic response experienced by Laura MacGregor and notes that there are at least two components to the injury done by not acknowledging medical error with at least an apology. The client is a primary injured party, but so too is the caregiver who lives with the guilt of what s/he has done. Apologising, even without acknowledging guilt, can go far to allowing that caregiver to move on with at least greater awareness of the impact of their actions on their clients and their families.[429]

The situation in Canada is somewhat different as Canada does not facilitate legal compensation for "pain and suffering." While legal compensation can be sought in a court of law this is generally limited to reimbursement of the costs associated with the outcomes of malpractice. In addition, the medical association that defends caregivers has largely unlimited financial resources compared to those of most individuals who might chose to take a caregiver to court. This association also appears to prioritize the integrity of the profession over the needs of the client. The result is that it is extremely difficult to sue for malpractice in this country.

Perceptions of professional incompetence may contribute to the likelihood of taking legal action. In the Canadian MES, as many as 25% of respondents rated their caregiver competence as less than ideal.[430] More than half (52%) of Canadian women with previous experience of Female Genital Mutilation rated the doctor who assisted their delivery as not competent to do so.[431] Such ratings of perceived caregiver in/competence by women following birth suggest that, at least, clarifying potential misunderstandings about their care might be valued.

It is, however, unacceptable that questions of law should determine appropriate medical practice as, for example, may currently be the case regarding the excessively high caesarean section rate (to cover oneself in case of negative outcomes) in some countries. Whether a legal system based on trial by jury as opposed to trial by judge is more, or less persuaded by clinical or pharmaceutical argument is also unknown. Juries are, however, less likely to be able to comprehend the nuances of medical treatments: expert testimonies are not always understood as scientific information or evidence-based care may not be well understood by lay persons. Especially when medical professionals themselves disagree on preferred treatment courses, jurors may not be able to assess medical responsibility reliably.[432] The result is that it is difficult for women to successfully plead their cases relating to medical mistreatment in jury-based trials. Resolution of the conflicting needs of legal, financial, psychological, and healthcare issues is needed urgently to prevent the further direction of, and in some instances, misdirection of, medical care arising from legal concerns.[433]

Listening to Women

In perinatal care, the voices of all women and their families should be heeded.[434] Ongoing quality assurance assessments through asking women and men about the care they wish to and/or have received should be a normal and routine part of healthcare services. The concept of feedback regarding educational programs is well recognized, integrated and accepted in technologically sophisticated societies. No conference or educational course ends without delegates completing an evaluation form. Why is this, similarly, not integrated into healthcare services? Is it because women's (and men's) voices are still not acknowledged as an integral part of the healing process and are weighted as of far less, or even of no, significance than the biological basis of their illness, or their clinical outcomes? Even if surveys are undertaken, the reports of families need to be carefully reviewed, discussed and changes implemented where appropriate, for them to be useful or effective tools for improvement. Becoming partners in care, rather than simply clients, is still the challenge for the future.

Satisfaction with Care

Although reactions to the use of specific practices in pregnancy and birth care are the usual focus of these surveys, perhaps the most overarching outcome is women's ratings of their satisfaction with their care. Satisfaction is, however, difficult to assess and is only a partial step towards evaluating cognitive and emotional contentedness. Numerous issues contribute to satisfaction ratings including: a positive birth outcome; congruence between expectations and reality regarding pregnancy, labour, and birth; the number and nature of medical interventions used; postpartum care; type of caregiver and continuity of caregiver; place of birth; social support in pregnancy, labour, birth, and the postpartum period, from the partner and other family members; previous birth experiences; and the newborn itself, among others. Despite the difficulties of measuring satisfaction, surveys of this kind can provide telling information: for example, that a little over half of Canadian women (54%) were "very positive" and a further (26%) "somewhat positive" about their overall experience of labour and birth. Satisfaction levels among the 4% of Canadian mothers who were attended in labor and birth by midwives, averaged 71% with ratings of "very positive," compared with those of obstetricians (52%) and family doctors (58%).[435] This situation is not unique to Canada: Only 35% of women in the USA rated the quality of their maternity care system as "excellent."[436] In 2023, one in five women reported mistreatment in maternity care, and a third faced discrimination in the USA according to a Centre for Disease Control report. Mistreatment occurred more often among Black (30%), Hispanic (29%) and multiracial (27%) women.[437] In Australia, in a 2021 survey of over six thousand women, over 85% wished to do something different during a future pregnancy.[438] It appears that a significant proportion of women are not fully satisfied with their childbirth care. Viewed in a different context, any business where one of every two or three customers was not fully satisfied with their service would soon cease to exist, as customers would simply go shopping elsewhere.

Ideally, a very positive rating should be the goal to achieve for all women, regardless of birth outcome. Women with adverse pregnancy outcomes might give lower ratings, although, in an ideal world, well managed and supported pregnancy distress could be rated reasonably well by women whose psychological as well as physical needs at birth are supported.[439]

Privacy

In some countries, where women's rights and independence have not been seriously considered, conducting surveys may require the approval of their partners. Although such patterns of conduct may seem strange and unacceptable in the western world, these practices are common in many societies. Researchers need to be respectful of these differences and take care when seeking women's opinions that such responses are collected in private and remain confidential.

In eastern Europe, caregivers never sought women's opinions of their care. Even when I was regularly visiting mothers in their postpartum wards in the 1990's and 2000's (making trips to these countries about ten times a year for approximately fifteen years after the collapse of the Soviet Union), I would ask mothers questions about their birth experiences only to have my escort, the chief of Obstetrics and Gynaecology or similar, move to stand between me and the mother, and answer on her behalf. These officials clearly thought that their opinions on the woman's birth experiences were more important than were hers. Or, they did not want me to hear what mothers had to say about their care. As far as I am aware, no surveys of women's experiences of birth were undertaken under Soviet rule, or prior to my own.

Home Birth

Why do some mothers – in countries like Canada where (predominantly hospital-based) birth outcomes are very good – choose to give birth at home with midwives in attendance? Why do some women in Canada and the USA even consider, or actually choose, to give birth at home without *any* skilled birth attendants? In 2006, 36% of 24,970 home births in the USA were not attended by a physician or midwife according to the USA Centre for Disease Control and Prevention.[440] By 2020 this figure had risen to 45,646.[441] About two-thirds of these were reported as "planned."[442] More recent USA data are not readily available. Although comparable Canadian figures do not exist, Vogel reported that on April 5, 2011, 15,000 active discussions on unassisted childbirth appeared on a popular website.[443] Reasons for this increasing interest in, and willingness to have a "freebirth" as unassisted births are termed, include women's belief that they are safer giving birth alone than attended by any of the licenced professionals available to them, even when they are fully aware of the risks attendant on home births without formal medical care. Indifference, disrespect, abuse, and the lack of informed consent contribute to this belief, with healthcare provider assisted birth considered to be a greater risk of injury or death than going it alone. Such concerns were exacerbated during the Covid-19 pandemic due to the even harsher restrictions placed on birthing women in hospital care, such as excluding partners from the birth experience. The increasing limitations on women's ability to control and make decisions about their own bodies and health care in the USA (and in some other countries), emerging from the controversial debates about the right to abortions and, more recently, about some aspects of assisted reproductive technology, in the USA, is possibly, or even probably, contributing to this rejection of formalized medical care. Women who wish to avoid the cascade of interventions in birth that appears to occur in hospitalized care settings may do so by giving birth at home, unattended by trained birth attendants.

Whatever the contributing factors to women's interest in "freebirth," this movement has been exploited by some to create a very lucrative business. The "Free Birth Society," led by Emilee Saldaya from Canada, and Yolande Norris-Clarke, in North Carolina, USA, ex-doulas turned social media influencers, has gained a global following through podcasts that have been downloaded millions of times.[444] They profit from sales of instructional videos as well as membership in a group for pregnant women. They run two online courses that train "radical birth keepers" and "authentic midwives" to support women at birth. Almost 1,000 students have "graduated" from their Radical Birth School, which charges $6,000 for a three-month Zoom course for birth attendants. A year long "gold standards online intensive course" costs $12,000. The business is estimated to have generated more than $13 million in revenues since 2018.

Many of the Free Birth Society's claims conflict with evidence-based standards, including that there is "zero risk" of infection when cutting the umbilical cord, incorrect guidance on how to resolve shoulder dystocia, and taking a passive approach to newborn resuscitation.[445] A review of the Society revealed forty-eight cases of late-term stillbirths or neonatal deaths involving mothers or birth attendants who have attended their courses or appeared in the Society's podcasts. Most of these cases involve mothers in the USA and Canada, but some include births in Switzerland, France, South Africa, Thailand, India, Australia, the UK, and Israel.[446] Not surprisingly, the Society promotes an extreme version of "Freebirth" called "wild birth" and "wild pregnancy," advocating for both to occur without the attendance of professional birth attendants.[447]

While this development is extreme, its widespread and apparently growing influence may be indicative of a growing loss of trust in professional caregivers and care systems. It highlights the imperative for caregivers to provide treatment that is respectful and sensitive to the emotional needs of women in addition to appropriate, but only essentially interventionist treatment that leaves women satisfied with their care. Not doing so will likely encourage increasing numbers of women to seek "free/wild births."

Blame

While blame is not a useful concept in most discussions, for change to happen, it is necessary to identify where responsibility lies. The blame for the current state of overmedicalized and under-sensitive perinatal care can be attributed to many factors.[448] We readily blame mothers for not listening to the doctor's advice when it results in their baby's death, thus justifying a medicalized approach to birth. We also blame mothers for increasing the rates of caesarean sections and other interventions when they comply with our endorsement of medicalized care by requesting caesareans, epidurals, inductions, or even nursery-based infant care. We can even blame current evidence-based medicine that emphasizes a "scientific" or technologically biased approach.

We avoid blaming ourselves – the caregivers – for what might actually be the underlying reasons why some mothers are so dissatisfied with their care that they even choose unassisted home births.[449] Caregivers are comfortable with a medicalized approach: they are taught that is how births should occur. We also view technology as more important than sensitive care. *Good intervention is seen as good medicine.* Yet mothers in the Canadian MES clearly showed that, for vaginal births, the more interventions they experienced, the lower their ratings of satisfaction with their birth experiences.[450] Similarly, in a comparative survey of mothers in the UK and the Netherlands, the absence of complications and a spontaneous vaginal birth were related to positive childbirth experiences.[451] A recent, large-scale, national Swedish study of over 34,000 births, also reported that women who have instrumental births, compared to those with spontaneous vaginal births, reported inadequate support, insufficient information, and a lack of involvement in decision making, all factors contributing to less respectful care.[452] Caregivers may view being emotionally supportive and empathetic as unimportant, time consuming or not authoritative. Only two-thirds (65%) of Canadian women in the MES gave "very positive" ratings of their caregivers' compassion and understanding.[453] Many women who have caesarean sections choose to have a vaginal birth for their next birth: some report such negative and traumatic experiences of impersonal and disrespectful care during their in-hospital birth care that they opt for a home birth after caesarean section for their next birth.[454] Opting for an unassisted home birth is simply the next step.

Of great concern, and only recently receiving the attention it deserves, is that women may regard over-medicalization of perinatal care as abusive, exemplified in the Society of Obstetricians and Gynaecologists of Canada publication on *Improving Sexual and Reproductive Health: Integrating Women's Empowerment and Reproductive Rights*.[455] The document lists the right to health, free from non-consensual medical treatment, from violence, and from harmful practices, as second only to the right to life.[456] The Covid-19 pandemic has contributed even more to the wish of many mothers/parents to give birth at home, away from the potentially infectious and more restrictive world of the hospital. Rather than seeing the maternity care centre as a safe place for birth it has, to some extent, become something to be feared.

Researchers have pointed to serious shortcomings in current maternity care and to some guidelines that have encouraged caregivers to use possibly unsafe interventions and practices, such as, for example, routine caesarean sections for breech births.[457] In addition, even when fully informed choice may be feasible, caregivers may disregard women's preferences for less intervention, and adhere to these guidelines. Caregivers should heed the messages from these authors and others[458] that value women's feedback, and take greater responsibility themselves rather than blaming a multitude of other sources, including women, or guidelines, for the excessive use of many obstetric practices. They need to explore an evidence-based, less interventionist, individualized, humanistic, and holistic basis for how they teach and practice if they want to improve both the safety and satisfaction of women's birth experiences. They also need to seriously listen to what mothers say they want, and to earnestly endeavour to heed these requests. Simply going through the motions of listening to mothers and then ignoring their requests is abusive.

Stress

Psychological concerns or stresses arise during pregnancy, birth and in the days and months after birth, even when this is a normal, healthy experience. Mothers and partners, and probably caregivers too, could benefit from debriefing some time after the birth. The MES examined the stress experienced by Canadian women in the year before giving birth. About one-fifth (17%) of women reported experiencing three or more stressful life events during this period. Almost 13% reported that most days were very stressful. The majority (87%) did have support available to them all or most of the time during their pregnancy which assists in coping with such pressures.[459]

For many pregnant people, birth itself looms large on the horizon and imagining the newborn or contemplating caring for the newborn during pregnancy is difficult. Although prenatal preparation classes offer information for families on breastfeeding and newborn care, the reality of looking after a new baby may only become apparent once the newborn arrives. On top of this is the need for families to deal with the events of birth, especially if these were difficult, traumatic, or disappointing experiences.[460] For many, if not most, new parenthood is stressful. Emotional distress such as postpartum blues, affecting up to 80% of women, or depression, emerging in approximately 10 - 20% of new mothers, or, more severely, and rarely, psychosis (in fewer than 1% of women), can be difficult to manage.[461] Fathers too, may experience pregnancy and postpartum related depression.[462] Most significant in this respect is the importance of coming to terms with a pregnancy loss, or birth of a baby with disabilities or medical conditions. Pre-existing psychological or psychiatric concerns including depression, or addictions to alcohol, drugs, or other substances make adjustment even more challenging. Physical, emotional, or sexual abuse before, during or after pregnancy also makes the transition to parenthood more difficult. The MES revealed that 11% of Canadian women reported physical or sexual abuse in the year before giving birth with younger, less educated, and lower income women reporting abuse more often.[463]

Families may benefit from debriefing emotionally regarding their experiences. Supporting families emotionally during the pre-conception, pregnancy, birth, and early postpartum months is central to promoting infant mental health as well as parental mental health. Parental stress and mental health pathologies during the perinatal period can adversely affect the parent-infant relationship leading to later infant mental health development concerns.[464] In the absence of any specific professionals dedicated to caring for psychological concerns during pregnancy, at birth, and in the postpartum period, these concerns become the responsibility of any or all professionals (and/or family members) caring for new families during their transition to parenthood, with more debilitating disturbances requiring referral to specialist caregivers. These caregivers also need the appropriate training, on psycho-social and cultural aspects of childbearing as well as on respectful care, and resources, such as perinatal psychologists, to be available to them to cope with such demands. Clients need funding support to access these services.

Perinatal Psychologists

In all cases, discussing the birth and its outcomes with a mother, and encouraging, but not forcing, her and/or her partner to talk about their birth experiences can go a long way to relieving anxiety and releasing pent up emotions. Psychological and psycho-social forms of postpartum care are helpful in reducing the severity of these emotional experiences.[465] Accepting what happened compared to what was hoped for is a major psychological milestone that must be achieved to allow the couple to move on with their lives. Reassurance that she, personally, was not able to control the actions of her body's largely involuntary activities during birth; or her baby's development, size or positioning; or the routines in place in the institution in which she gave birth; or indeed the preferences and practices of her caregivers; can serve to ease the (often inappropriate) personal responsibility that women may assume (and are encouraged to undertake by many), when they are pregnant or give birth. Offering an opportunity to debrief after giving birth, with a chance to discuss what happened and how this compared with expectations may contribute to a family's ability to reconcile prior hopes with possible feelings of disappointment. Families require validation that their thoughts and feelings are normal and justified. Perinatal psychologists can play an immensely important role in providing this supportive care. Sometimes these discussions are best held shortly after birth. In other situations, and particularly with a pregnancy loss, or when women are seriously upset by their experiences, discussions may be needed on a number of occasions in the weeks or months after birth.[466] Such discussions need to occur when the people in question are ready for them: for some this might be soon after the birth while for others the need may arise some weeks or even months later. As with any aspect of clinical care, psychological health concerns need to be treated in the strictest confidence. Health care services that do not provide such psycho-social support services are neglecting their responsibilities. Appointing well trained perinatal psychologists to the maternity health care team in every birthing facility is a first step towards meeting this need.

Community-Based Supports

Society can help families move into parenthood with happiness. Encouraging families to avail themselves of community-based social networks can be immensely helpful. If they do, local community support networks provide extensive opportunities to learn from, and to share with other families facing similar experiences.[467] Some prenatal classes continue to meet and share parenting experiences for years after their first meeting. Extended families can provide much of this support, if they are close, but in today's highly mobile world, many may not have such traditional support systems in place.

Discussing unexpected negative emotional reactions after having a baby can be difficult. Society emphasizes the wonderful, beautiful, joyous, exciting experience of having a baby. Family and friends are filled with good wishes and congratulations. Faced with this array of positive reactions the mother or parents who are struggling with tiredness, discomfort and/or pain, anxiety about their ability to care for the newborn, insecurity about their knowledge of baby care, and faced with a totally dependent and seemingly fragile, helpless life to care for, many find it incredibly difficult to acknowledge that they do not feel overjoyed. Someone to talk to about their concerns and feelings, who can reassure them that these reactions are normal and common, can be an immense help.

Spiritual Needs

Spiritual needs require consideration with regard to both normal pregnancy and pregnancies with adverse outcomes. For some this might involve support from religious personnel in times of need, such as when a pregnancy loss occurs. For others this need may manifest as wearing or maintaining contact with some symbol of spiritual importance, or the following of traditional rituals or practices. Whatever spiritual needs women have should be considered, particularly when they may contribute to enhanced emotional adjustment.

Principles and Values

The above issues are not exhaustive of the psycho-social concerns of families' experiences of obstetric and gynaecological care today. Nor do they necessarily reflect the current interests of researchers as published in Journals such as *Birth,* the JRIP (*Journal of Reproductive and Infant Psychology)* or the *ISPOG* journal (*Journal of the International Society of Psychosomatic Obstetrics and Gynaecology),* all of which tend to focus on questions regarding reproductive healthcare practices and women's or families' experiences compared to the more clinically focused journals such as the *BJOG* (*British Journal of Obstetrics and Gynaecology*), the *AJOG (American Journal of Obstetrics and Gynecology)* or the *BMC Pregnancy and Childbirth.* In contrast, this chapter highlights some of the critical issues surfacing in healthcare services of low-, middle-, and high-income countries. It highlights some of the underlying principles regarding offering non-abusive, psychologically sensitive, but also evidence-based, care that pervade our work in this field.

Long held values underscore the importance of these issues, such as: concern for the whole person and not only the body, i.e., holistic and humanistic care; respect for women and their families and for their perceptions and needs when undergoing medical care; a sincerely gentle and concerned approach to care, with sensitivity rather than routine politeness being the order of the day; all combined with evidence-based clinical practice. It is apparent that although we have long recognized the importance of providing respectful care and have gone far in introducing systems that encourage such approaches, we are still grappling with the effective application of this fundamental tenet in many parts of the world. At the very least, the integration of this approach into educational programs for caregivers is a first step. Continuing to teach a primarily physiologically-based curriculum in medical schools, that largely excludes consideration of psychological care during the transition to parenthood, is simply malpractice and will result in abusive treatment.

The inclusion of psycho-socially sensitive concepts into the United Nations Agencies for Health recommendations will help raise awareness of these issues. Recognition of their importance in health has emerged in the publications of United Nations agencies in recent years. Concerns with issues such as women's and children's reproductive healthcare rights, violence against children and in families, bullying in teenagers, child employment, human trafficking, child sex abuse, the reproductive health plight of immigrants, refugees, and displaced persons, and the dilemmas of street kids are now given equal if not even greater weight than the traditional healthcare indicators of morbidity and mortality. The academic and professional world would do well to follow these directions.

Humanizing Care

Why are we so surprised that well designed studies confirm what we have known for decades: that women wish to be cared for with sensitivity, respect for their dignity, concern for their cultural, religious, or ethnic needs, and with gentleness as well as with evidence-based care? Have we become so engrossed with science that we have separated it from humanity? As a scientist, I am aware of the importance of randomization, reducing bias, testing hypotheses, and checking beliefs. As a psychologist, I know that emotional integrity is central to well-being. As a human being, I realise that when I am afraid, I want to be with those I love and trust, who understand me and who will protect me from harm, or at least look out for my interests. As Maslow said many decades ago: safety and love needs are primary, especially when these are threatened.[468] Why do we continue to ignore or neglect these messages?

During an academically sound, recently presented paper on women's mental health issues during pregnancy and birth, given by a (female) medical resident in North America, the presenter referred to "patients" dozens of times without once referring to them as "the woman," "the person," or as "the mother." I was, sadly, reminded of Soviet style perinatal care where being official, technical, scientific, and aloof, were valued highly, rather than being a warm, caring, and knowledgeable person. Although it was most admirable that this topic was addressed as part of the obstetrical staff educational program, it is a pity that especially at this senior level there is still a need to distance oneself from the "humanness" in the birthing person. Why are we so awed by the medicalization of birth that we have lost the ability to accept that psychological sensitivity during pregnancy and birth is just as important as technological advances, if not more so? Why are we reluctant to express sensitivity when caring for people? Do we perceive this as weakness? Or is it too threatening to allow ourselves to delve into feelings? Or are such emotions regarded as extraneous to good clinical care? Why are we afraid to *not* intervene? In the modern North American hospital, most women cannot give birth spontaneously without multiple medical and/or surgical interventions. Although some are essential at times, none is routinely required.[469] But all require explanation, understanding of women's and their family's perceptions of them, and gentle sensitivity. It is time to seriously rethink perinatal care.

Preparing Families

Obtaining information about their transition to parenthood and making decisions about these events are central issues for all childbearing families. The importance of preparation, not just for birth (e.g., pregnancy care, labour, birth, mother-infant contact and feeding, partners' needs, roles, and support), but also for parenthood (e.g., early child development, infant nutrition, marital adjustment, motherhood, conflict resolution, child discipline, employment and parenthood, and other questions) cannot be underestimated. Providing information about pregnancy, birth, and parenthood prior to pregnancy, during pregnancy, and after birth, is an integral component of family-centred care and is a necessary component of including families as partners in decision-making about their care.

Birth and Parenthood

Families rely on a number of resources, both formal and informal, to assist them to learn about childbearing, including healthcare providers, family and friends, the internet, books, TV, prenatal preparation classes and, for women having their second or later babies, their previous pregnancy experiences. The Canadian Maternity Experiences survey revealed that of these options, the most useful sources of information for women were health care providers (32.2%), books (22.3%) and a previous pregnancy (17.1%).[470] Among women attending prenatal education classes, 19.4% reported them as major sources of information.[471] Childbirth educators focus, primarily, on preparing women and their partners or family members for birth, although there is an enormous need for them to extend this care into the postpartum period.[472] Preparation for parenthood is possibly even more important than preparation for birth and is a sadly neglected part of education globally. Although most people enter the profession of parenting, there is no preparation for it other than the example set by one's own family. This may, or may not, be a satisfactory model.

Prenatal Preparation

In most countries, there is no specific training provided for prenatal educators, and little or no standardization of the content of programs. Classes became popular at a time when childbirth moved from the home environment to the less emotionally supportive hospital setting. They also achieved prominence as families moved from an extended to a nuclear structure, depriving women of the benefit of family/ community members' own experiences of pregnancy, birth, and parenthood. Classes initially promised some relief from pain as well as some preparation for the unknown and more fearful hospital setting. Later, classes added further goals of increasing knowledge about pregnancy and birth; physical preparation for the event; techniques to assist women to cope with labour, such as relaxation, controlled breathing, or even hypnosis; knowledge about baby care and breastfeeding; and psychological adjustment to parenthood. Programs were initially directed towards women and later included their partners. They are offered by professionals with varying qualifications as well as by those without any tertiary level training. Some are offered by mothers without training but with experience (good or bad) of birth. They may be offered by hospitals, public health units, or by private educators, may be short or long, and may be accompanied by exercise programs, baby care meetings, and postpartum get-togethers. Gaps in preparation programs exist, such as a paucity of preparation for unexpected outcomes including caesarean sections or pregnancy loss, despite a considerable number of women in technologically advanced societies experiencing surgical delivery and many infants requiring a period of NICU care, if not experiencing morbidity, or more rarely, mortality. Monitoring of the outcomes and effectiveness of courses may not always confirm their value[473] and is hampered by the wide variability among them regarding content, objectives, format, and trainers.[474] Evaluation of their effectiveness may also be masked by a focus on physiological outcomes of the research such as reduced length of labour or type of birth rather than psychological and social outcomes such as families' increased satisfaction with the pregnancy-birth experience, or their adjustment to parenthood. For many women in a nuclear family setting, the first baby they hold may be their own, especially if they were the youngest of their own family network. Unless they have siblings or cousins who have had babies before them, and with whom they have extensive contact, becoming a parent can be a frightening, even though exciting experience.

Training Prenatal Educators

Given the wide variety of subjects that could, and probably should, be included in such courses, it is unlikely that educators with only one professional training background could do justice to these expectations. What is needed is a specialized expert, well trained and capable of guiding new couples and their families through their multifaceted transition to parenthood.[475] The Lamaze International, and National Childbirth Trust in the UK and the International Childbirth Education Association of the USA, go some way towards meeting this need by offering extensive training for childbirth educators. These are not, typically, college or university level programs. Shifting them to the level of higher education might offer an approach to standardising the level of knowledge required and might provide some level of quality assurance for prospective participants. Expanding them to include holistic and humanistic content, and a longer-term perspective including parenthood, in addition to providing knowledge of the physiology of pregnancy and birth, is necessary. At present, there is little in the way of global, standardized content, teaching approach, or evaluation of such courses or their proponents.

In 1989, my colleagues and I were tasked with developing a graduate diploma in Childbirth Education by the University of the Witwatersrand Medical School, in South Africa. The resulting graduate diploma was approved by the Medical School/Health Faculty of that University, but never implemented due to funding restrictions.[476] This program would have facilitated students from a variety of disciplines including medicine, nursing, midwifery, physiotherapy, psychology, social work, and others, to undertake the program. It allowed course credits to be granted, exempting students from further study in the subject of their undergraduate training but allowing them to develop expertise in subjects of importance for childbirth education to which they had not yet been exposed. The worthwhile intention was to provide a standard of excellence for childbirth educators and their course contents: still a goal worthy of pursuit.

Emotional Support from Classes

Prenatal preparation classes for families provide an additional value beyond the specific information conveyed in them. The emotional support that can be derived from sharing their pregnancy and birth experiences with others, often friends or neighbours going through the transition to parenthood, can be both reassuring (if these confirm the couple's own doubts or concerns) as well as disheartening (if they provoke previously unconsidered fears). Yet, for most, the ongoing benefit of sharing both the vicissitudes of becoming a parent, before their baby is born, and for some groups, for many years after birth, probably outweigh any potential negative moments.

Sources of Information

Sources of information about pregnancy, birth, and parenthood extend beyond childbirth preparation programs. These include healthcare providers, books, previous pregnancies, families and friends, the media, and the internet. In all likelihood, there is some benefit (and likely misinformation as well) to be gained from most if not all of them, although the websites of most professional organizations are likely to prove more trustworthy than others, at least regarding clinical components if not psycho-social ones. Health and healthcare have become enmeshed in the web, so that medical information and knowledge is moving more readily into the hands of the layperson than ever before. Medical practitioners are now expected to share their knowledge with their clients, (and were the most relied on source of knowledge in the Canadian survey[477]) raising issues such as shared decision making, collaborative care, information and knowledge exchange, confidentiality, and informed choice by recipients of care. In our increasingly web-based world, these avenues provide exciting opportunities to explore.

There is an explosion of information available on the internet for families embarking on parenthood. Similarly, there are hundreds of books on pregnancy, birth, babies, and parenting. Many of these provide good information and some provide misinformation. In addition, caregivers may differ in the advice they provide and all of this may differ from what the woman's mother or other family members tell her. It is frequently difficult to decide what information is best to believe. These contradictions probably arise because of the passionate feelings that birth and babies evoke in us all – professional and non-professional. They also reflect the fact that every family is different and that parents differ each time they have another baby because of increased learning and experience. So too is every caregiver different. Knowledge is changing day by day as new research is undertaken and new findings emerge, some of these taking many years to disseminate across all caregivers. Parents are best advised about these contradictions and to choose caregivers, websites, and family and friends whose opinions they respect and trust, and to listen most closely to these. In addition, they need to consider that one of the basic principles of perinatal care is that of "individualized care" meaning that what is best is what suits each family during each pregnancy and that there is no universal "right" way to give birth or be a parent.

Decision Making

Regardless of their sources of knowledge, decision making by women and their families regarding their care during pregnancy, birth, and the postpartum period, needs to be based on unbiased information and evidence. Facilitating "informed choice" has long been a foundational component of family-centred care. Care choices should be offered to the woman/family in an objective manner, based on the best available evidence, and should be devoid of coercion, or "informed coercion." Despite its appealing face value, this goal may be difficult to implement, as information provided by a caregiver will be influenced by their personal approaches, practices, or biases. Ideally, objective information should also be available from sources other than the primary caregiver, with the primary caregiver available to respond to questions and supplement the evidence-based information. Information should preferably be offered in formats that families can access at home, in their own time, giving them the opportunity to consider, research, and thoroughly evaluate it before making decisions about their care. It should be provided in multiple formats to accommodate people with varying linguistic, accessibility, and literacy needs/ capacities.

Informed consent should be obtained without discrimination based on caregivers' biases for or against women's/families' biographical characteristics. Social determinants of health such as race, education level, and socio-economic class have long been known to influence caregivers' practices.[478] Whether or not caregivers seek consent from women for their perinatal practices is also affected by such factors.

Refusing Treatment

Involvement in decision-making incorporates the concept that women and families have the right to refuse consent for care. In most cases, this right should be respected, although at times a conflict of interest between the rights of the mother, the baby, the partner, or the family arises. In family-centred care, the needs and expectations of the mother are a priority with respect to her care. Once the baby is born, the needs of the newborn become a priority with regard to the baby's care. Individualized care advocates that "each childbearing woman and her family should be treated as if they are extraordinary."[479] Although professional guidelines and the best available evidence can indicate what approach to care is generally best, those guidelines are based on evidence for the majority of people, and typically exclude outliers or people in unique situations. Consequently, each individual woman's and family's needs may require that alternative practices be followed.

Conflicts may also occur between a person's decision or request for a particular form of care and their caregiver's own professional, philosophical, or religious commitment. Giving priority to the mother's needs and expectations may give rise to issues of crucial importance in questions of life or death, but also applies to less crucial, or non life-threatening, situations such as facilitating skin-to-skin care at birth or not using stirrups to support the woman's legs. In emergencies, the hierarchy of needs may change so as to give priority to a caregiver's needs in order to provide optimal, and possibly life-preserving, care for the mother and newborn. Although there has long been a value on individualized care, the meaning of this, and how this value is implemented, requires renewed attention. Conflicts between the woman's/family's wishes and those of her caregivers sometimes arise leading to legal consultation. The resolution of such cases is often controversial, giving rise to debates about the value of life of the mother or baby, the importance of respecting mother's or families' beliefs or choices, and sincere, but contradictory, ethical dilemmas.

Women's Voices

Women's decisions regarding their perinatal care are not limited to their own pregnancy, labour, and birth experiences. Their voices need to be heard by maternity care services, including organizations and the professionals who work within these organizations.[480] Some maternity and newborn centres are increasingly including women and parent advocates in their decision-making processes, with a few national centres such as the UK's NICE involving women directly in their globally, highly respected, national policy and standard setting programs. Ideally, an overarching national organization including one branch that represents families' perspectives on the process of becoming parents and another that represents inter-professional viewpoints is needed to ensure widespread dissemination of family-centred concepts to both. Close collaboration, if not full integration, between these branches is optimal. The lack of implementation of such an organization in most places, and especially in the industrialized world, reflects the considerable gap that still exists between current systems and truly family-centred and respectful approaches.

Attending to the needs of parents for appropriate and evidence-based information about their pregnancy and birth experiences, and facilitating their participation in decision making about their own or their baby's care, is respectful, and central to meeting the family's needs for knowledge about their transition to parenthood.

Multi-Professional Care

It is best to choose the caregivers with the most appropriate skills needed for the level of care required.[481] Primary care practitioners such as midwives or family physicians ideally care for normal pregnancies and births: the development of complications requires referral to specialists. Choice of caregiver is affected by the availability of types of caregivers and maternity care centres, geographical limitations, financial restrictions, transport facilities in case of need, and families' personal choices. Whatever option is decided upon by the woman and her family, inter-professional collaboration is needed to facilitate optimal maternal and newborn safety, particularly as care is transferred to or shared with alternate professional caregivers. The sometimes-conflicting roles of obstetricians and midwives, and the emerging roles of psychologists, as well as family and community members are discussed in this chapter.

Alternative/Complementary Care

An emerging issue relates to the rapidly growing use of alternative, so-called traditional, complementary, natural, or herbal therapies in both everyday life and maternity care.[482] A recent literature review identified the need for greater respect and cooperation between conventional and alternative practitioners as well as communication between all maternity care practitioners and their clients about the use of complementary and alternative medicine.[483]

I served as a member of the Health Science Research Ethics Board for about a decade at the University of the Witwatersrand, South Africa.

Occasionally, proposed research projects sparked heated debate among our approximately twenty-member group. One of these was a proposal to study the value of alternative remedies such as the use of cabbage leaves to reduce breast engorgement after birth.[484] Some members of the board feared that conducting research into such practices would grant them validity as potential treatment methods. Others argued that unless we test them, we would never know if they were, in fact, helpful. Ultimately, the Ethics Committee granted permission to undertake such studies. A randomized trial revealed that women who placed cabbage leaves over their breasts in the hope that this would reduce their engorgement, tended to report less swelling but not statistically significantly so. These women were, however, more likely to be breastfeeding at six weeks after birth, and to breastfeed for longer. Their greater breastfeeding success may have been due to the use of cabbage leaves, or may have been secondary to the reassurance and confidence they gained by this intervention. Or, indeed, that women who are likely to try using cabbage leaves to reduce engorgement are those most interested in breastfeeding despite any pain or discomfort. Regardless of its outcome or the difficulty of interpreting the findings, this study helped legitimize the importance of studying less conventional practices.

The underlying principle emerging from this is not that alternate treatment programs are valuable, or viable, but that an open-minded, inquiring approach to alternate ideas that are often proposed by lay groups and by mothers or their families are worthy of consideration and examination. When discussing traditional medicine from differing cultural backgrounds, it is necessary to recognize that many of these practices (such as upright positions for birth) have been used for centuries longer than western medicine. It is unlikely that they would have continued to be practiced if they did not have value. Outright rejection of alternate approaches is disrespectful, and may result in interesting and valuable ideas being lost. Had we not chosen to study the value of companions at birth, or skin-to-skin care of mother and baby at birth, both psycho-social and so-called "soft" interventions, we would likely never have introduced these remarkably valuable clinical care practices.

Midwives and Obstetricians

For decades there has been both overt and covert conflict between midwives and obstetricians regarding their value or place in maternity care, with family doctors providing an intermediate role offering some elements of both professions.[485] In some parts of the world, and particularly in Scandinavian countries and the UK, the midwife's role is well recognized and they are responsible, as the WHO advocates, for the care of normal birth. Obstetricians in this context provide specialized care for complications – an entirely appropriate use of resources. Yet in other parts, and particularly in North America, battles have long raged over the place of midwifery in perinatal care[486] with the majority of births being assisted by obstetricians. Midwives have been excluded and, some would say, persecuted, at times, for their approach to care. Yet midwives are welcomed by most mothers who use them, as they provide continuity of care and caregiver, and holistic, supportive care. In Canada, for example, almost three quarters of women cared for by midwives rated their overall pregnancy and birth experience as "very positive" compared to a little over half cared for by obstetricians, family doctors, or nurses.[487] Despite this, the majority of women are still cared for by obstetricians with, to date, a paucity of midwives having been qualified.

Types of Caregivers

Midwives offer a personal and holistic approach to perinatal care, regarding themselves as responsible for preparing the woman and her family, both emotionally and intellectually, for all aspects of birth and new baby parenting, in addition to providing clinical care, whereas physicians do so to a much lesser extent. Family doctors provide continuity of caregiver particularly if they offer care at birth and after birth as well as during pregnancy but may take a less holistic approach to care than midwives. Obstetricians (57%) and family doctors (36%) are most likely to regard birth as dangerous, although few midwives agree (4%).[488] Randomized trials have clearly shown that intervention rates for similar kinds of mothers with similar levels of risk/

complication are far higher among physicians than among their midwifery colleagues. Not surprisingly, outcomes of such midwifery managed births tend to be better than outcomes for physicians.[489] Despite this, in many countries, including Canada and the USA, fewer than about 10% of women have access to midwifery care.[490]

The conclusion to be reached is not necessarily that midwives should care for all normal births but that the quality of care that is needed by women is the same, no matter who the caregiver is.[491] Holistic, humanistic, caring support, together with respectful treatment that is considerate of biological, emotional, and intellectual needs of women and their family members should be offered by all caregivers for all pregnant and birthing women regardless of the normality of their birth experiences or the degree of complication they develop. There is no theoretical or practical justification for condoning differences in this regard. Anything less is inappropriate, may be insensitive, and might be inadequate. Health care systems, and caregiver remuneration packages, do not facilitate similar approaches to care, however, with midwives able to spend far more time with clients and to treat them at home, than obstetricians or family medicine caregivers. Such limitations clearly restrict the resources available for care for some professions.

Psychologists

In addition to preparation for birth and parenthood through prenatal education classes, psychological support is needed at many stages of the perinatal and parenting period, although with the exception of Dr. Adik Levin's NICU care model, discussed earlier, this is not often acknowledged or provided.[492] Difficulties regarding adjustment to pregnancy can happen for any family in any circumstances, and psychological support could be invaluable for helping those families. In addition, women experiencing more severe unwanted or traumatic outcomes should have access to specialist, clinical psychological care.

At a less severe level of disturbance, every maternity care setting should have easy, and readily available, access to trained, perinatal psychologists to provide support and care for women, their families and their healthcare providers.[493] Such care is also known to be cost-effective.[494] Even when all goes well, adjusting to pregnancy, the events surrounding birth, as well as the postpartum period, creates demands on women and their families that are not always well met without professional support. The finding that postpartum depression is reduced by the presence of a supportive companion during labour and in the postpartum period reinforces the importance of emotional support during emotionally challenging experiences.[495]

Supporting Caregivers

It is not only women and their families that could benefit from the support of psychologists, but healthcare providers as well.[496] In particular, those caring regularly for babies or parents in difficulty, such as with newborns in NICUs, or those coping with a stillbirth, birth of a baby with anomalies, or infant death, may value assistance.[497] Psychologists can play an important role in easing the pressures on these healthcare providers. Although this need is often recognized, it has not always led to the creation of positions for perinatal psychologists, although it is standard practice in Levin's, Estonian, neonatal care centre, and in all maternity care centres in the Republic of Moldova.

The normal concerns of adjusting to parenthood are not generally regarded as the purview of healthcare providers, but are considered the responsibility of parents or their family members. Whereas, in an ideal world, healthcare providers would alleviate emotional concerns related to any biological events, this is not, and probably never will be, reality. Consequently, some other resource is needed to assist parents emotionally. Perinatal psychologists can fill this gap.[498]

Training Perinatal Psychologists

As can be expected, due to the lack of recognition of their importance globally, there is little formal training for perinatal psychologists.[499] Psychologists with an interest in healthcare can, and do, choose to specialize in one or other aspect of medical practice, including perinatal care. Traditionally clinical psychologists, as opposed to perinatal psychologists, focus on counseling for more extreme cases of emotional distress such as, in the perinatal world, postpartum depression or psychosis. Referral to specialist clinical psychologists may be difficult as they may be a relatively scarce resource. Psychologists familiar with perinatal care issues are rarely integral members of the perinatal team. We are advocating to include, as part of the perinatal care team, psychologists with a thorough knowledge of perinatal practices, who focus on the emotional, intellectual, and spiritual challenges faced by couples when negotiating through the current day, medicalized experience of a normal transition to parenthood. These are both rare and urgently needed.

The Terms of Reference for Perinatal Psychologists developed in the Republic of Moldova provide an excellent blueprint, and starting point, for determining the role of Perinatal Psychologists in maternity care settings.[500] Their specifications are listed below, but have been adapted here to reflect current thinking.

Terms of Reference for Psychologists

In General:

- All healthcare providers should respect the privacy, dignity, and confidentiality of people in perinatal care.
- All healthcare providers should avoid emotional or physical violence or abuse when caring for people.
- Psychologists will support women, families, and healthcare providers.
- Psychologists will work with families when necessary or when requested to do so by the family.
- Healthcare providers should refer clients for psychological assistance when this is perceived to be needed or when requested.
- The psychologist should be regarded as an integral member of a multidisciplinary perinatal team and should attend and contribute to clinical case review meetings within perinatal departments.

- The psychologist should work together with social workers and other specialists in collaborating with local authorities such as welfare agencies.
- Psychologists should assist with conflict between healthcare providers and patients.

In Prenatal Services Psychologists Should:

- Contribute to antenatal preparation for women and their families regarding pregnancy, birth, and the postpartum period, together with other members of the healthcare team.
- Provide counseling for any family/women who request it, or who have been referred by their physician.

Intrapartum Services:

- Psychologists should endeavour to ensure the presence of a companion at birth for all women.

In Postpartum Services Psychologists Should:

- Provide counseling for women who experience unwanted or traumatic pregnancy outcomes.
- Offer support services to families after birth (for example, "would you like to talk to someone about your birth experiences?").
- Assist women and their families in the event of neonatal death or newborn anomalies.
- Assist the mother and family of babies in the NICU.
- Conduct discussion groups with new parents in postpartum units to discuss issues of psycho-social concern, such as the birth experience, difficulties with breastfeeding or baby care, integrating the new baby into the family, marital concerns etc.
- Provide counseling for women with unwanted babies, surrogate mothers, or those intending to give up their children for adoption.
- Provide counselling for adoptive parents.

- Assist individuals or families who have psychological concerns.
- Assist those with postpartum depression.

Educational Needs to Achieve the Above:

- Healthcare workers need knowledge and skills in counseling.
- Psychologists should be trained about perinatal care.
- Training is needed for those providing antenatal preparation for women and their families.
- Healthcare workers should be educated about the role of the psychologist in perinatal care.

Inadequate Training

Schools of Psychology do not usually provide training for perinatal psychologists, resulting in a dearth of trained professionals able to fill this void. Such barriers to inter-professional collaboration in perinatal care are, however, being identified, and methods of overcoming these being postulated. Exploratory steps towards inter-professional perinatal education are in place at some universities, showing some success. Fortunately, those involved in education for healthcare providers are increasingly receptive to new inter-professional developments. The WHO has recently taken up the challenge of directing attention to inter-professional models of education, practice, and policy across healthcare specializations and has developed a framework within which to consider local initiatives for greater, and more successful inter-professional practice. New developments along these lines, with a particular focus on respectful perinatal care should be encouraged and welcomed.

Sharing Information

Most caregivers recognise the importance of sharing accurate records between caregivers, and ensuring that all caregivers have access to relevant client information. What is less frequently recognised is that sharing case notes across disciplines requires client consent. This not only requires client approval, and involves questions of confidentiality of sensitive information, but is also often physically difficult to do. Paper-based records mean that information about a person is held separately in every facility that cares for this person. This can create obstacles to both sharing essential client information with other caregivers, as well as with ensuring clients have access to their own information.

In some parts of the world where access to paper-based records is often difficult (for example, where clients attend geographically distant clinics) and where digital records are not yet available, client-carried records provide the only sure way of accessing health care information for each person.

This has long been endorsed by the WHO[501] and is supported by randomized trials[502] as resulting in increased maternal satisfaction as well as increased likelihood of a woman's records being accessible at the time of birth.[503] At the very least, women's records should be accessible either in hard copy format or as electronic files, whenever and wherever she gives birth. Mother-held electronic access cards or documents would facilitate this, although currently are not frequently used. Part of the reluctance to provide women with their own case notes is an attitude of disrespect that implies that women are not responsible enough to care for them. Most people take their medical care seriously. In Ethiopia, for example, I observed patients in a crowded, Mother Theresa hospice care setting – without a penny to their name, and only the clothes they had on as possessions – clutching scraps of cardboard (corrugated cardboard) on which their medicine and dosage, most often for HIV/AIDS, were recorded. Every one held on to this precious piece of paper: none had lost it. Women who are pregnant also take extra care of themselves at this time and most are trustworthy enough to carry their records. Far more records are lost in transition from prenatal care settings to labour and birth places than when they are held by mothers themselves.[504]

An alternate interpretation of why women are not entrusted to carry their health records is that caregivers may not want mothers to read them. Impolite comments or remarks included in such records are potentially offensive. Comments such as "Mediterranean syndrome" indicative of a more emotionally expressive personality are insulting. Comments intended for follow-on caregivers may also serve to bias later caregivers towards, or against, the client and should not find a place in clinical records. Yet they do. When health care systems impose restrictions on care providers making such derogatory comments in patient records, then noting the patient is "a pleasant person" may be even more telling, if *not* included in the notes. To eliminate derogatory personal comments being included in case notes, all clients should have easy and immediate full access to their own records, test results, and notes, on demand, and in a format they can access. They should have an easy way to report errors, delete insulting comments or inaccuracies, and report inappropriate content to someone who will resolve the problem, while preventing retribution being taken against clients by their potentially aggrieved caregivers.

Today, with an increasing reliance on digital facilities, medical information is increasingly open to shared access across caregivers, facilities, and time periods. In these contexts, however, the client herself is not included in this data sharing. There is no reason she should not have access to her medical records. Aside from the basic principles involved – control over one's own information, and recognition of the client as a partner in care – including clients in the dissemination and management of their own records creates an opportunity for them to correct errors and discuss and resolve misunderstandings and miscommunications. Clinical caregivers are as prone as anybody to misunderstandings, misinterpretations, or simple errors. Including clients in access to records provides a necessary check to improve their accuracy. Accuracy of records is crucial when sharing clinical issues across caregivers.

That same accuracy becomes additionally important when faced with legal challenges to care received. While providing respectful care is not simply about avoiding a lawsuit, there are any number of contexts in which medical records can become part of legal proceedings. In this context, lawsuits are based on written records and the only lasting record of any interaction between caregivers and clients is made by the caregiver. This makes the doctor the final arbiter of what is believable in a court of law. This can be problematic for the client, if the doctor's records are inaccurate or misleading. Digitally based, and comprehensive medical records that are shared with clients also allows for easy access to records by the client when these are needed for insurance purposes, access to care services such as Medical Assistance in Dying (MAiD), or other services that require a review of medical records. They can also provide support for a doctor defending their record-keeping accuracy; if a client has had consistent and complete access to records, and those have been discussed and agreed upon, it makes it significantly more difficult to challenge their accuracy later.

Respecting clients' interest in their own health care is fundamental to accepting that providing health information to both caregivers and to the client personally is optimal.

Inter-Professional Education

Education to prepare for a multicultural, psycho-socially sensitive, and evidence-based approach to health should be mandatory for all caregivers. Traditionally, the teaching of obstetrics, neonatology, nursing, and other disciplines involved in childbirth, in Medical Schools, has been separated along disciplinary lines.[505] Some components of care are not included at all, particularly those relating to social science issues such as social work, psychological counselling, and childbirth education. A concentration on pathology in medical training may overshadow the care of the normal birth and normal newborn.[506] We do little to encourage medical students to take courses in the humanities applied to medicine or in psycho-social-cultural issues. Banaszek reports that only sixty-nine of 133 accredited medical schools in the USA required students to take courses in the medical humanities.[507] Few, if any, of the seventeen medical schools in Canada require a similar course, although a few offer an elective option.[508] Many of these programs, particularly if they are based in Psychology or

Behavioural Science departments rather than medical schools, or if they are limited to pre-clinical years and focus on theory rather than clinical application, have failed or are likely to fail. They may be perceived by students as programs to be endured, or which are undemanding “bird courses” (so named because one “flies” right through them) and not central to their ability as future doctors. When offered at a graduate level, within the medical curriculum, as students face the challenge of caring for people in clinical practice, they are perceived as more valuable.

Integrating Training

Inter-professional, psycho-social, and cultural issues involved in clinical practice should be integrated into mainstream medical teaching programs. For example, when clinical management of a fetal death is taught, both the psychological impact of the experience and diagnostic and treatment procedures should be considered. Teaching should be shared by physician and social scientist (and/or other related professionals involved) concurrently. Joint teaching programs of this nature, when tried, have shown promise of a new and better model for educational success.[509]

The University of the Witwatersrand, Johannesburg, set an early model of integrated education in the 1970’s. Medical students generally scorned taking courses in Human Behavioural Science that were offered as options. Disillusioned with offering courses for only a handful of students, I refused to continue the program and recommended to the Dean of Medicine (Health Sciences) that the School allocate this teaching time to courses that the faculty obviously valued highly, such as Anatomy and Physiology, rather than pay lip service to the idea that they were teaching medical students about humane care. In response, the School decided that students would be required to take, and pass, the Medical School’s Human Behavioural Science course before being allowed to progress to their fourth year of study and the start of their clinical training. This requirement was implemented, to the mortification of a few students who were required to write a supplementary examination after their year-end vacation, or repeat a year, and led to full classes and serious students.

Combined Care and Teaching

Problem-based learning models require that the somewhat artificial distinctions between disciplines be minimized. Instead of teaching obstetrics separately from neonatology, the care of the mother during birth as well as the baby immediately after delivery and the interaction between the two, requires a more closely integrated teaching model. The traditional distinctions between these disciplines in the classroom allowed for the customary separation of mother and baby into postpartum wards for mothers (cared for by obstetricians and obstetric nurses), and nurseries for the babies (cared for by paediatricians/ neonatologists and paediatric nurses). The need to integrate these disciplines academically has made itself clear in the architecture of the clinical setting. Combined care requires combined teaching models. Changed healthcare services today encourage rooming-in for all mothers as well as early, if not immediate, contact between mother and baby at delivery without separation from this moment on. To achieve this goal, close cooperation between obstetricians (or other delivery assistants) and neonatologists is required. It seems logical that the teaching of these disciplines should likewise be closely associated as it is in the model followed by WHO training programs.

In many hospitals around the world the structural layout of delivery rooms includes a separate area to which the baby is removed almost immediately after birth and cared for by a neonatologist or neonatal nurse rather than an obstetrician, obstetric nurse, or the mother. Often this is in a completely separate room adjacent to the birthing room. The separate teaching model followed for obstetric and paediatric education has, in these settings, become built into the physical layout of the maternity hospital. In eastern European settings, this structural divide was taken even further: "women's consultations" (women's hospitals) cared for mothers after delivery, whereas infants were cared for in separate buildings by different caregivers ("children's polyclinics").

Similarly, women gave birth in "maternity houses" while their newborns, if requiring neonatal intensive care, were sent to separate hospitals for sick children. Such models of care prevent continuity of both care and caregiver and neglect to see the mother-baby pair (and ideally also including the partner) as the focus of maternity care.

Hospitals may address the complexities of inter-professional care in different ways, including through education and quality assurance programs. Many (in Canada, 67%) regularly schedule interdisciplinary meetings (which may include mortality and morbidity rounds) that include multiple professionals, such as nurses, midwives and physicians.[510] In Canada, many (75%) have also established systems for resolving problems between nurses, midwives, obstetricians and family doctors that might arise.[511] Although these may represent the major categories of maternity healthcare providers, they do not often include the full array of professionals, typically excluding experts such as perinatal psychologists, social workers, and breastfeeding consultants. Adopting an integrated, multidisciplinary approach to teaching about perinatal care would, in all likelihood, prevent many of the problems of disrespectful care from arising in clinical practice, rather than trying to resolve them after they have emerged.

Culturally Appropriate Care

The world is increasingly multicultural, revealing diversity of ethnic origin, religion, race, and language. Global population movements have allowed for, and even encouraged, the intermingling of cultures through migration, and political upheavals and war in multiple countries have resulted in major demands for refugee relief.[512] Climate crises are increasingly making demands for alternate living spaces for some population groups a priority. Perinatal care must meet the needs of this changing, cultural mosaic.

Cultures differ significantly in their beliefs regarding health and illness, as well as in their attitudes and practices regarding childbearing.[513] Biological functioning is considered to be paramount in western societies. In contrast, significant sections of the global village regard this level of functioning as of least importance with spiritual, social, cultural, and psychological concerns playing a primary role in illness aetiology, treatment, and prognosis.[514] It is as unacceptable in these cultures to neglect spiritual or cultural rites, as it is to omit checking blood pressure in pregnancy in the West. Misunderstanding the cultural expectations of pregnant or birthing women regarding their care can be hurtful, disappointing and anxiety provoking for them. Neglecting to learn about, understand, and respect the cultural expectations of women from cultures different from that of caregivers, leads to abusive and insensitive treatment and is disrespectful.

Differences and Similarities

The lowliest woman in the poorest country gives birth in the same way as royalty. Childbirth is the greatest leveler we have; we are all equal in this experience.[515] There are, however, significant variations in birth practices based on cultural, economic, social, religious, or medical factors. These include, for example, choice of caregiver as midwife, obstetrician, family physician or traditional birth attendant; position adopted for birth ranging from lithotomy to a supported, standing position, squatting position, or kneeling on all fours; place of delivery as hospital, birth unit or home; presence or absence of a partner/ companion during delivery; and breast- or bottle-feeding practices, to name only some. Variations in approaches are evident world-wide.[516] There are variations in childbirth practice from place to place, from hospital to hospital within the same city, and from doctor to doctor within the same hospital.[517] In many parts, there is no doctor at birth and it does not take place in a hospital: the mother, in her home attended by the midwife or traditional birth attendant, is the central focus. There is enormous variability in the world and people differ widely in knowledge, attitudes, values, expectations, beliefs, societal conditions, and economic levels. The birth experience can vary within the same mother from birth to birth just as it varies for different mothers with different social, cultural, and psychological backgrounds.

While it may be easy to accept that countries' approaches to birthing may vary widely such as in Africa compared to Europe, or North America compared to Russia, it is even more striking to consider that approaches to birth may vary widely within any one country. Canada, for example, is an extremely multicultural society including over 250 ethnic identities.[518] Even within the dominant culture in the country, there are vastly differing needs regarding perinatal care among sub-groups of society such as among LGBTQ+ communities, among men/partners, among those who have babies that need NICU care, among women of vastly differing cultural origins such as African. Indian, Asian and others. Although there is a standardized set of guidelines for perinatal care that apply to all birthing people across the country, variations within such subgroups (and others) can be immense. In Canada, for example, the majority of women experience over-medicalized, evidence-based care, yet the experiences of some subgroups of women, such as Indigenous women and those with prior experience of Female Genital Mutilation, are often vastly inferior.[519]

Sensitivity is called for when caring for multicultural differences within any one society as well as when working in countries or cultures beyond one's own borders. The assumption that their way is the best way is implicit in any country's educational system regarding maternity care, and every caregiver's practice, but this may not apply equally to all subcultures within any one society or to any other country. What then is the "right" way to "do" birth? Until recently, eastern European doctors and mothers were convinced that their doctor-centred, highly medicalized approach offered the best deal. Their northern European counterparts regard midwifery attendance as superior whereas rural Black African women respect traditional birth attendants. Canadians believe that their universal health care system is far superior to all others. Who has the right to say which approach is best? And does a supposedly universal approach to birth apply equally in rural settings as it does in the urban home, and modern tertiary care centres?

Challenges

Cross-cultural challenges regarding perinatal care occur both when caring for women who come from different countries or who belong to differing subcultures withing our own country, and when working in countries other than our own.

Cultural Diversity

There are many pitfalls to be avoided when attending to women from differing cultural groups or subgroups than the dominant culture in our own countries. Language differences combined with status inequalities may make it difficult for foreigners' healthcare needs to be met or, indeed, understood in their adopted country.[520] Assistance with translation, at least, is essential. Although this is a necessary first step, the intimate nature of maternity care provides a particular challenge for translators. Expecting children in the family to translate – as they are often the first to acquire a new language when immigrating– is clearly inappropriate given the subject to be discussed.[521] The partner – who in many cultures plays no part in pregnancy or birth – may also be inappropriate and unacceptable. Making sure that the client's physical symptoms are discussed (which itself may be an unacceptable diagnostic procedure, such as in some traditional Black cultures[522]) or that the elements of the treatment procedures are understood, are challenging but are only the minimum level of communication that is needed. Greater understanding of the woman's culturally determined needs should also be discussed. Community members can facilitate translation and communication and written information sheets can sometimes be helpful. Ignoring these needs is disrespectful and may lead to abusive care.

Respecting Cultural Practices

Sensitivity, respect and tolerance is needed when considering traditional customs or practices (such as wearing protective amulets during birthing or traditional methods of disposal of the placenta), and should be encouraged unless evaluated as harmful, such as Female Genital Mutilation.[523] Condemning or disallowing such practices because they are different is inappropriate for although they may not contribute to biological health (in the caregiver's eyes) they might be essential for psychological wellbeing. They should be evaluated as biologically beneficial, neither beneficial nor harmful, or harmful. Only the latter forms of traditional care (such as giving newborns honey, or rubbing ash, dung, or oil on the severed umbilical stump) need to be discouraged.

Among many Southern African Black women, it is customary to tie a piece of string, cut from the same ball, around the abdomen of all family members when one of them leaves home, providing spiritual continuity when separated. In labour, ignorant of its psychological role, western doctors may remove the string as it is "dirty," causing immense distress at a particularly vulnerable time. This is not unique to traditional Black women. In the western world, an item of jewellery or other personal trinket – in my case a necklace holding a set of charms given to me by each member of my family when I first began to travel extensively apart from them - may be carried as a symbol of connectedness with loved ones, with reluctance to remove this in times of stress – such as childbearing. Similarly, religious symbols – such as a crucifix – may take on protective meaning for some women and will be relinquished with distress, leaving the woman feeling insecure and fearful.

Overcoming distrust in different cultural practices is difficult. While many are willing to tolerate these practices, understanding them may not occur, and silent disapproval may well be expressed non-verbally at least, and be abundantly, and hurtfully, clear. Disapproval is not always silent, however. Regardless of one's views on Female Genital Mutilation, the treatment of women who have experienced it is often egregious. A Canadian study of over 400 women's experiences of childbirth following previous experience of Female Genital Mutilation, showed women's dissatisfaction with care and a perceived lack of knowledge and ability by health practitioners to care for them appropriately during birth.[524] As one woman reported "The doctor told me I don't have a vagina and he cannot take the risk to care for my pregnancy." Another doctor said to his nurse "Put on a glove and find out if she has any vaginal or urethral hole." He asked her how she passed urine and where she urinated. Another multiparous woman was told "You are like a time bomb that can explode. Please seek one of your [own] people who can handle your birth." But he suggested she never gets pregnant again or she would lose her life.[525]

Harmful Traditional Practices

Abhorrent though Female Genital Mutilation might be to caregivers, the care of any individual woman in pregnancy and childbirth requires sensitivity and respect, that, according to women's reports, was often lacking. Most women (88%) participating in the Canadian survey reported hurtful comments being made at some stage during their care.[526] Comments were made such as "The labour room nurses were very mean, no support. They laughed at me and made jokes" and "The nurse asked me how I would raise a daughter?" I asked "Why?" and she said, "you will be causing hurt and a foster mother would be better for her."[527] Women indicated that doctors did not provide the kind of birth procedures (such as vaginal delivery rather than caesarean section) that they would have preferred. The caesarean section rate of over 50% for this sample is excessively high compared to the national average of less than half this figure at the time of the survey and way beyond the 0.5% of women who wanted a caesarean.[528] While the perineal area of women with Female Genital Mutilation does require special care during birthing (such as either or both anterior and lateral episiotomies) the pelvis, vaginal canal and uterus are no different from women without Female Genital Mutilation and should therefore, be at no greater risk for caesarean section.

Even when cultural practices are regarded as harmful, caregivers still need to be sensitive when caring for women for whom the practices have meaning. For example, women from countries where Female Genital Mutilation is normal practice may be convinced that caesarean section means death.[529] In many of their countries of origin, admission to hospital only occurs after prolonged and/or obstructed labour and frequently results in death. Particularly supportive care needs to be provided, rather than brusquely discounting fears, or simply ignoring the issue altogether through ignorance. Even in a country such as Canada where cultural differences are purportedly valued and respected in society, ignorance and disrespect for women that do not conform to the dominant ethic still play a disconcertingly large role and are frequently abusive.[530]

Harmful Societal Impositions

Socio-economic marginalization and poor health status characterize many First Nation, Inuit, and Métis women in Canada, if not in many countries where Indigenous women live. First Nations, Métis, and Inuit people continue to be adversely affected by a long history of residential schools, and colonization, both of which included unethical and abusive treatment as well as medical experimentation and so-called research. This brutal history, including the practice of separation from families, forced adoption of a different language, culture and religion, physical, emotional and sexual abuse, and enduring systemic discrimination, has understandably resulted in mistrust in all colonial systems, including the medical and educational system.[531] Healthcare providers, when working with Indigenous women and their communities, must be aware of and sensitive to these issues, making respect, information sharing, partnership and collaboration essential components of appropriate and ethical care practices.

The abuses experienced by children in residential schools, together with the breakdown of traditional family life resulting from their forced assimilation, have left their mark on many Indigenous families of today, and include disruption of traditional pregnancy and birth related events. There is tension, as relocating women from their homes to give birth in technologically based and interventionist hospitals has been widespread in past decades due to less sophisticated healthcare facilities closer to home,[532] a problem exacerbated by Canada's vast geographical spread and sparse Indigenous populations. Evacuation of women for childbirth, usually without any supportive family member, to hospitals far from their homes, has deleterious psychological, social, and cultural effects.

Systemic discrimination against Indigenous people is pervasive in Canada, including in the medical profession,[533] leading to distrust of the medical and reproductive health care professions. An extensive survey in British Columbia reports that there is widespread Indigenous-specific stereotyping, racism, and discrimination in the health care system (and likely across the county). Stereotyping, prejudice, and racist treatment are common experiences. Clients experience unacceptable personal interactions including disparaging and racist comments, long wait times or denial of services, a lack of communication or being shunned, or not believed, or have their concerns minimized including being accused of "faking."[534] They receive inappropriate or no pain management sometimes with explicit reference to the stereotype that Indigenous people were drug-seeking or somehow felt pain differently. They get rough treatment – disrespectful and "manhandling" treatment, at times resulting in physical harm and chronic pain. Medical misdiagnoses and mistakes occur, often related to falls, and based on the belief that a patient was under the influence of alcohol or drugs. There is a lack of recognition or respect regarding cultural protocols: health care workers are not open to hearing about traditional medicine, often deny permission for clients to practise cultural protocols and ceremonies, and are intolerant of the involvement of family and community.[535]

As if these indignities were not enough, some aspects of Indigenous women's reproductive health are even more egregious. Horrific as it is to acknowledge, coerced tubal ligation of Indigenous women has recently been reported in Saskatoon, Canada. At least sixty women have joined a class action suit against their caregivers, the hospital in which this occurred, the provincial health authority overseeing the hospital, and the Canadian Government. Women were coerced into having a tubal ligation by caregivers and many were led to believe that it was simply birth control that could be reversed.[536]

These actions do not occur in a vacuum. In 2015, over 30,000 children who were physically and/or sexually abused in residential schools, filed suits against the government, and were awarded damages. Coerced tubal ligation also occurred in parallel with the cultural genocidal policy of the residential school system. Historically, large numbers of Indigenous people were sterilized as "mentally unfit." Between 1929 and 1972, approximately 2,800 people were sterilized in Alberta alone. Such events justify the distrust that Indigenous people have for health care providers. Healing racism in Canadian health care remains an ongoing challenge and continues to impose cruelly abusive treatment for pregnant Indigenous women in particular.[537]

Respecting Spiritual Differences

Providing for the spiritual needs of clients, concurrently with physiological needs, is both possible and beneficial.[538] In South Africa, physicians were advised to encourage traditionally oriented clients who feared surgery to seek the blessing of their *sangoma* (traditional healer) before entering hospital. Conviction that surgery kills does little to support recovery. Praying for one's own or another's recovery is also a global practice.

Healthcare services that cater for multicultural clientele need to develop innovative approaches to incorporate these needs into their healthcare services.[539] Encouraging healthcare facilities to offer clients contact with others of similar cultural background and similar healthcare needs may provide a stronger voice for the expression of these needs to the healthcare authorities. Establishing contact with local community groups and liaison through cultural representatives is another possibility to explore to provide mutually beneficial, two-way information exchanges. Alternative and/or complementary treatment paradigms should be considered in addition to western pharmacopoeia. Finally, it is essential to monitor how well the health needs of clients are being met. This monitoring may involve formal research, utilizing techniques such as focus group discussions or survey type assessments, and should be an integral and continuous part of the healthcare services offered.[540]

The examples of culturally diverse perinatal practices among the Indigenous peoples of Canada, and women with prior experience of Female Genital Mutilation, highlight the importance of recognizing cultural diversity within any one country, and in many cases highlight abusive, and sometimes extremely cruel, perinatal care. They are by no means representative of varying cultural practices in Canada, or exhaustive of them, nor of abusive perinatal care. They emphasize the importance of understanding and exploring the background and cultural practices of women that caregivers may encounter in their practices. They also emphasize the value of understanding women's knowledge, expectations, and perceptions when providing perinatal care so as to incorporate a truly respectful, and family-centred approach. Above all, they indicate the importance of questioning our approaches to care as not necessarily being universal, or superior, or optimal.[541]

Working in Other Countries

There are numerous difficulties involved in working with childbirth across cultures.[542] One of these is the obvious and often difficult-to-avoid problem of seeing things through the eyes of one's own culture, and judging all others as inferior instead of as simply different.

A second difficulty emerges when trying to assess – usually through research - which approach is clinically "better."[543] Western evaluations call for "scientific facts" when trying to determine which birth practices are most beneficial. Yet, data regarding the outcome of birthing procedures in different countries are, unfortunately, not often available and, when they are, may not always be reliable, or comprehensive. Records may be hand written and filed, and data aggregation is done manually, slowly, and sometimes inaccurately. Less "hard science" evidence of birth outcomes, such as assessments of patient satisfaction, are not routinely collected in most parts of the world, due partly to the challenges of doing so, but, more often because women's opinions are not valued. In addition, many of the so-called "safe" birth practices of western medicine (e.g., routine, continuous, fetal heart monitoring, induction, epidurals, routine multiple ultrasound scanning, caesarean sections, and the lithotomy position for birth), have come under fire from evidence-based studies. What was regarded as good practice is now being discarded as harmful in the light of evidence-based research. What practices should then be used to assess appropriate birth procedures? And will these still be seen as best practice in a few years time?

Which is Best?

Working extensively in the international cross-cultural milieu has raised a number of academic and ethical challenges for me. Questions such as what right do we have to suggest that our, or an alternate, healthcare system is superior to one already in place in a country in which we consult? How can we assess that what we offer is appropriate for our host country? Could we actually do harm by transforming one system of care into another? How do we avoid the ethical issue of coercion when offering suggestions for alternate systems of care to a country when this advice is offered in the name of international agencies such as the WHO or UNICEF or when it is associated with benefits such as educational opportunities? There are no easy answers to these concerns other than to remain sensitive to the implications of our work and to remain scrupulously honest at all times.

Misuse of Technology

A third difficulty arises in that sophisticated technology may be used inappropriately.[544] Is a "half-baked" application of western technology at times more harmful than the traditional way? For example, in parts of eastern Europe, routine prenatal ultrasound became available in the late 1990s. Research evidence suggests that, on a routine basis, multiple screening is not beneficial for mother or baby, or cost-effective, and that, if used at all, one or two routine scans is all that could reasonably be routinely justified. Clinically indicated scanning is, of course, not questioned by this research. In eastern Europe, however, multiple screening was usually introduced as soon as equipment became available with screening even being done at every prenatal visit. Combined with insufficiently skilled technicians and poor-quality equipment, this misapplication likely led to unnecessary, or harmful, interventions. Even in Canada, with its high regard for evidence-based clinical care, and at a time when only one routine ultrasound was recommended clinical care, women surveyed by the Maternity Experiences Survey, reported an average of three scans during pregnancy, and some many more.[545]

Optimal Practices

In our efforts to reform other countries' health practices, we may not readily recognize what aspects of their systems are good and may be even better than our own. For example, some former Soviet practices were valuable. The immensely supportive, systematic, postpartum follow-up of infants (called "patronage") was beneficial, not only for its clinical usefulness but also for the psychological support it gave parents.[546] The western birth environment leaves this aspect of maternal-child care less well attended, and the eastern European model could be of value for other countries. Yet this system was dismantled in the rapid overhaul of Soviet healthcare systems – with western assistance – in the 1990s. Simultaneously, specialist paediatricians were forced to re-train as family doctors – a "missing" category of healthcare provider under the Soviet Union where all medical students chose a speciality early on in their studies – resulting in intense dissatisfaction among these now "demoted" caregivers. Local dissatisfaction with this change was not heeded. The "gung-ho" imposition of our "superior" models of care on this culture was, at times, breathtaking, and harmful.

International Consultants

Local voices must be heard and attended to when making recommendations for changing birth practices. How often is lip service paid to this? How easy is it to influence countries in the name of science and with the authority attributed to the "foreign expert" especially if wearing a WHO or other United Nations agency hat? How often too, are practices changed only because locals wish to gain prestige (and income) through collaboration with international consultants?

During my hundreds of visits to multiple countries, I often observed how tempting it was for locals to introduce changes that were advocated because their collaboration with "international experts" enhanced their prestige - or their pockets. Sometimes this was harmful, such as distributing free formula samples to new mothers on behalf of international formula industries, in return for personal payments by the industry. While appearing to be a magnanimous gesture this action virtually ensured that mothers would fail to breastfeed successfully if they utilized the products.

Which practices are regarded as harmful, harmless, or beneficial also have to be judged against the alternatives that are available in any community.[547] For example, in countries where tight swaddling of babies from head-to-toe was practiced, we advocated abandoning such swaddling and encouraged skin-to-skin contact to promote breastfeeding. Although our advice was followed and the tight swaddling was removed, it was replaced by thick towels wrapped around the infant's neck to support the newborn's head as a "floppy" baby's head (never seen when babies heads were tightly swaddled) was regarded as pathological. In addition, our advice created a need for infant clothing – not available in these countries – as they had hitherto not been necessary with a tightly swaddled baby. Finding the right balance between encouraging practices that are potentially harmless or beneficial and discouraging those that are truly dangerous can be challenging![548]

Cross-Cultural Misunderstandings

Cross-cultural misunderstandings also present challenges.[549] Translators vary in quality and do not always understand your perspective. For example, when working with a colleague in St Petersburg we entered a WHO-Euro promoted, healthcare centre for teenagers. We were met with a print of the famous Leonardo da Vinci *Madonna and Child*, the original of which has pride of place in the city's Hermitage Museum. My colleague, the late Marsden Wagner (then the Regional Advisor for Maternal and Child Health in the WHO Regional Office for Europe) was proudly shown this picture and told it had been introduced in response to his suggestion, made months earlier, to liven up the walls: to make the place more attractive to teenagers by decorating it with pictures of "Madonna." Cross-cultural misunderstandings do occur but are not always as harmless or humorous as this. For example, some well-intentioned international consultants donated "snugglies" (soft padded surrounds for the naked NICU baby) to replace the practice of swaddling these babies in incubators, in eastern Europe. We arrived some time later and were proudly shown the tightly swaddled babies lying peacefully in the centre of the "snugglies" in the incubators, but far from their padded, comforting edges.

We have much to learn about how best to work when striving to improve birth globally.[550] The challenge is to find out how to satisfy the childbirth needs of women and their families within the woman's own cultural group. Simply applying what works in one's own family and culture may be inappropriate and unacceptable in another, as for example, when we eradicated swaddling practices. Misuse of technologies may also occur. For example, abuse of prenatal ultrasound with consequent termination of female fetuses in countries like China and India has been prevalent. The resulting gender imbalance is already leading to crimes of kidnapping, child brides, and sale of increasingly scarce women.[551]

International Health Consulting

Some principles of international health consulting may serve to inform more respectful family-centred caregivers who work with women from differing cultural backgrounds within their own society, or who encounter women from differing backgrounds when working in other countries.[552] These include:

- Recognizing whose needs are being met by practices proposed – those of the woman and her family or those of the consultant.
- Providing a collaborative approach to care that involves the woman and her family in decision making about her care.
- Being flexible about clinical care guidelines so as to offer individualized care that suits the woman's particular cultural background but still complies with evidence-based recommendations.
- Acknowledging that some of the woman's or her family's wishes may, at times, offer better options than those of the consultant or caregiver.
- Remaining sensitive to cultural differences.
- Providing respectful care that is non-abusive.
- Ensuring that advice is sustainable by the woman and her family (and not, for example, too costly for her economic situation, or too contradictory to her cultural practices).
- Following up on advice to assess compliance/agreement.
- Offering a holistic and humanistic approach to care and not simply biologically-based advice.
- Removing social barriers to collaboration such as following acceptable local dress codes.

- Fostering a trusting and honest caregiving relationship, and remaining committed to the care of the woman and her family within their cultural framework.[553]

These characteristics of care are essential, not only for inter-cultural care, but also for care provided for all women and their families.

It is also important to follow local customs as far as is possible. Following acceptable dress codes in order to be acceptable to women of differing cultural practices from one's own is often necessary, even if challenging. While working in Tajikistan in an Islamic fundamentalist community, it was essential to wear long-sleeved clothing, full length dresses, and head coverings at all times. The women in our team also had to be sure that they never moved out of our Medicine Sans Frontières "safe house," where we lived during our mission, without a male escort, for fear of being stoned by conspicuously present elders who were watching our street and house. Whether one agrees with these restrictions or not is irrelevant if one wants to be effective in providing healthcare advice – and, at the very least, to remain safe!

The need for respect, dignity, self-esteem, and emotional support during pregnancy and particularly during childbirth is universal. How these needs are met during childbearing can vary from culture to culture and are linked to such issues as privacy, decision-making responsibility, and continuity of care. Discerning what healthcare services and practices could enhance each woman's reaction to birth within the confines of a "safe" birth, and her culturally determined expectations, is the challenge faced by today's caregivers.

Abusing Data

An efficient system of global, national, and regional perinatal data collection that is reliable, timely, and standardised is necessary for effective monitoring and evaluation of perinatal care and the development of guidelines for care. Ensuring that we have reliable data on which to base appropriate care decisions is an essential component of care that is respectful and does not abuse either the women who participate in the research or the caregivers that implement it.

The WHO's European Regional Office maintains an ongoing database (*The Health for All Database*[554]) that coordinates key indicators of health, including perinatal health, across all its member states. Although this is exceptionally valuable and provides a means of global inter-country comparison, as well as within-country progress over time, the vast health framework that it covers limits the number of indicators that can be followed, as well as the depth of inquiry that can be made into perinatal issues. Individual countries also retain ongoing data collection systems that include perinatal indicators such as the Public Health Agency for Canada's Perinatal Surveillance System,[555] and the American PRAMS[556] and Listening to Mothers[557] surveys. Many, if not most, of these programs need to expand their perinatal health surveillance coverage to give a broader understanding of family-centred perinatal care issues.

Abuse of perinatal data and of data collection methods occurs in multiple ways ranging from delays in data integration, suppression of vital information ostensibly to preserve privacy, deliberate and/or unintentional inaccuracies in recording data, and limitations of data collection to clinical rather than psycho-social indicators. All these practices can result in data abuse.

Data Collection

A major challenge to national perinatal database collection is obtaining data in a timely fashion. Frequently data collected at the hospital level has to be collated and forwarded to regional authorities before being sent to national data collection centres. The integration of these multiple sources of data is then required, together with validation that data submitted is accurate. This is often a lengthy process, resulting in several years old data being the most up-to-date available. Real time data collection is still not the norm, although with an increasing application of web-based technology, assessment and integration of current perinatal events should become the gold standard. BORN, the Ontario, Canada, Better Outcomes Registry and Network, is a rapidly expanding, perinatal monitoring system designed with this goal in mind.[558] In addition, databases vary from one centre, region, or country, to another, making integration of disparate measures difficult or impossible. The need for a nationally agreed, perinatal data collection method is obvious, even though reaching agreement across a country (and across the globe) as to just what indicators should be included and when they should be recorded is challenging. Thirty years ago, when working with the WHO Regional Office for Europe, I was asked to contribute to the development of a global perinatal indicator list: yet it is still not in evidence.

Privacy of Information

Even when such information is collected, the use and dissemination of national perinatal data is hindered by concerns for privacy of the information. The result may be that local planning services do not obtain the necessary information they need on which to base predictions of services required, particularly when these refer to remote areas or infrequently occurring health events, as such events must often be amalgamated with other information in the database to protect privacy. Rare events such as those requiring suppression in order to preserve the privacy of the individual involved, may be the most severe, or life threatening and could be the most important to have available for evaluation and future preventive planning. Much as such suppressions and omission of data are made in the name of privacy, they are likely to be abusive and negligent of any other individual facing similar challenges who will not be able to benefit from this data.

Corrupt Data

In addition, data collection is open to corruption and manipulation. When conducting hospital assessments in some countries I frequently asked to examine the monthly records of maternity hospital wards or other hospital records. In many places, records were hand written and frequencies amalgamated without any arithmetical aids such as calculators or computers. I frequently uncovered errors in these calculations when I checked them. I soon realised that such miscalculations may not have always been accidental. Hospital budgets were allocated to care for a fixed number of specific incidences. For example, "pathological wards" were expected to have a certain number of women (or neonates) in them each month. If the records indicated that fewer pathologies had occurred than were anticipated, funding for these (often more lucrative wards) was cut. The result of this may have been a "fudging" of numbers so that reports conformed to the expected estimates set by the health authorities. Hence the correct entry of cases into records, but the incorrect totalling of some pathological incidents when amalgamating these records. While I cannot prove that this did occur, certainly the temptation was there to encourage such misrepresentations. An alternative practice was to allocate "physiological" ("normal") mothers and babies to pathological wards to ensure that the numbers looked "appropriate." Systems that encourage or, in reality, demand such distortion of data in order to be allocated budgets, are simply dishonest.

Data distortions may not be quite so obvious but may be more subtly introduced. Failing to report on issues that are embarrassing to a government is abhorrent. Even when data is collected about controversial healthcare practices, such as, for example, the extent of, and support for, midwifery care in a country where midwifery is not well endorsed, can be misleading because of errors of omission rather than errors of commission. Not reporting on such data publicly, even if it is known and collected, is a more subtle means of suppressing information.

Incomplete Data

So too is having incomplete datasets. An egregious example comes from Canada, otherwise a highly respected health care provider. According to the WHO and UNICEF, Canada's maternal mortality rate, while still low, is as much as 60% higher than what is reported by Statistics Canada.[559] Contributing factors to these inaccuracies include varying definitions of what counts as a maternal death, both across provinces and territories within Canada, and from global indicator definitions, as well as a lack of maternal death reviews in seven of the thirteen provinces and territories in the country. In contrast, the UK has tracked maternal deaths and near misses since 1952 using a monitoring system titled MBRRACE that follows up all deaths of women during their childbearing years to explore whether these were linked to a birth in the year prior to her death. WHO-Euro advocated for this program to be introduced across the European region in the WHO/UNICEF teaching programs that were implemented after the fall of the Soviet Union, and for decades thereafter.

Indicators

The lesson that has been learned from the analysis of the importance of social support in labour and birth, lends urgent support to the need to develop psycho-social perinatal indicators. Outcomes of studies regarding labour support acknowledge the emotional, cognitive, social, and cultural needs of parents as well as their biological/medical requirements. Perinatal data collection has, however, traditionally focussed on clinical events or practices. Psycho-social and cultural issues are not usually included in large scale perinatal databases either routinely or even at all. However, data monitoring approaches can, and should, contribute to family-centred care. Even more egregious is a failure to collect and report on abusive clinical practices and women's reports of them at a local, provincial or state, and national level.

Women's Experiences

Some countries have, occasionally, conducted national surveys of women's experiences of their perinatal care through federal government agencies, for example, the national Maternity Experiences Survey (MES) in Canada,[560] the USA surveys of women's birth experiences encompassing about 78% of all births in that country (the Listening to Mothers surveys[561]), the Pregnancy Risk Assessment Monitoring System (PRAMS)[562] and a number of surveys conducted in the UK.[563] Other countries have, at times, supported regional or local surveys of experiences of perinatal care.[564] Assessing women's (and sometimes men's[565]) satisfaction with their care is commonly a central focus of such surveys although multiple issues, including clinical events, are also explored. While repeated surveys of this nature have occurred in Australia, the UK and the USA, Canada has not supported a recent follow up study to either their MES[566] or their Hospital Policies and Practices Survey.[567] It is now about twenty years since women's reports of their birth experiences were systematically followed up at national level. This despite the fact that repeated attempts have been made to initiate a further survey and that there is clear evidence of considerable academic and professional impact of such surveys. Over forty peer-reviewed publications were based on the 2009 MES and three Canadian healthcare policies have incorporated its findings, including the latest revision of the Canadian National Guidelines for Family-Centred Maternal and Newborn Care.[568] Clearly, such surveys are valuable sources of information for both clinical and psycho-social perinatal care analysis and should become regular occurrences.

Adverse Perinatal Outcomes

The MES examined normal birth experiences among Canadian women. This is admirable, but is insufficient. We need similar surveys among a plethora of families with differing life experiences as well. We need surveys of father's or partner's experiences if we are to call ourselves truly respectful of family-centred and non-abusive care. What are the experiences of parents with multiple births? We need surveys of families' experiences when things go wrong: what happens to them if their baby requires NICU care? What kind of birth experiences do women with Disabilities have? Or women in any equity-owed groups such as LGBTQ+ people, or Indigenous families? What are families' experiences of maternal or neonatal morbidity, or worse, mortality? What is the care like for families with babies who are born with anomalies? Do we know how families are cared for in these situations? Do we want to know? Providing supportive care for these families is essential and respectful. Why do we apparently not want to undertake such analyses? Of course, if we ask these questions, we might expect some changes to be made to improve care if the data warrants this. It is always easier to simply not ask the questions if we do not really want to know the answers or to make any needed changes.

Standardized Questionnaires

Comparing perinatal practices across countries also poses several challenges. Primary among these is that questionnaires used in each country/survey are different and not often comparable. Even when similar issues are explored questions regarding them vary as do methods of response analysis. In addition, the items not reported in these comparisons may be even more valuable to address than those that are included. For example, some interventions such as pushing on the top of the abdomen to help push the baby down in labour were only included in the Canadian and USA surveys and not those of many other countries. In Canada and the USA, reported rates were, surprisingly, as high as 15% and 17% respectively. No surveys included questions regarding routine cervical examination after birth, or even exteriorizing the cervix for this purpose, as was widespread traditional practice some time ago, and may or may not be continuing in some places. Nor were questions regarding routine sweeping of the membranes before or during birth, or routine artificial rupture of membranes, commonly included in all surveys. Women's reactions to such practices were, consequently, also not examined. There is clearly a need for the development of a uniform, international, perinatal assessment process including a careful analysis of the family-centredness and non-abusiveness of this care from the perspective of women and their families.

Psycho-Social Indicators

The nature of issues that are addressed when comparing perinatal indicators across countries is a further concern. It is likely that agreement could be reached regarding traditionally measured indicators of clinical care. However, we should be developing indicators of successful birthing beyond the biological level to include social, psychological, and cultural implications. Can we adequately determine when technology is truly beneficial – in a family-centred and holistic sense - and when it leads to more harm than good when we do not assess its psycho-social impact? Evaluating psycho-social and cultural issues in perinatal care is difficult but that does not justify their omission. Given that many issues, and particularly psycho-social issues, can often not be addressed through randomized controlled trials, how valuable is our current – almost exclusive - emphasis on such trials as the primary basis for our practice? What is the real, holistic, evidence for the use of technology in maternal and child healthcare? We need to consider, and value, alternate research paradigms to randomized controlled trials if we are to measure the complexity of psycho-social outcomes, particularly when randomization to psychologically differing groups is unethical.

We also need to incorporate research findings into a model that emphasizes an individualized approach to care. This is difficult to do when the application of quantitative research findings in care relies on an average group response to an intervention rather than more individualized, qualitative findings. Quantitative research analyses focus on finding the mean, median, or modal response to any intervention and deciding on the optimal application of any intervention based on this. But what about the individual outliers at either extreme under the bell curve? How well do we consider or address their needs?

Agreement regarding which psycho-social issues to explore in perinatal surveys is difficult to reach. In addition, the range of items that can be included, the variety of ways such questions can be asked and the lack of unanimity as to just which of these are crucial indicators of psycho-social, perinatal health, make it extremely difficult to reach agreement on a universal set of indicators.

Limitations of Trials

It is also not always possible to test potential clinical care practices through randomized control trials, sometimes for psychological reasons. For example, current attempts to study the value of inositol in addition to folic acid on reducing neural tube defects in women who have already experienced this adverse outcome in a previous pregnancy are almost impossible to undertake. Women are, understandably, unwilling to be randomized to a placebo group when inositol appears to be potentially protective and harmless, based on animal research and some human case studies.[569] Obtaining adequate/randomized control trial evidence of its value or potential harm, may never be possible. Data on the value of inositol in preventing neural tube defects may be possible to obtain using population-based case-control studies such as that exploring over 23,000 births included in the National Birth Defects Prevention Study. This study revealed the value of inositol in preventing cardiac heart defects when taken in addition to folic acid.[570]

Assessing Respect

Of most importance today, is the need to assess respectfulness of care. For decades women have anecdotally reported dissatisfaction with their birth experiences, and many have reported downright abusive care. Some are turning away from the formal health care system to embrace home birth, sometimes even declining to have a "skilled" birth attendant with them. Academics have long discounted surveys reporting women's satisfaction with their birth experiences as inaccurate and unreliable indices. We can no longer ignore these calls for consideration of women's subjective birth experiences as failing to do so is abusive.

It is not only the mother's experiences that are of importance in family-centred data monitoring, but also those of her chosen family support persons. Just as some countries have begun to examine women's perceptions of their care, a few are becoming concerned about partners' views as well.[571] In a family-centred approach, the experiences of extended family members, who are an integral part of many families' experiences at this time, should also be considered.

The benefits that can be gained from conducting national and international comparisons of perinatal practices are immense. On the one hand, such surveys provide a global standard against which any country, city or even maternity service can compare itself so that it can identify areas in need of improvement as well as areas of strength. On the other hand, such comparisons reveal intriguing differences across regions, such as the higher rates of partner support in labour in North America and the UK compared to lower rates in many other countries, or the higher proportion of Baby Friendly Hospitals in European centres compared to those in North America.[572] Comparisons may also facilitate monitoring changes in rates over time if surveys are repeated. They may also stimulate adoption of more effective care practices.

Local Data Collection

In addition to national or regional perinatal data collection, it is important for maternity hospitals to conduct local surveys of women's and their partner's experiences of their perinatal care in order to monitor and evaluate their own particular policies and practices. Findings are crucial for hospital self-improvement. Assessing women's or families' satisfaction and the respectfulness, or family-centredness of care offered – through follow-up evaluations of their hospital experiences - should be as much a part of such surveys as the medical procedures routinely documented by hospitals such as how many caesarean sections were done, and the occurrence of adverse pregnancy outcomes. Ideally, all these variables will be considered in evaluating hospitals' and caregivers' effectiveness. Failing to assess the impact of hospital or caregiver practices on women's experiences of care is disrespectful and inadequate care.

Health Promotion vs. Research

The conflict between health promotion and research has been prominent in my work, particularly in eastern Europe. While research has remained a primary interest, the ethical question of whether it is appropriate to indulge in academic research when countries are struggling with basic educational, technical, and clinical needs is paramount. United Nations Health Agencies support health promotional programs and are not directly concerned with research unless this is clearly beneficial for the host country. When resources are scarce, bringing existing knowledge to countries that desperately need it is far more important than answering new questions. Once basic priority issues (such as reducing maternal and infant mortality) are managed reasonably well, then there can be time for more academic research pursuits. Notwithstanding these accepted priorities, combining the two approaches of health promotion and of research has remained a challenge for me throughout my career.

Is Research Health Promotion?

Data collection globally is not only for the purposes of monitoring and evaluation, but is also essential for research. Contrary to common belief, research into health issues – whether international or local - does not necessarily result in or imply health promotion. Such research may also be unethical. In the international arena, the ideological value of "contributing to the improvement of global health" does not always justify exploiting the resources of developing countries by means of research without the host countries/organizations receiving any benefit.

In theory, local researchers can gain from participating in international research trials through obtaining knowledge of hitherto unknown research methodologies, employment income, and (possibly) some academic credit. However, they seldom gain sufficient understanding of the research methods followed to enable them to replicate or generalise the methods, report or publish the research findings locally (or internationally), or offer any direct benefit to study participants. The study findings may also lack any relevance to the countries participating in the research, or may fail to be implemented locally to benefit the population. It is possible too, that some research could put local collaborators at risk, particularly if governments are not sympathetic to the research outcomes or proposed changes. This is not health promotion; it is research exploitation.

Priorities

International perinatal research often fails to address health concerns that are a priority for developing countries. Multicentre studies that include developing countries should address both their needs as well as those of the developed world. For example, the Term Breech Trial,[573] one of the largest multi-national, randomized, controlled trials to be undertaken in recent decades in perinatal care, addressed the issue of the optimal method of delivering babies presenting in a breech position at term – about 4% of births. In some of the participating countries in this trial, where maternal and neonatal mortality rates are at extremely high levels due to a multitude of unrelated challenges, this issue was, although still relevant for them, likely not a priority. The conclusions of this trial, which have contributed significantly to increased caesarean section rates worldwide, raise concerns about the applicability of the findings and the resulting promotion of caesarean sections in developing countries.

In rural African communities, a woman having a caesarean section may find the experience so unpleasant and unwanted that she might avoid seeking medical care for her next pregnancy, choosing instead to give birth at home with support from local, untrained, traditional birth attendants. She may thereby increase her chances of potential mortality or morbidity, especially if the previous caesarean section was essential and the reasons for it likely to recur. In some cases, even if she were willing to seek medical care, her lack of access to healthcare facilities (common in the vast tracts of rural African lands) will increase her risk. Increasing the rate of caesarean section for all but the most essential indications in such environments can, therefore, have life-threatening consequences. The applicability of the Term Breech Trial to rural African countries was a concern for me. Although I participated in the initial study, when I requested that this issue be followed up and assessed following the trial, I was told this was not important for the Study Team and should be investigated further by the countries themselves if they wished to. In consequence, I withdrew from further affiliation with the study group – long before the findings of the study led to considerable controversy in academic circles.

In considering whether or not to participate in such trials, countries need to fully explore the consequences of potential findings on their own healthcare settings. Ethics committees that review such trials, and researchers developing such studies, need to be aware of, and consider, these implications. While the research itself may be admirable and even well conducted, the implications of the findings for the development of local guidelines for practice that address the needs of local families, need to be carefully considered within each cultural context. Failure to do so is unethical and irresponsible.

Implementing Research

Donor and local health systems frequently differ in their systems of change and reform.[574] While democratic decision-making processes may be the standard of the donor country or consultants, the hosts may be more familiar with autocratic decision-making. Integrating such different models can be a challenge. International consultants should consider both the ethical and psychological effects of trying to change these differing approaches. For example, healthcare providers accustomed to autocratic approaches may find western ethical research requirements foreign, at best, if not needlessly constraining. Requirements such as those for informed consent, the freedom to refuse participation without fear of reprisal, and to fully inform participants of the requirements of participation may be viewed as unnecessary in some host countries. They may even be perceived as challenging to the authority of healthcare providers, or signalling their apparent weakness. Family-centred and respectful treatment in such an authoritarian setting is unlikely to be established. Research protocols need to incorporate a value of family-centred and respectful care, and involvement in both understanding and consenting to the research process, as well as to the clinical intervention being offered. In former Soviet countries, for example, when I asked for every woman giving birth in a unit to be asked to participate in my survey research I was often told "Oh, you do not want that woman to answer your questions! She's not helpful! We'll ask this woman instead." It took some time and effort to explain the importance of including everyone, and especially those women who were not happy or "helpful."

The globally significant Promotion of Breastfeeding Intervention Trial in Belarus was confronted with a different challenge: that of conducting research respectfully, with consideration for women's and hospitals' rights to refuse to participate. Local researchers were accustomed to "ordering" patients to do whatever they wished. In this case, as the study had the backing of the Ministry of Health, non-compliance with it was frowned upon. The research team, on the other hand, emphasized that women had the right to refuse to participate in the study without penalty, and devoted a great deal of time to this issue in the training of our research collaborators. We also made it clear that we did not expect any centres potentially eligible for inclusion in the trial to comply with it against their wishes, and one or two did withdraw before randomization, as they were not willing to be potentially allocated to the control arm of the study. Bridging this cultural difference was challenging but essential.

Conflicting Goals

Combining research and health promotion can be difficult.[575] It may easily be possible to test the effects of an intervention in a randomized controlled trial where one arm of the trial contains the "new" intervention and the other does not. Research grants will usually support the application of the "new" approach to the experimental group. If this treatment proves beneficial, there is, however, no provision in the usual research grant to provide the intervention for the control group as well. Nor is there funding available to ameliorate the effects of an unsuccessful or even harmful intervention.[576] From a health promotional and ethical point of view, this is unacceptable, as both groups should benefit from the research findings. From an ethical perspective viewpoint, this is potentially harmful for those participating in the study. Reversing any negative effects of research interventions in the experimental group at the conclusion of the study, as well as applying the findings to the control group if found to be beneficial, should be built into all research grants. At present this does not occur. Some rethinking of the ethical consequences of grant funding policy is needed. Study populations – meaning women and their families in perinatal care – continue to be viewed simply as guinea pigs and are expected to be willing to contribute to lofty ideological goals such as "the betterment of care in future"[577] – or to somewhat less ideological goals of advancing the individual researcher's career aspirations. This is abusive and should not be permitted going forward.

It is rare, but not impossible, to conduct major international, health research studies differently, by (unusually) incorporating the potential outcomes of the study into its intervention program. For example, the Promotion of Breastfeeding Intervention Trial[578] did consider the ethical implications of manipulating populations for the purposes of gaining research findings. This study, of over 17,000 Belarusian mother-baby pairs, revealed clear infant health benefits to being born in a Baby Friendly Hospital. We did not ask the granting agencies that supported the trial for funding to provide the intervention to the control group in the event of a positive impact of the intervention, (or withdrawal of the intervention from the experimental group should the intervention have been shown to be harmful). A request of this nature would have been regarded as "beyond the scope of the proposed research" and may have resulted in the entire study being refused funding. I, however, was not willing to agree to collaborate with the study without implementing the appropriate intervention as a consequence of the findings. We chose, in response, to seek further funding for follow-up interventions. As a result, we provided training for hospitals that had agreed not to implement the BFHI during the trial (the control group hospitals) after the conclusion of the study, supported by additional funding that we obtained from the WHO Regional Office for Europe.[579]

Interim Analyses

We accept that a trial should be stopped if an interim analysis reveals clear negative consequences if it were to be continued. Yet a positive interim analysis does not always result in a decision to apply the findings to all.[580] One could also argue that completed research without implementation of its findings is of little value. A significant body of work has been published with the altruistic hope that others will read about it and apply it in practice. Sadly, we have learned that dissemination and application of research findings is a neglected area as well as a generally unsuccessful or, at least, lengthy one. If research grants required implementation of positive research outcomes – thus blending research and health promotion – this would be far more effective. At present, women provide the data collected in much perinatal research, researchers publish this data and enhance their careers, professional bodies disseminate guidelines based on research findings to their members; and few if anyone assesses whether these findings have been implemented to benefit either the mothers who provided the data in the first place or indeed, any mothers. This is hardly a woman- or family-centred approach. Or an ethical one.

Research and health promotion programs raise thorny ethical issues. Conflicts between the goals and methods of research, and their health promotion consequences, remain.[581] Going forward we owe it to all women and their families to rethink our approach to both endeavours to ensure that research and health promotion activities are ethical, respectful, and never cause harm.

Opposing Abuse

People in all health care settings, including those encountering perinatal care, are currently being advised to advocate for themselves to oppose the abuse they experience. While appearing to empower patients, this advice is nonsensical in the obstetric environment and could even be harmful. There are several reasons why this is a harmful suggestion. Firstly, families cannot be expected to become experts about maternity care in order to oppose incompetent treatment offered by their obstetricians, midwives, doulas, or other care providers. Encouraging this only serves to further undermine their faith in the medical profession. While Dr. Google may be a very helpful resource for families, many do not have the tools to evaluate the quality of the medical information they find online or from family and friends, and when even the medical profession is saying "do not trust us, advocate for yourself," it becomes impossible for the average person to access genuinely expert care. Additionally, even those who are willing and able to review and interpret evidence-based care recommendations, such as those published in reputable peer-reviewed journals, cannot easily access that information because most medical research is published in journals that require significant financial resources to access. Even graduates of some universities (in Canada at least, such as the University of British Columbia) are unable to access on-line library services if they are no longer registered as students or are not staff/faculty at the university.

Secondly, there is a notable power imbalance between a physician and a client. As stated previously, physicians and their notes are the last legal word in what happens in any given appointment, meaning that any conflict that arises between a patient and a physician will only ever be viewed through the lens created by the physician. Moreover, those notes get transferred to other caregivers and other legal contexts. A client with a legitimate complaint against a physician who attempts to advocate for themselves may fear retaliation from the physician in the form of a note in their medical records that they are non-compliant, adversarial, or potentially an unfit parent. Clients have no recourse against such accusations, and have no way of knowing if their choice to advocate for themselves might result in a caregiver retaliating (or perhaps covering their own behind) in that way.

Even when care is appropriate and evidence-based, the manner in which it is given may be disrespectful or abusive: but this does not make it any easier for women to oppose. Complaints about disrespectful treatment are far too easy to dismiss with the usual gaslighting responses, such as "you are being too sensitive" or "you are overreacting." These are particularly notorious when women are being cared for, as "hormones" are blamed and emotional responses discounted.

Expecting families to demand respectful and sensitive interactions with their caregivers during labour or at delivery is even more preposterous. The expectation that women, while lying naked on a bed with their legs spread, are in any psychologically or physically safe space from which to advocate for more sensitive or effective care is asinine. Being naked, lying down while interacting with a standing caregiver, with intimate bodily areas blatantly exposed, is a psychologically significantly vulnerable position, even absent the experience of being in labour. Expecting women to stand up for themselves while so disadvantaged is simply unrealistic. Advising women to employ a doula to advocate for them is also unreasonable given that doulas are likely to rank low on the maternity care power hierarchy and may be equally unable to oppose the actions of obstetricians, midwives, or nurses. Such advice also ignores the fact that many families do not have the financial capacity to hire a doula or other advocate.

In addition, advising women to advocate for themselves, implies that there is something amiss with the care they are being offered that justifies their need to advocate for themselves. Women and their families should be the central team member/s in their caregiving team. They should also, however, be able to trust that their caregivers are competent, acting in their interests, and will treat them with respect and dignity. Caregivers should be held to a far higher standard than they currently face: they should be expected to provide expert, respectful, sensitive, and professional care to every single client; they should be held accountable whenever they do not meet any of these standards; and they should recognize that client and family centred care is the minimum acceptable standard and not simply something "nice to have." Rather than being taught to act as though they respect their clients, caregivers should actually respect them and act accordingly.

Institutional Opposition

Over the past decade or so, social movements have arisen in a number of countries shedding light on mistreatment of women in childbirth. Recognition of such abuse is growing, albeit slowly. New social movements demanding rights for women in childbirth have arisen in several countries including Italy, Croatia, France, the Netherlands, Hungary, and Finland.[582] In Finland, the launch of the program resulted in 150 accounts of violence, human rights violations, and inappropriate conduct in maternity care being reported within two weeks. In Ireland, following the death of a mother and her baby in a maternity ward in 2019, a woman telephoned her local radio station to report her own experience of mistreatment, neglect and unsafe labour and birth conditions. Following this, more than 1,000 women contacted the program leading to an in-depth discussion of such practices.[583] In Sweden, a non-governmental organization highlighted the failure of the government to provide out-of-hospital birthing facilities and reported this as resulting from misogyny and the lack of priority given to women's immediate and long-term mental and physical health.[584]

Opposing violence against childbearing women is not a new concern. In 2007, for example, Venezuela published a new *Organic Law on the Right of Women to be Free from Violence* that included legislation against violence in the obstetric care setting.[585] The law defines obstetric violence as "the appropriation of the body and reproductive processes of women by health personnel, which is expressed as dehumanized treatment, an abuse of medication, and to convert the natural processes into pathological ones, bringing with it loss of autonomy and the ability to decide freely about their bodies and sexuality, negatively impacting the quality of life of women."[586] According to this act, obstetric violence includes:

- Untimely, and ineffective, attention to obstetric emergencies.
- Forcing the woman to give birth in a supine position, with legs raised, when the necessary means to perform a vertical delivery are available.
- Impeding the early attachment of the newborn with his/her mother without medical cause, thus preventing early attachment and the possibility of holding, nursing, or breastfeeding immediately after birth.
- Altering the natural process of low-risk delivery by using acceleration techniques, without obtaining voluntary, expressed, and informed consent of the woman.
- Performing delivery via caesarean section when natural childbirth is possible, without obtaining voluntary, expressed, and informed consent from the woman.[587]

WHO too, has taken active steps to address the problem of disrespect and abusive maternity care. The WHO statement on this subject, states "Every woman has the right to the highest attainable standard of health, which includes the right to dignified, respectful health care."[588] WHO has called for "greater action, dialogue and advocacy on this important topic and human rights issue."[589] A WHO funded systematic review of what constitutes respectful maternity care revealed several domains of care that should be offered.[590] These include:

- Being free from harm and mistreatment.
- Maintaining privacy and confidentiality.
- Preserving women's dignity.

- Prospective provision of information and seeking informed consent.
- Ensuring continuous access to family and community support.
- Enhancing quality of physical environment and resources.
- Providing equitable maternity care.
- Engaging with effective communication.
- Respecting women's choices that strengthen their capabilities to give birth.
- Availability of competent and motivated human resources.
- Provision of efficient and effective care.
- Continuity of care.

Application of these standards of care is urgently called for. I would add supportive care of women's psychological and emotional health. Truly respecting women would result in their more considerate care. A caregiver who respects each woman seeking his care would not mistreat them, breach their privacy, treat them in undignified ways, communicate with them as inferiors, not consider their choices, provide them with inequitable treatments, or deny them access to their chosen family supports. In my professional work, I have been advocating for respectful perinatal care for over fifty years; we have still not learned this lesson.

Contributing Factors

Overall, factors contributing to abuse include the normalization of disrespect and abuse during labour as part of standard care that reflects systemic components of the health care system, lack of community engagement and oversight, financial barriers, lack of women's empowerment or autonomy, lack of national laws and policies regarding human rights and ethics, and lack of respect for some types of clients and care providers.[591] These issues manifest in multiple ways, some of which are highlighted here:

Systemic problems that lead to a normalization of disrespectful treatment include: remuneration systems that reinforce increased interventions in birthing such as higher fees for caesarean sections than vaginal births; only allowing clients to present one problem at a time in any medical consultation as occurred in British Columbia, Canada; encouraging caregivers to spend no more than ten minutes at a time at any one consultation; paying caregivers the same amount for seeing a complex patient compared to a client with few or simple concerns leading healthcare providers to selectively accept less complex clients into their practices; lack of choice of care provider by clients due to shortages of providers; and difficulties in changing caregivers due to such shortages. Historical ideological trends, based on misogyny, colonialism, etc. and their subsequent influence on medical research has led to poorer care for those who are not White, wealthy, Christian, straight, cisgendered women. There are also power dynamics influenced by these ideological trends, which reinforce the fallacy that the doctor is the expert and the patient needs to be compliant.

Individual level factors contributing to abuse include: racism, colonialism, bias and stigma, sexism, poor training, few or any professional requirements to practice evidence-based care, no repercussions for poor care, and biased research methodologies and interpretations that are clearly evident in the perinatal treatment of women with high BMI, or those that practice cultural traditions like Female Genital Mutilation.[592]

Lack of oversight allows abusive care to flourish. There are few, if any, externally moderated standards of care for professional groups. When a complaint is filed, it is only reviewed internally, by the professional group being challenged. Even where standards of care are clearly outlined, they are often not enforced. Arms length reviews of complaints against caregivers are rare, with the exception of legal proceedings, which in turn are biased towards those who can afford them, and in some countries, like Canada, almost impossible to pursue given the virtually endless resources of professional associations to defend against them, and restrictions on compensation for victims to loss of income and direct expenses incurred, rather than for pain and suffering.

We need to go beyond simply preventing or avoiding abusive treatment to actively promoting respectful care. This work needs to be done at every level of the healthcare system, from legislation and administration, through individual care providers and how we educate them, to research methodologies and interpretations. We need to examine the beliefs, behaviours, and research that are at the foundation of our practices, and determine whether they are supporting effective, competent, and respectful care, or undermining our aspirations towards those goals.

Perinatal healthcare providers need to consider whether they are contributing to abuse or whether they actively promote respectful care in their practice. Cultivating respectful care as the default approach is needed: it should not be considered as a "nice add-on" to care or an aspirational goal; it is the minimum standard to meet. Strengthening healthcare provider training to mandate care that is respectful, with increased awareness of psychological and social issues in childbearing, follows a rights-based approach to care, and includes legal, professional and accountability interventions, are some of the changes needed to eliminate disrespect and abuse during obstetric and gynaecological care.[593] Simply working towards offering more respectful care than we offer at present is insufficient as the bar is currently set far too low. We need respectful care, not simply *more* respectful care. The WHO, in association with other United Nations Aid Agencies, has issued a statement endorsing the importance of preventing the mistreatment of women during childbirth, and at the same time, promoting respectful care.[594] It is hoped that the needs of all women and families and especially those from equity-owed groups are considered in the future developments of standards and indicators of respectful care, and interventions to eliminate mistreatment. It is also hoped that simply offering non-abusive care is insufficient. This is the minimum standard to aim for, not the ultimate goal.

Notes

1 Beverley Chalmers, *Family-Centred Perinatal Care: Improving Pregnancy, Birth and Postpartum Care* (Cambridge: Cambridge University Press, 2017).
2 Chalmers.
3 WHO, *Essential Antenatal, Perinatal and Postpartum Care Course* (Copenhagen: WHO Regional Office for Europe 2002), Department of Reproductive Health and Research, *Managing Complications in Pregnancy and Childbirth: A Guide for Midwives and Doctors*, by WHO et al., WHO/RHR/oo.7 (Geneva: World Health Organization, 2000), B Chalmers, and K Omer-Hashi, *Female Genital Mutilation and Obstetric Care* (Vancouver, BC, Canada: Trafford Publishers, 2003), B Chalmers, and A Levin, *Humane Perinatal Care* (Tallinn, Estonia: TEA Publishers, 2001).
4 P Sellers, *Midwifery* vol. 1 and 2 (Cape Town: Juta & Co, 1993).
5 Beverley Chalmers, *Pregnancy and Parenthood: Heaven or Hell* (Sandton, South Africa: Berev Publications, 1990).
6 Ellen Tilden et al., "One Hundred Yeas of Seeking Respectfiul Maternity Care: History and Evolution," *Birth* (2024), https://dx.doi.org/Httpe://doi.org/10.1111/birt.12876.
7 Robbie Davis-Floyd, ed., *Birthing Techno-Sapiens: Human Technology Co-Evolution and the Future of Reproduction*, First ed. (USA: Routledge, 2020).
8 The Lancet, "Empowering Women during Childbirth.," *The Lancet,* 406, no. 10498 (2025), Beverley Chalmers, and Dana Solomon, "Actually Empowering Women during Childbirth," *The Lancet* 406 (2025).
9 Chalmers, *Family-Centred Perinatal Care: Improving Pregnancy, Birth and Postpartum Care.*
10 B Chalmers, and V Mangiaterra, "Appropriate Perinatal Technology: A WHO Perspective," *Journal of the Society of Obstetricians and Gynaecologists of Canada* 23 (2001).

11 UNICEF, *The State of the World's Children* (2014). http://www.unicef.org/sowc/.
12 Beverley Chalmers, *Child Sex Abuse: Power, Profit, Perversion* (UK: Grosvenor House Publishers 2022).
13 D Bowser, and K Hill, *Exploring Evidence for Disrespect and Abuse in Facility-Based Childbirth: Report of a Landscape Analysis* (Washington, DC: USAID-TRAction Project. Harvard School of Public Health and University Research Co, 2010), http://www.tractionproject.org/sites/default/files/Respectful_Care_at_Birth_9-20-101_Final.pdf. .
14 Meghan Bohren et al., "The Mistreatment of Women during Childbirth in Health Facilities Globally: A Mixed-Methods Systematic Review," *PLOS Medicine* 12, no. 6 (2015), https://dx.doi.org/10.1371/journal.pmed.1001847.
15 Ronald Lamont et al., "Obstetric Trauma Due to Abuse and Preventable Events: A Commentary on Definition, Classification and Qualitative Research," *BJOG An International Journal of Obstetrics & Gynaecology* 132 (2025), https://dx.doi.org/doi.org/10.1111/1471-0528.18316.
16 Elizabeth Kukura, "Obstetric Violence," *The Georgetown Law Journal* 106 (2018): 728.
17 Dybravka Simonovic, *A Human Rights-Based Approach to Mistreatment and Violence against Women in Reproductive Health Services with a Focus on Childbirth and Obstetric Violence*, ed. UN Human Rights Council (New York: United Nations General Assembly, 2019). https://digitallibrary.un.org/record/3823698?ln=en.
18 Simonovic.
19 Sarah Moxon et al., "Nothing About Us without Us: Consolidating Experiences of Maternity Care to Advance Equity," *BJOG* 0 (2025), https://dx.doi.org/doi.org/10.1111/1471-0528.18300.
20 Kukura 724.
21 Lamont et al.
22 Kripalini Patel et al., "A Simultaneous Concept Analysis to Provide Clarity between Obstetric Violence and Birth Trauma," *Birth* 0 (2025).
23 The Lancet.
24 Chalmers, and Solomon.
25 The Lancet.
26 Chalmers, and Solomon.
27 The Lancet.
28 Chalmers, and Solomon.
29 Chalmers, and Solomon.
30 Beverley Chalmers, "Psychosomatic Obstetrics and Gynaecology in the New Millenium: Some Thoughts and Observations," *Journal of Psychosomatic Obstetrics and Gynaecology* 19 (1998), Chalmers, and Levin.
31 Simonovic.

32 Simonovic.
33 Simonovic.
34 Chalmers, and Omer-Hashi.
35 Simonovic.
36 Kukura 737.
37 G J Hofmeyr et al., "Companionship to Modify the Clinical Birth Environment: Effects on Progress and Perception of Labour and Breastfeeding," *British Journal of Obstetrics and Gynaecology* 98 (1991).
38 Bohren et al.
39 Bohren et al.
40 M Enkin, M Keirse, and I Chalmers, *A Guide to Effective Care in Pregnancy and Childbirth* (Oxford: Oxford University Press, 1989).
41 Chalmers, "Psychosomatic Obstetrics and Gynaecology in the New Millenium: Some Thoughts and Observations.", Chalmers, and Levin.
42 Stephanie Batram-Zantvoort et al., "The Association between Women's Perception of Birth during the Pandemic, Companion of Choice and Support from Health Professionals: A Cross-Sectional Study in 20 Countries in the WHO European Region," *Birth* 52 (2025), https://dx.doi.org/doi.org/10.1111/birt.12915.
43 Sanjana Ratakonda et al., "Wait, What? What's Going On?— Pregnancy Experiences of Deaf and Hard of Hearing Mothers Who Do Not Sign," *Birth* 52, no. 2 (2024), https://dx.doi.org/doi.org/10.1111/birt.12881, Monika Mitra et al., "Pregnancy, Birth, and Infant Outcomes among Women Who Are Deaf or Hard of Hearing," *American Journal of Preventive Medicine* 58, no. 3 (2020), https://www.ajpmonline.org/article/S0749-3797(19)30477-5/abstract.
44 Gunnel Hensing et al., ""Brave Men" and "Emotional Women": A Theory-Guided Literature Review on Gender Bias in Health Care and Gendered Norms Towards Patients with Chronic Pain," *Pain Research & Management* 2018 (2018), Mika Guzikevits et al., "Sex Bias in Pain Management Decisions," *Proceedings of the National Academy of Sciences* 121, no. e2401331121., 33 (2024).
45 Lesley Tarasoff et al., "Prenatal Care Experiences of Childbearing People with Disabilities in Ontario, Canada," *Journal of Obstetrics, Gyanaecology, and Neonatal Nursing* 52 (2023), https://dx.doi.org/doi.org/10.1016/j.jogn.2023.02.001, Karli Swenson, Sydney Comstock, and Darah Briley, "Reducing Stigma among Providers Caring for Pregnant People with Substance Abuse Disorders: A Systematic Review of Interventions.," *Birth* (2025), https://dx.doi.org/doi.org/10.1111/birt.70027.
46 Chalmers, "Psychosomatic Obstetrics and Gynaecology in the New Millenium: Some Thoughts and Observations.", Chalmers, and Levin.

47 B Chalmers, and J McIntyre, "Integrating Psychology and Obstetrics for Medical Students: Shared Labour Ward Teaching," *Medical Teacher* 15, no. 1 (1993).
48 Bowser, and Hill.
49 Kukura 750.
50 Kukura 747-50.
51 Bohren et al, Kukura.
52 Bohren et al, Kukura.
53 Simonovic.
54 Susan Bell, "Quebec Indigenous Groups Collecting Stories of Forced Sterilization," (Canada)2021, https://www.cbc.ca/news/canada/north/indigenous-forced-sterilization-quebec-study-cree-1.6186212, Sylvie Fournier, "Black, Indigenous Mothers Say They Were Sterilized without Full Consent at Quebec Hospitals," CBC, 2021, accessed 30 September, 2021, https://www.cbc.ca/news/canada/montreal/quebec-hospital-sterilization-1.6188269.
55 Derek Cai, "Japan Sterilisation Law Victims Included Nine-Year-Olds," BBC, 2023, accessed 20 June, 2023, https://www.bbc.com/news/world-asia-65958119.
56 Simonovic, 9.
57 Cai
58 Beverley Chalmers, *Birth, Sex and Abuse: Women's Voices under Nazi Rule* (UK: Grosvenor House Publishers, 2015), 29.
59 Open Society Foundation, "Against Her Will: Forced and Coerced Sterilization of Women Worldwide," Open Society Foundation, 2011, accessed 20 June, 2023, https://www.opensocietyfoundations.org/publications/against-her-will-forced-and-coerced-sterilization-women-worldwide#:~:text=Women%20worldwide%20have%20been%20forced,Africa%2C%20Asia%2C%20and%20Europe.
60 Open Society Foundation
61 Open Society Foundation
62 Open Society Foundation
63 Open Society Foundation
64 Christy Cooney, "Greenland Women Seek Compensation over Involuntary Birth Control," BBC News, 2023, accessed 3 October 2023, https://www.bbc.com/news/world-europe-66990670.
65 Open Society Foundation
66 Open Society Foundation
67 S Singh, and G Posner, "Doctors Behaving Badly and the Tyranny of Peer Pressure," *Journal of Obsterics and Gynaecology of Canada* 37, no. 12 (2015).
68 Anonymous, "Our Family Secrets," *Annuls of Internal Medicine* 163, no. 4 (2015), https://dx.doi.org/10.7326/M14-2168.

69 Anonymous.
70 Singh, and Posner.
71 Singh, and Posner 1114.
72 Simonovic.
73 Jason O'Neale Roach, and Gavin Yamey, "Witnessing Unethical Conduct: The Effects," *Student BMJ* 322, no. 011022 (2201), www.studentbmj,com/current_issue/editorials/2.html.
74 Roach, and Yamey.
75 Phoebe Frieson, Wan-Li Sun, and Sarah Towle, "Consent and Educational Sensitive Exams on Anaesthetized Patients: Experiences of Medical Students across Canada," *Education* 46, no. 11 (2024).
76 Bowser, and Hill.
77 Abirami Kirubarajan et al., "Pregnancy and Childbirth during Incarceration: A Qualitative Systematic Review of Lived Experiences," *BJOG* 129, no. 9 (2022), https://dx.doi.org/ https://doi.org/10.1111/1471-0528.17137.
78 Simonovic.
79 American College of Obstetricians and Gynecologists, "Sexual Misconduct: ACOG Committee Opinion 796," *Obstetics and Gynaecology* 135, no. 1 (2020), https://www.acog.org/en/clinical/clinical-guidance/committee-opinion/articles/2020/01/sexual-misconduct.
80 Idan Zonshine, "Gynecologist Gets 18 Months in Prison after Sexually Assaulting Patients," *Jerusalem Post* (Israel), Aprtil 21, 2021, https://www.jpost.com/israel-news/gynecologist-gets-18-months-in-prison-after-sexually-assaulting-patients-665887.
81 Praveena Somasundaram, "Hospitals to Pay Nearly 150 Patients Who Say Gynecologist Abused Them," *Washington Post* (Washington), October 8 2022, https://www.washingtonpost.com/nation/2022/10/08/columbia-university-doctor-sexual-abuse/.
82 Emma Gadeski, "Dozens More Women Say Provo Ob-Gyn Sexually Assaulted Them," *The Daily Universe* (Utah), March 24 2022, https://universe.byu.edu/2022/03/24/dozens-more-women-say-provo-ob-gyn-sexually-assaulted-them/.
83 Brianna Keilar, Isabelle Khurshudyan, and Haley Britzky, "Exclusive: What Led the Army to Investigate Gynecologist Described in Lawsuit as a 'Predator in Uniform'," *CNN* (USA)2025, https://www.cnn.com/2025/11/21/politics/army-investigation-gynecologist-sexual-misconduct.
84 Bowser, and Hill.
85 Bohren et al.
86 Marit S. G. van der Pijl et al., "Disrespect and Abuse during Labour and Birth Amongst 12,239 Women in the Netherlands: A National Survey,"

Reproductive Health Matters 19, no. 160 (2022), https://dx.doi.org/https://doi.org/10.1186/s12978-022-01460-4.

87 Sarah Yahr Tucker, "A Growing Number of Women Allege Doctors Abused Them during Childbirth," *Vice* (Canada), Ocxtober 16 2019.

88 Moxon et al.

89 Heather Murray, Christopher Gillies, and Armand Aalamain, "Physician Incivility in the Health Care Workplace," *CMAJ* 196, no. 9 (2024), https://dx.doi.org/doi.org/10.1503/cmaj.231377.

90 Murray, Gillies, and Aalamain.

91 James Gallagher, Natalie Truswell, and Jonathan Sumberg, "Female Surgeons Sexually Assaulted While Operating," BBC News, 2023, accessed 12 September, 2023, https://www.bbc.com/news/health-66775015.

92 Gallagher, Truswell, and Sumberg

93 Gallagher, Truswell, and Sumberg

94 P Simkin, "Non-Pharmacological Methods of Pain Relief during Labour.," in *Effectiveness and Satisfaction in Pregnancy and Childbirth*, ed. M Enkin I Chalmers, M Keirse. (Oxford: Oxford Medical Publications, 1989).

95 J Rush, "A Randomized Control Trial of the Effects of the Bath in Labour" (PhD, University of Toronto, 1999).

96 G J Hofmeyr, "50 Years of 'Active Management of Labour' Is Enough.," *BJOG* (2023), https://dx.doi.org/10.1111/1471-9528.17377.

97 Bowser, and Hill.

98 Bowser, and Hill.

99 Bowser, and Hill.

100 Juliet Dobson, "Ignoring Women's Experiences Led to the NHS's Biggest Maternity Scandal," *BMJ* 377, no. 0899 (2022), https://dx.doi.org/https://doi.org/10.1136/bmj.o899.

101 Pijl et al.

102 Bohren et al.

103 Bohren et al.

104 Simonovic.

105 Priya Fielding Singh, and Amelia Dmowska, "Obstetric Gaslighting and the Denial of Mothers' Realities.," *Social Science and Medicine* 301, no. 114938 (2022).

106 Singh, and Dmowska.

107 Sophie Isobel, "Trauma and the Perinatal Period: A Review of the Theory and Practice of Trauma□Sensitive Interactions for Nurses and Midwives," *Nursing Open* 10, no. 12 (2023), https://dx.doi.org/doi:10.1002/nop2.2017

108 Chalmers, *Child Sex Abuse: Power, Profit, Perversion.*

109 WHO, *Global and Regional Estimates of Violence against Women: Prevalence and Health Effects of Intimate Partner Violence and Non-Partner Sexual Violence* (Geneva: World Health Organization, 2013).

110 Chalmers, "Psychosomatic Obstetrics and Gynaecology in the New Millenium: Some Thoughts and Observations.", Chalmers, and Levin.

111 Isobel.

112 Isobel.

113 Isobel.

114 D Midmer et al., *The ALPHA Form - Antenatal Psychosocial Health Assessment Form*, 2nd edition ed. (Toronto: University of Toronto, Faculty of Medicine, Department of Family and Community Medicine, 1966).

115 Chalmers, "Psychosomatic Obstetrics and Gynaecology in the New Millenium: Some Thoughts and Observations.", Chalmers, and Levin.

116 C L O Schachter et al., *Handbook on Sensitive Practice for Health Care Practitioners: Lessons from Adult Survivors of Childhood Sexual Abuse.* (Ottawa Public Health Agency of Canada., 2008).

117 Mollie C. Marr et al., "Creating a Trauma-Informed Multidisciplinary Clinic," (2025), https://dx.doi.org/doi.org/10.1111/birt.70032.

118 Schachter et al.

119 Alison Gemmill et al., "Infant Deaths after Texas' 2021 Ban on Abortion in Early Pregnancy," *JAMA Paediatrics* 178, no. 8 (2024), https://dx.doi.org/doi:10.1001/jamapediatrics.2024.0885.

120 Andrea Suozzo, Sophie Chou, and Lizzie Presser, "Texas Won't Study How Its Abortion Ban Impacts Women, So We Did," Propublica, Propublica, 2025, accessed 7 November 2025, https://www.propublica.org/article/texas-maternal-mortality-analysis-methodology.

121 Simonovic.

122 Bowser, and Hill.

123 B Chalmers, J McIntyre, and D Meyers, "South African Obstetricians' Views on Caesarean Section," *South African Medical Journal* 82 (1991).

124 Chalmers, McIntyre, and Meyers.

125 Magan Solomon et al., "A Health Care System Divided: How Apartheid's Lingering Effects Harm South African Maternal Health," *McGill Journal of Global Health* 9 (2020), https://mghjournal.com/2020/09/24/vol-ix-a-health-care-system-divided-how-apartheids-lingering-effects-harm-south-african-maternal-health/.

126 M Price, and J Broomberg, "The Impact of Fee-for-Service Reimbursement System on the Utlization of Health Services: Part III. A Comparison of Caesarean Section Rates in White Nulliparous Women in Private and Public Sectors," *South African Medical Journal* 78 (1990).

127 Solomon et al.

128 T Morris, K McNamara, and C Morton, "Hospital-Ownership Status and Cesareans in the United States: The Effect of for-Profit Hospitals," 44 (2017), https://dx.doi.org/10.1111/birt.12299.

129 B Chalmers et al., "Rates of Interventions in Labor and Birth across Canada: Findings of the Canadian Maternity Experiences Survey.," *Birth* 39, no. 3 (2012).

130 Elizabeth Rivelli, "How Much Does It Cost to Have a Baby?," Forbes, 2025, accessed 4 May, 2025, https://www.forbes.com/advisor/health-insurance/how-much-does-it-cost-to-have-a-baby/.

131 Rivelli

132 B Chalmers, *African Birth: Childbirth in Cultural Transition.* (Sandton, South Africa: Berev Publications, 1990), B Chalmers, "Maternity Care in the Former Soviet Union," *British Journal of Obstetrics and Gynaecology* 112 (2005), Chalmers, and Omer-Hashi.

133 Bohren et al, Bowser, and Hill.

134 Frances Fornah, "The Childbirth Experiences and Perceptions of Sierra Leonean Women Relating to Basic Maternal Rights." (Walden University, Minneapolis, 2022).

135 Elizabeth O'Brien, and Miriam Rich, "Obstetric Violence in Historical Perspective," *The Lancet* 399, no. June (2022).

136 O'Brien, and Rich.

137 Chalmers, *Birth, Sex and Abuse: Women's Voices under Nazi Rule.*

138 B Chalmers, *Birth, Sex and Abuse: Women's Voices under Nazi Rule* (UK: Grosvenor House Publishing, 2015).

139 Chalmers, *Birth, Sex and Abuse: Women's Voices under Nazi Rule.*

140 Elaine Jung, "Doctors Fitted a Contraceptive Coil without My Consent," *BBC News* (UK)2022, www.bbc.com/news/world-europe-63863088.

141 Caroline Pukall, *Human Sexuality: A Contemporary Introduction*, Third ed. (Canada: Oxford University Press, 2020).

142 The Associated Press, "China Forces Birth Control on Uighurs to Suppress Population," *The Associated Press* (Canada), 29 June, 2020, https://www.voanews.com/a/east-asia-pacific_china-forces-birth-control-uighurs-suppress-population/6191919.html#:~:text=The%20Chinese%20government%20is%20taking,majority%20to%20have%20more%20children.

143 Yvonne Boyer, and Judith Bartlett, External Review: Tubal Ligation in the Saskatoon Health Region: The Lived Experience of Aboriginal Women, 2017, Health Region Saskatoon, Canada, https://www.saskatoonhealthregion.ca/DocumentsInternal/Tubal_Ligation_intheSaskatoonHealthRegion_the_Lived_Experience_of_Aboriginal_Women_BoyerandBartlett_July_22_2017.pdf.

144 Boyer, and Bartlett.

145 O'Brien, and Rich.
146 Amy Mackinnon, "What Actually Happens When a Country Bans Abortion?," *Foreign Policy* (USA), May 16 2019, https://foreignpolicy.com/2019/05/16/what-actually-happens-when-a-country-bans-abortion-romania-alabama/, P Stephenson et al., "Commentary: The Public Health Consequences of Restricted Induced Abortion--Lessons from Romania.," *American Journal of Public Health* 82, no. 10 (1992), https://dx.doi.org/doi: 10.2105/ajph.82.10.1328.
147 Mackinnon.
148 Mackinnon, Stephenson et al.
149 H Morton, and P Simkin, "Can Respectful Maternity Care Save and Improve Lives?," *Birth* 46, no. 3 (2019), https://dx.doi.org/ DOI: 10.1111/birt.12444.
150 United Nations, *Reproductive Rights* (2014). http://www.un.org/en/development/desa/population/theme/rights/index.shtml.
151 United Nations.
152 Family Care International, *Action for the 21st Century: Reproductive Health and Rights for All* (New York: Family Care International, 1994).
153 United Nations, *LGBTQ+ People* (Geneva: United Nations, 2024). www.un.org/lgbtiq-people.
154 *Draft Outcome Document of the United Nations Summit for the Adoption of the Post-2015 Development Agenda*, by United Nations General Assembly, A/69/L.85 (New York, 2015), .
155 A Starrs, "A Lancet Commission on Sexual and Reproductive Health and Rights: Going Beyond the Sustainable Development Goals," *The Lancet* 386, no. 9999 (2015): 1112.
156 *The Respectful Maternity Care Charter: The Universal Rights of Childbearing Women* by White Ribbon Alliance (2011).
157 Childbirth Connection, *The Rights of Childbearing Women.* (USA: Childbirth Connection, 2012), http://www.childbirthconnection.org/article.asp?ck=10084&ClickedLink=0&area=27.
158 Department of Health, *Breastfeeding Mothers' Bill of Rights* by New York State Department of Health (State of New York, 2010).
159 *US Center for Reproductive Rights Declarations*, by Center for Reproductive Rights (1992-2013).
160 Society of Obstetricians and Gynaecologists of Canada, *International Women's Health Program. Sexual and Reproductive Rights and Health* vol. 2013 Mar 12 (Ottawa, ON: SOGC, 2009). http://iwhp.sogc.org/index.php?page=sexual-reproductive-rights&hl=en_US.
161 *The United Nations Convention on the Rights of the Child*, by United Nations (1989).

162 G Bevilacqua et al., "The Parma Charter of the Rights of the Newborn," accessed 13 February, 2016, http://www.uenps.com/media/Parma%20 Charter%20Rights%20of%20the%20newborn.pdf.

163 Bevilacqua et al.

164 Public Health Agency of Canada, *Family-Centred Maternity and Newborn Care Guidelines* (Ottawa, Ontario: Government of Canada, 2021).

165 The Transforming Maternity Care Vision Team, "2020 Vision for a High-Quality, High-Value Maternity Care System," *Women's Health Issues* 20, no. 1 (2010), http://transform.childbirthconnection.org/vision/ high-quality-high-value/.

166 J Smith, F Plaat, and N Fisk, "The Natural Caesarean: A Woman-Centred Technique," *BJOG: An International Journal of Obstetrics and Gynaecology* 115, no. 1037-42 (2008), http://www.ncbi.nlm.nih.gov/ pmc/articles/PMC2613254/.

167 J R Roudebush et al., "Patient- and Family-Centered Perinatal Care: Partnerships with Childbearing Women and Families " *Journal of Perinatal & Neonatal Nursing* 20, no. 3 (2006).

168 B Chalmers, and S Dzakpasu, "Interventions in Labour and Birth and Satisfaction with Care: The Canadian Maternity Experiences Survey Findings," *Journal of Reproductive and Infant Psychology* 33, no. 4 (2015).

169 E Zwelling, and C R Phillips, "Family-Centered Maternity Care in the New Millennium: Is It Real or Is It Imagined?," *Journal of Perinatal and Neonatal Nursing* 15, no. 3 (2001).

170 WHO, *Having a Baby in Europe* (Copenhagen: World Health Organization, 1985).

171 Chalmers, *Family-Centred Perinatal Care: Improving Pregnancy, Birth and Postpartum Care*, 11.

172 WHO, "Safe Motherhood: Mother-Baby Package: Implementing Safe Motherhood in Countries " World Health Organization, Maternal Health and Safe Motherhood Programme, 19962013 http://whqlibdoc.who.int/ hq/1994/WHO_FHE_MSM_94.11_Rev.1.pdf.

173 UK National Collaborating Centre for Womens and Childrens Health., "Antenatal Care. Routine Care for the Healthy Pregnant Woman.," (2008), www.nice.org.uk/nicemedia/live/11947/40145/40145.pdf.

174 National Collaborating Centre for Womens and Childrens Health.

175 Caroline Shenouda et al., "Labour Progression in Obese Women: Are Women with Increased Body Mass Index Having Unnecessary Cesarean Sections?," *Journal of Obstetrics and Gynaecology of Canada* 42 no. 3 (2020), https://dx.doi.org/DOI:https://doi.org/10.1016/j.jogc. 2019.04.014.

176 Beverley Chalmers, "Psychosocial Factors and Obstetric Complications" *Psychology and Medicine* 13 (1983).

177 Chalmers.

178 Past president of the International Federation of Obstetricians and Gynaecologists (FIGO) and former Director of the United Nations Development Programme/ United Nations Family Planning Association/ WHO/ World Bank Special Program of Research, Development and Research Training in Human Reproduction

179 Tarasoff et al.

180 WHO, "Safe Motherhood: Mother-Baby Package: Implementing Safe Motherhood in Countries "

181 B Chalmers, and R Porter, "Assessing Management of Normal Labour: The Bologna Score," *Birth* 28, no. 2 (2001).

182 GJ Hofmeyr et al., "WHO Next-Generation Partograph: Revolutionary Steps Towards Individualised Labour Care," *BJOG* 128, no. 10 (2002), https://dx.doi.org/htttps://doi.org/10.1111/1471-0528.16694.L

183 Pilli Rajani, and Manjula Pathri, "A Comparative Evaluation of the Paperless Partograph and the Modified WHO Partograph in Labor Management," *Journal of Contemporary Clinical Practice* 11, no. 7 (2025), https://dx.doi.org/doi:10.61336/jccp/25-07-15.

184 Society of Obstetricians and Gynaecologists of Canada, "Joint Policy Statement on Normal Birth.," *Journal of Obstetrics and Gynaecology of Canada* 30, no. 12 (2008).

185 Royal College of Obstetricians and Gynaecologists, Royal College of Midwives, and National Childbirth Trust, *Making Normal Birth a Reality: Consensus Statement from the Maternity Care Working Party* (London: Maternity Care Working Party 2007). http://www.rcog.org.uk/womens-health/clinical-guidance/making-normal-birth-reality.%20Accessed%206%20March%202013.

186 Royal College of Obstetricians and Gynaecologists, Royal College of Midwives, and National Childbirth Trust.

187 B Chalmers, V Mangiaterra, and R Porter, "WHO Principles of Perinatal Care: The Essential Antenatal, Perinatal and Postpartum Care Course," *Birth.* 28 (2001).

188 B Chalmers et al., "Breastfeeding Rates and Hospital Breastfeeding Practices in Canada: A National Survey of Women.," *Birth* 36, no. 2 (2009).

189 Beverley Chalmers, "Breastfeeding Unfriendly in Canada?," *Canadian Medical Association Journal* 185, no. 5 (2013), https://dx.doi.org/10.1503/cmaj.121309.

190 B Chalmers et al., "Cesarean and Vaginal Birth in Canadian Women: A Comparison of Experiences," *Birth* 37, no. 1 (2010).

191 J Winberg, "Mother and Newborn Baby: Mutual Regulation of Physiology and Behavior— a Selective Review," *Developmental Psychobiology* 47 (2005).

192 E R Moore et al., "Early Skin-to-Skin Contact for Mothers and Their Healthy Newborn Infants.," *Cochrane database of systematic reviews* 5 (2012).

193 D Affonso et al., "Reconciliation and Healing for Mothers through Skin-to-Skin Contact Provided in an American Tertiary Level Intensive Care Nursery," *Neonatal Network* 12 (1993), G C Anderson, "Current Knowledge About Skin-to-Skin (Kangaroo) Care for Preterm Infants," *Journal of Perinatology* 11 (1991), S M Ludington, "Energy Conservation during Skin-to-Skin Contact between Premature Infants and Their Mothers," *Heart and Lung* 19 (1990).

194 WHO/UNICEF, *Protecting, Promoting and Supporting Breastfeeding: The Special Role of Maternity Services* (Geneva: World Health Organization and UNICEF, 1989).

195 WHO, *WHO Recommendations: Intrapartum Care for a Positive Childbirth Experience* (Geneva: World Health Organization, 2018).

196 WHO, "Appropriate Technology for Birth.," *Lancet* 8452 (1985).

197 Cochrane Library, "The Cochrane Database of Systematic Reviews," John Wiley and Sons, 2015, accessed 17 April 2015, http://www.cochranelibrary.com/cochrane-database-of-systematic-reviews/index.html.

198 WHO, *Having a Baby in Europe*.

199 WHO, "Appropriate Technology for Birth."

200 Beverley Chalmers, "WHO Appropriate Technology for Birth Revisited," *British Journal of Obstetrics and Gynaecology* 99 (1992).

201 Chalmers, "WHO Appropriate Technology for Birth Revisited."

202 Cochrane Library

203 UK National Institute for Health and Clinical Excellence, *Nice Guideline: Routine Care for the Healthy Pregnant Woman* vol. PMID: 21370514. (CG 62 update: repr., London: RCOG Press, March 2008).

204 WHO, *Workshop on Perinatal Care Proceedings: Venice* (Copenhagen: World Health Organization, 1998), *Second Meeting of Focal Points of Reproductive Health/Health of Women and Children in the European Region* by WHO (Copenhagen: World Health Organization, 1998).

205 Chalmers, and Mangiaterra.

206 WHO, *Workshop on Perinatal Care Proceedings: Venice*

207 Enkin, Keirse, and Chalmers.

208 Enkin, Keirse, and Chalmers, Murray Enkin et al., eds., *A Guide to Effective Care in Pregnancy and Childbirth* (Oxford: Oxford University

Press, 2000), Murray Enkin et al., *A Guide to Effective Care in Pregnancy and Childbirth*, 2nd ed. (Oxford: Oxford University Press, 1995).

209 Public Health Agency of Canada.

210 Enkin et al.

211 Enkin et al.

212 Enkin et al.

213 *The Global Numbers and Costs of Additionally Needed and Unnecessary Caesarean Sections Performed Per Year: Overuse as a Barrier to Universal Coverage*, by L Gibbons et al. (Geneva World Health Report, 2010).

214 A P Betran et al., "WHO Statement on Caesarean Section Rates.," *BJOG* 123, no. 5 (2016), https://dx.doi.org/10.1111/1471-0528.13526, *WHO Statement on Caesarean Section Rates*, by WHO, WHO/RHR/15.02 (Geneva: WHO Human Reproduction Programme, 2015).

215 Betran et al, *WHO Statement on Caesarean Section Rates*.

216 *WHO Statement on Caesarean Section Rates*.

217 *WHO Statement on Caesarean Section Rates*.

218 E Declercq, and B Chalmers, "Mothers' Reports of Their Maternity Experiences in the USA and Canada.," *Journal of Reproductive and Infant Psychology* 26, no. 4 (2008).

219 Beverley Chalmers, "Childbirth across Cultures: Research and Practice," *Birth* 39, no. 4 (2012).

220 Klein MC et al., "Epidural Analgesia Use as a Marker for Physician Approach to Birth: Implications for Maternal and Newborn Outcomes.," *Birth* 28, no. 4 (2001).

221 Hofmeyr.

222 F Althabe et al., "Cesarean Section Rates and Maternal and Neonatal Mortality in Low-Middle- and High-Income Countries: An Ecological Study.," *Birth* 33, no. 4 (2006), J Villar et al., " Caesarean Delivery Rates and Pregnancy Outcomes: The 2005 WHO Global Survey on Maternal and Perinatal Health in Latin America " *Lancet* 367, no. 9525 (2006).

223 Villar et al.

224 PHAC Public Health Agency of Canada, *Perinatal Health Indicators for Canada 2011* (Ottawa, ON: Public Health Agency of Canada, 2012). http://www.phac-aspc.gc.ca/rhs-ssg/phi-isp-2011-eng.php.

225 M J.K. Osterman, and J A. Martin, "Primary Cesarean Delivery Rates, by State: Results from the Revised Birth Certificate, 2006–2012.," *National Vital Statistics Report* 63, no. 1 (2014), http://www.cdc.gov/nchs/fastats/delivery.htm.

226 S Hellerstein, S Feldman, and T Duan, "China's 50% Caesarean Delivery Rate: Is It Too High?," *BJOG* (2014), https://dx.doi.org/10.1111/1471-0528.12971.

227 *WHO Statement on Caesarean Section Rates.*
228 *WHO Statement on Caesarean Section Rates.*
229 Chalmers, "Childbirth across Cultures: Research and Practice."
230 L F Beck et al., *PRAMS 1999 Surveillance Report* (Atlanta, GA: Division of Reproductive Health, National Center for Chronic Disease Prevention and Health Promotion, Centers for Disease Control and Prevention, 2003).
231 E Declercq, C Sakala, and M Corry, *Listening to Mothers II: Report of the Second National US Survey of Women's Childbearing Experiences* (New York: Childbirth Connections, 2006), E R Declercq, C Sakala, and M P Corry, *Listening to Mothers: Report of the First National U.S. Survey of Women's Childbearing Experiences* (New York: Maternity Center Association: Maternity Center Association, 2002).
232 PHAC Public Health Agency of Canada, *What Mothers Say: The Maternity Experiences Survey* (Ottawa, ON: Public Health Agency of Canada, 2009).
233 J Garcia et al., *First Class Delivery: A National Survey of Women's Views of Maternity Care* (London: Audit Commission, 1998), J Green, V Coupland, and J Kitzinger, "Expectations, Experiences and Psychological Outcomes of Childbirth: A Prospective Study of 825 Women," *Birth* 17 (1990), J M Green et al., *Greater Expectations: The Inter- Relationship between Women's Expectations and Experiences of Decision Making, Continuity, Choice and Control in Labour, and Psychological Outcomes. Summary Report* (Leeds: Mother & Infant Research Unit, University of Leeds, 2003), J M Green, V A Coupland, and J V Kitzinger, *Great Expectations: A Prospective Study of Women's Expectations and Experiences of Childbirth*, 2nd ed. (UK Books for Midwives Press, 1998), Scottish Programme for Clinical Effectiveness in Reproductive Health, *Maternity Care Matters: An Audit of Maternity Services in Scotland 1998* (Aberdeen: Douglas Baird Centre for Research on Women's Health, 1999), M Redshaw et al., *Recorded Delivery: A National Survey of Women's Experience of Maternity Care* (Oxford: National Perinatal Epidemiology Unit, University of Oxford, 2007).
234 S Brown, and J Lumley, "Satisfaction with Care in Labour and Birth: A Survey of 790 Australian Women," *Birth* 21 (1994).
235 U Waldenstrom et al., "A Negative Birth Experience: Relevance and Risk Factors in a National Sample," *Birth* 31 (2004).
236 B Chalmers et al., "What Women Say About Antenatal Care in St Petersburg, Russian Federation," *Journal of Psychosomatic Obstetrics and Gynaecology* 20 (1999), B Chalmers et al., "Women's Experiences of Birth in St Petersburg, Russian Federation Following a Maternal-Child Health Intervention Program," *Birth* 25, no. 107-116 (1998),

B Chalmers et al., "What Women Say About Post-Partum Care and Breastfeeding in St Petersburg, Russian Federation," *Journal of the Society of Obstetricians and Gynaecologists of Canada* 21 (1999), B Chalmers et al., "Contraceptive Knowledge, Attitudes and Use among Women Attending Health Clinics in St Petersburg, Russian Federation," *Canadian Journal of Human Sexuality* 7 (1998), E Heiberg et al., "Women's Experiences of Giving Birth in Northwest Russia in 2000 and 2002 and in Northern Norway 2000," *Acta Obstetrica et Gynecologica Scandinavica* 86, no. 3 (2007).

237 B Chalmers, and D Jeckaite, "Giving Birth in Two Maternity Hospitals in Lithuania.," *Birth* 37, no. 2 (2010).

238 P Stratulat et al., "Evaluarea Rezultatelor Implementarii Technologiilor Programului National De Ameliorare a Asistentei Medicale Perinatale in Republica Moldova," *Buletin de Perinatologie* 3 (2002).

239 B Chalmers, and D Qulieva, "A Report of Women's Birth Experiences in Baku, Azerbaijan," *Journal of Psychosomatic Obstetrics and Gynaecology* 25 (2004).

240 Chalmers, "Childbirth across Cultures: Research and Practice."

241 Beverley Chalmers, "Over-Reliance on a Medical Approach to Care: Some Thoughts for Consideration," *Journal of the Society of Obstetricians and Gynaecologists of Canada* 21, no. 11 (1999), M Wagner, *Pursuing the Birth Machine: The Search for Appropriate Birth Technology* (Australia: ACE Graphica, 1994).

242 Declercq, and Chalmers.

243 Roosa Tikkanen et al., "Maternal Mortality and Maternity Care in the United States Compared to 10 Other Developed Countries," The Commonwealth Fund, 2020, accessed 14 September, 2023, https://www.commonwealthfund.org/publications/issue-briefs/2020/nov/maternal-mortality-maternity-care-us-compared-10-countries.

244 Declercq, and Chalmers.

245 V A D S Rodrigues, Abreu Y R, and Santos C A G et al., "Nonpharmacological Labor Pain Management Methods and Risk of Cesarean Birth: A Retrospective Cohort Study," *Birth* (2022), https://dx.doi.org/doi:10.1111/birt.12617.

246 Chalmers et al.

247 F Bragg et al., "Variation in Rates of Caesarean Section among English NHS Trusts after Accounting for Maternal and Clinical Risk: Cross Sectional Study," *British Medical Journal* 341 (2010).

248 J Nagpal et al., "Widespread Non-Adherence to Evidence-Based Maternity Care Guidelines: A Population-Based Cluster Randomised Household Survey," *BJOG* (2014), https://dx.doi.org/10.1111/1471-0528.13054 (http://dx.doi.org/10.1111/1471-0528.13054).

249 Chalmers, McIntyre, and Meyers.

250 Public Health Agency of Canada.
251 Public Health Agency of Canada.
252 Chalmers et al.
253 Chalmers et al.
254 Simonovic.
255 Kim Robin van Daalen et al., "Racial Discrimination and Adverse Pregnancy Outcomes: A Systematic Review and Meta- Analysis," *BMJ Global Health* 7, no. e009227 (2022), https://dx.doi.org/10.1136/bmjgh-2022-009227.
256 S M Phelan et al., "Impact of Weight Bias and Stigma on Quality of Care and Outcomes for Patients with Obesity," *Obesity Reviews* 16 (2015), R Puhl, and K D Brownell, "Bias, Discrimination, and Obesity," *Obesity Research* 9, no. 12 (2001).
257 S B De Joy, and K Bittner, "Obesity Stigma as a Determinant of Poor Birth Outcomes in Women with High BMI: A Conceptual Framework," *Maternal Child Health Journal* 19, no. 693-9 (2015), https://dx.doi.org/10.1007/s10995-014-1577-x.
258 J S Mercer et al., "Evidence-Based Practices for the Fetal to Newborn Transition.," *Journal of Midwifery & Women's Health* 52, no. 3 (2007).
259 A M Romano, and J A Lothian., "Promoting, Protecting and Supporting Normal Birth: A Look at the Evidence," *Journal of Obstetric, Gynecology and Neonatal Nursing* 37 (2008), H Goer, and A Romano, *Optimal Care in Childbirth: The Case for a Physiologic Approach* (USA: Classic Day Publishing, 2012).
260 UK National Institute for Health and Care Excellence, "Weight Management before, during and after Pregnancy. Quick Reference Guide.," (2010), www.nice.org.uk/nicemedia/live/13056/49929/49929.pdf.
261 I Chalmers, M Enkin, and M Keirse, *Effective Care in Pregnancy and Childbirth* (Oxford: Oxford University Press, 1989).
262 Chalmers, and Mangiaterra.
263 NICE National Institute for Health and Care Excellence, "Intrapartum Care: Care of Healthy Women and Their Babies during Childbirth.," (2014), www.nice.org.uk/guidance/cg190, Neel Shah, "A Nice Delivery-the Cross-Atlantic Divide over Treatment Intensity in Childbirth," *The New England Journal of Medicine* 372, no. 23 (2015), https://dx.doi.org/DOI: 10.1056/NEJMp1501461.
264 M L DeRegil et al., "Effects and Safety of Periconceptional Folate Supplementation for Preventing Birth Defects," *Cochrane database of systematic reviews* 10 (2010).
265 Tilden et al.
266 Editorial, "Cancer Care : Beyond Survival," *The Lancet* 399, no. 10334 (2022), https://dx.doi.org/https://doi.org/10.1016/S0140-6736(22)00698-5.

267 V Berghella et al., "Preconception Care.," *Obstetrical & Gynecological Survey* 65, no. 2 (2010), M C Lu, "Recommendations for Preconception Care.," *American Family Physician* 76, no. 3 (2007).
268 J Scott, "Folic Acid Consumption Throughout Pregnancy: Differentiation between Trimesters," *Annals of Nutrition & Metabolism* 59, no. 1 (2011).
269 Taniya S Nagpal et al., "Are Pre-Pregnancy Weight Fluctuations and Adherence to Prenatal Nutrition and Exercise Recommendations Related to Excessive Gestational Weight Gain?," *Journal of Behavioral Medicine* 43, no. 6 (2022).
270 Berghella et al.
271 M Whitworth, and T Dowswell, "Routine Pre-Pregnancy Health Promotion for Improving Pregnancy Outcomes," *Cochrane database of systematic reviews* 4 (2009), S F Posner et al., "Where Are the Data to Drive Policy Changes for Preconception Health and Health Care?," *Womens Health Issues* 18, no. 6 (2008).
272 Francesco Rubinoa et al., "Definition and Diagnostic Criteria of Clinical Obesity," *The Lancet Diabetes and Endocrinology* 13, no. 3 (2025).
273 Nagpal et al.
274 Shenouda et al.
275 Mark V Roehling, Patricia V. Roehling, and Shaun Pichler., "The Relationship between Body Weight and Perceived Weight-Related Employment Discrimination: The Role of Sex and Race.," *Journal of Vocational Behavior* (2007).
276 Obesity Canada, "Overcoming Weight Bias: Do You Have It in You," Obesity Canada, 2024, accessed 19 February, 2024, https://obesitycanada.ca/wp-content/uploads/2022/07/Overcoming-Weight-Bias-11x17-May-2018-Eng-Fr4-4.pdf.
277 K Melzer et al., "Effects of Recommended Levels of Physical Activity on Pregnancy Outcomes.," *American Journal of Obstetrics and Gynecology* 202, no. 266 (2010).
278 M I Cedergren, "Maternal Morbid Obesity and the Risk of Adverse Pregnancy Outcomes," *Obstetrics and Gynaecology* 103, no. 2 (2004).
279 Shenouda et al.
280 Francesco Rubino et al., "Joint International Consensus Statement for Ending Stigma of Obesity," *Nature medicine* (2020), https://dx.doi.org/https://doi.org/10.1038/s41591-020-0803-x, Shenouda et al.
281 Meredith Evans et al., "Disability Justice and Collective Access to Labour and Delivery Care: A Qualitative Study," *MBC Pregnancy and Childbirth* 24, no. 832 (2024), Https://bmcpregnancychildbirth.biomedcentral.com/articles/10.1186/s12884-024-07036-3.
282 E Abalos et al., "Antenatal Care for Healthy Pregnant Women: A Mapping of Interventions from Existing Guidelines to Inform the

Development of New WHO Guidelines on Antenatal Care," *BJOG* (2015), accessed 23 December 2015, https://dx.doi.org/DOI: 10.1111/1471-0528.13820.

283 Davis-Floyd, Beverley Chalmers, and Robbie Davis-Floyd, "Birthing Techno-Sapiens in Disruptive Times," in *Birthing Techno-Sapiens: Human Technology Co-Evolution and the Future of Reproduction*, ed. Robbie Davis-Floyd (USA: Routledge, 2021), Beverley Chalmers, "Family-Centred, Evidence-Based, Psycho-Socially Sensitive, and Culturally Respectful Perinatal Care," in *Birthing Techno-Sapiens;: Human Technology Co-Evolution and the Future of Reproduction*, ed. Robbie Davis-Floyd (USA: Routledge, 2021).

284 G Novick, "Women's Experience of Prenatal Care: An Integrative Review," *Journal of Midwifery and Womens Health* 54, no. 3 (2009).

285 S Downe et al., "What Matters to Women: A Systematic Scoping Review to Identify the Processes and Outcomes of Antenatal Care Provision That Are Important to Healthy Pregnant Women.," *BJOG* (2015), https://dx.doi.org/10:1111/1471-0528.13819.

286 Carina Vedeler et al., "What Women Emphasise as Important Aspects of Care in Childbirth - an Online Survey," *BJOG* Preprint (2021), https://dx.doi.org/https://doi.org/10.1111/1471-0528.16926.

287 A P Alio et al., "Feto-Infant Health and Survival: Does Paternal Involvement Matter?," *Maternal Child Health Journal* 14, no. 6 (2010).

288 P McNiven et al., "Midwives' Belief in Normal Birth: The Canadian Survey of Maternity Care Provider's Attitudes toward Labour and Birth," *The Canadian Journal of Midwifery Research and Practice* 10, 2 (2011).

289 Public Health Agency of Canada.

290 National Institute for Health and Care Excellence.

291 B Chalmers et al., *Essential Antenatal, Perinatal and Post-Partum Care Course* (Copenhagen: World Health Organization Regional Office for Europe, 1999).

292 Elizabeth Mitchell Armstrong, "Making Sense of Advice About Drinking during Pregnancy: Does Evidence Even Matter?," *Journal of Perinatal Education* 26, no. 2 (2017), https://dx.doi.org/10.1891/1058-1243.26.2.65.

293 C M O'Leary et al., "A Review of Policies on Alcohol Use during Pregnancy in Australia and Other English-Speaking Countries.," *Medical Journal of Australia* 186, no. 9 (2007).

294 M Enkin et al., *A Guide to Effective Care in Pregnancy and Childbirth*, 3rd ed. (Oxford: Oxford University Press, 2000).

295 Pelvic Obstetric and Gynaecological Physiotherapy, "Pregnancy-Related Pelvic Girdle Pain - for Health Professionals Formerly Known as Symphysis Pubis Dysfunction ", 2015, accessed 24 April, 2015,

http://pogp.csp.org.uk/publications/pregnancy-related-pelvic-girdle-pain-pgp-health-professionals, National Health Services, "Pelvic Pain in Pregnancy," UK Government, 2014, accessed 24 April, 2015, http://www.nhs.uk/conditions/pregnancy-and-baby/pages/pelvic-pain-pregnant-spd.aspx.

296 Novick, M Hatem et al., "Midwife-Led Versus Other Models of Care for Childbearing Women.," *Cochrane Database of Systematic Reviews.* (4):CD004667. (2008).

297 M P Austin et al., "The Antenatal Risk Questionnaire: Acceptability and Use for Psychosocial Risk Assessment in the Maternity Setting.," *Women Birth* 26, no. 1 (2013), https://dx.doi.org/10.1016/j.wombi.2011.06.002, Midmer et al.

298 Chalmers, Beverley Chalmers, "Types of Life Events and Factors Influencing Their Seriousness Ratings," *Journal of Social Psychology* 121 (1983), W P Witt et al., "Measuring Stress before and during Pregnancy: A Review of Population-Based Studies of Obstetric Outcomes," *Maternal Child Health Journal* 18, no. 1 (2014), https://dx.doi.org/10.1007/s10995-013-1233-x.

299 P Cavalli, and A J Copp, "Inositol and Resistant Neural Tube Defects," *Journal of Medical Genetics* 39, no. e5 (2002), https://dx.doi.org/DOI 10. 1136/jmg.39.2.e5.

300 S Harvey et al., "A Randomized Control Trial of Nurse-Midwifery Care.," *Birth* 23 (1996), W Hueston, and M Rudy, "A Comparison of Labour and Delivery Management between Nurse-Midwives and Family Physicians," *The Journal of Family Practice* 37 (1993), D Oakley et al., "Comparisons of Certified Nurse-Midwives and Obstetricians," *Journal of Nurse-Midwifery* 40 (1995), Hatem et al.

301 E D Hodnett et al., "Continuous Support for Women during Childbirth.," *Cochrane database of systematic reviews* 10: CD003766 (2012), M Klaus et al., "Effects of Social Support during Parturition on Maternal and Infant Morbidity," *British Medical Journal* 293 (1986).

302 Sylvia Csosz, "The Psychological and Physiological Effects of Social Support during Childbirth in African Women." (1992).

303 E Hodnett et al., "Continuous Support for Women in Childbirth.," *Cochrane Database of Systematic Reviews* 3 (2007).

304 S R. Magee et al., "Promotion of Family-Centered Birth with Gentle Cesarean Delivery," *Journal of the American Board of Family Medicine* 27, no. 5 (2014), Smith, Plaat, and Fisk, M S McClellan, and W A Cabianca, "Effects of Early Mother-Infant Contact Following Cesarean Birth.," *Obstetrics and Gynecology* 56 (1980).

305 Dubravko Habeka et al., "Modified Stark's (Misgav Ladach) Caesarean Section: 15 – Year Experience of the Own Techniques of Caesarean

Section," *European Journal of Obstetrics and Gynecology and Reproductive Biology* 247 (2020), Gunna Holmgren, MLennart Sjoholm, and Michael Stark, "The Misgav Ladach Method or Cesarean Section, Method Description," *Acta Obstetrica et Gynecologia Scandinavica* 78, no. 7 (1999).

306 Laura Radtke et al., "Charité Caesarean Birth Improves Birth Experience in Planned and Unplanned Caesarean Sections While Maintaining Maternal and Neonatal Safety: A Prospective Cohort Study," *CEOG* 49, no. 6 (2022-06-28 2022), https://dx.doi.org/10.31083/j.ceog4906124. individualized care

307 Chalmers, Enkin, and Keirse.

308 Rachna Bahl et al., "Assisted Vaginal Birth in 21st Century: Current Practice and New Innovations," *American Journal of Obstetrics and Gynecology*, no. March (2024).

309 Beck et al, B Chalmers et al., "The Maternity Experiences Survey: An Overview of Findings," *Journal of Obstetrics and Gynaecology of Canada* 30 (2008).

310 Beverley Chalmers, "Terminology Used in Early Pregnancy Loss," *British Jourrnal of Obstetrics and Gynaecology* 99 (1992).

311 P Simkin et al., "Roundtable Discussion on the Language of Birth," *Birth* 39, no. 2 (2012).

312 Simkin et al.

313 M Stewart, "Talking to, and About, Women in Labour. In Roundtable Discussion on the Language of Birth.," *Birth* 39, no. 2 (2011).

314 B Shearer, "Failure to Progress or Failure to Wait? In Roundtable Discussion on the Language of Birth.," *Birth* 39, no. 2 (2011).

315 M Keirse, "Just Roar-Rely on Acronym Rhetoric. Roundtable Discussion on the Language of Birth," *Birth* 39, no. 2 (2012).

316 Maternal, Child Health; Making Pregnancy Safer; Integrated Management of Childhood Illness, Family and Child Health.

317 Chalmers, "Terminology Used in Early Pregnancy Loss."

318 Chalmers, "Terminology Used in Early Pregnancy Loss."

319 Smitha Mundasad, and Tulip Mazumdar, "Baby Loss in Pregnancy: Pledge to Store Remains in Dignified Way," *BBC News* (UK)2023, https://www.bbc.com/news/health-66259223.

320 Zoe Clark-Coates, and Samantha Collinge, *.The Independent Pregnancy Loss Review - Care and Support When Baby Loss Occurs before 24 Weeks Gestation.* (UK: 2023).

321 Beverley Chalmers, *Early Parenthood: Heaven or Hell* (South Africa: Juta and Co., 1984).

322 Chalmers, *Early Parenthood: Heaven or Hell.*

323 B. Chalmers, and D. Meyers, "A Cross-Cultural View of the Psychosocial Management of Miscarriage," *Journal of Psychosomatic*

Obstetrics & Gynecology 13, no. 3 (1992), https://dx.doi.org/10.3109/01674829209019573.
324 *Miscarriage: A Crisis Discarded,* (1989).
325 Chalmers, *Early Parenthood: Heaven or Hell.*
326 D Bowen et al., "Discussions after Death," *South African Medical Journal* 78 (1990).
327 David Chazan, "Dutch Fertility Doctor Used Own Sperm to Artificially Inseminate Patients," *Daily Telegraph* (London, England)2019, https://www.telegraph.co.uk/news/2019/04/14/dutch-fertility-doctor-used-sperm-inseminate-patients/, Daniel Boffey, "Netherlands Fertility Doctor Used Own Sperm to Father 21 Children " *The Guardian* (Brussels)2022, https://www.theguardian.com/world/2022/feb/02/netherlands-fertility-doctor-jos-beek-father-21-children.
328 Nathan Hodson, and Susan Bewley, "Abuse in Assisted Reproductive Technology: A Systematic Qualitative Review and Typology," *European journal of obstetrics & gynecology and reproductive biology* 238 (2019), https://dx.doi.org/10.1016/j.ejogrb.2019.05.027.
329 Hodson, and Bewley.
330 Hodson, and Bewley.
331 Hodson, and Bewley.
332 Hodson, and Bewley.
333 Hodson, and Bewley.
334 Hodson, and Bewley.
335 Simon Weisenthal, *Justice Not Vengeance* (London: Weidenfeld and Nicolson, 1989), Ginia Bellafante, "JD Vance and the Age-Old Trope of 'Childless Cat Ladies'," *The New York Times* (New York)2024, https://www.nytimes.com/2024/07/25/nyregion/jd-vance-kamala-harris-cat-lady.html.
336 Y R Hong, and J S Park, "Impact of Attachment, Temperament and Parenting on Human Development.," *Korean Journal of Pediatrics* 55, no. 12 (2012), K Ma, " Attachment Theory in Adult Psychiatry. Part 1: Conceptualisations, Measurement and Clinical Research Findings.," *Advances in Psychiatric Treatment* 12 (2006), L A Sroufe, "Attachment and Development: A Prospective, Longitudinal Study from Birth to Adulthood.," *Attachment and Human Development* 7, no. 349-367 (2005), SL Warren et al., "Child and Adolescent Anxiety Disorders and Early Attachment " *Journal of the American Academy of Child and Adolescent Psychiatry* 36 (1997), H I Yoo et al., "Parental Attachment and Its Impact on the Development of Psychiatric Manifestations in School-Aged Children," *Psychopathology* 39 (2006).
337 Chalmers et al.
338 Chalmers et al, V Zanardo et al., "Elective Cesarean Delivery: Does It Have a Negative Effect on Breastfeeding?," *Birth* 37, no. 4 (2010).

339 Hodnett et al, Hofmeyr et al.
340 WHO, *Code of Marketing of Breastmilk Substitutes* (Geneva: World Health Organization, 1981), WHO/UNICEF.
341 N Rollins et al., "Why Invest, and What Will It Take to Improve Breastfeeding Practices?," *The Lancet* 387, no. 10017 (2016), C Victora et al., "Breastfeeding in the 21st Century: Epidemiology, Mechanisms and Lifelong Effect," *The Lancet* 387, no. 10017 (2016).
342 M S Kramer, and R Kakuma, "Optimal Duration of Exclusive Breastfeeding.," *Cochrane Database of Systematic Reviews* 8 (2012).
343 WHO/UNICEF, *Global Strategy for Infant and Young Child Feeding* (Geneva: World Health Organization; United Nations Children's Fund, 2003).
344 B L Horta et al., "Evidence on the Long-Term Effects of Breastfeeding.," *World Health Organization* (2007), http://www.who.int/maternal_child_adolescent/documents/9241595230/en/index.html, R A Lawrence, and R M Lawrence, *Breastfeeding: A Guide for the Medical Profession*, 7th ed. (USA: Elsevier, Mosby, 2011).
345 M Kramer et al., "Promotion of Breastfeeding Intervention Trial (Probit): A Cluster-Randomized Trial in the Republic of Belarus." *Journal of the American Medical Academy,* 285 (2001), M Kramer et al., "Breastfeeding and Child Cognitive Development: New Evidence from a Large Randomized Trial.," *Archives of General Psychiatry* 65, no. 5 (2008).
346 Victora et al.
347 Chalmers, *Early Parenthood: Heaven or Hell.*
348 Kramer et al, Kramer et al.
349 Public Health Agency of Canada.
350 Statistics Canada, *Overwhelming Majority of Canadian Women Start Breastfeeding Soon after Giving Birth, and More Than Half Stop within Six Months*, by StatCan (2022: Government of Canada, 2022).
351 Chalmers et al.
352 Rebekah Fox, Sara McMullen, and Mary Newburn, "UK Women's Extperiences of Breastfeeding and Additional Breastfeeding Support: A Qualitative Study of Baby Cafe Services.," *BMC Pregnancy & Childbirth* 15 (2015), https://dx.doi.org/10.1186/s12884-015-0581-5.
353 Chalmers, "Breastfeeding Unfriendly in Canada?."
354 Chalmers et al, Zanardo et al.
355 Chalmers, "Breastfeeding Unfriendly in Canada?."
356 WHO, *Ten Steps to Successful Breastfeeding* (Geneva: WHO, 2020). https://www.who.int/activities/promoting-baby-friendly-hospitals/ten-steps-to-successful-breastfeeding.
357 WHO, *Code of Marketing of Breastmilk Substitutes.*
358 WHO, *Code of Marketing of Breastmilk Substitutes.*

359 Beverley Chalmers, "Implementing the Baby Friendly Hospital Initiative.," *Journal of the Society of Obstetricians and Gynaecologists of Canada* 20 (1997).
360 Chalmers, "Implementing the Baby Friendly Hospital Initiative."
361 Beverley Chalmers, "The Baby Friendly Hospital Initiative: Where Next?," *British Journal of Obstetrics and Gynaecology* 111, no. 3 (2004).
362 Charlotte Hutting, "What Is a Kraamverzorgster and Where Can I Find One?," Amsterdam Mamas, accessed 30 May, 2023, https://amsterdam-mamas.nl/articles/what-is-a-kraamverzorgster-and-where-can-i-find-one/.
363 Daisy R. Singla et al., "Task-Sharing and Telemedicine Delivery of Psychotherapy to Treat Perinatal Depression: A Pragmatic, Noninferiority Randomized Trial," *Nature Medicine* 31 (2025), https://dx.doi.org/doi.org/10.1038/s41591-024-03482-w.
364 Bethany Atkins et al., "Is Care of Stillborn Babies and Their Parents Respectful? Results from an International Online Survey," *BJOG: An International Journal of Obstetrics & Gynaecology* (2022), https://dx.doi.org/ https://doi.org/10.1111/1471-0528.17138.
365 Susannah H. Leisher, "Respectful Stillbirth Care Is a Human Right," *BJOG* 22 March (2022), https://dx.doi.org/https://doi.org/10.1111/1471-0528.17157.
366 Chedda S et al., "Virtual Visitation in a Neonatal Intensive Care Unit: Insights from 5 Years Using a PDSA Model to Improve Family-Centred Care," *The Journal of Perinatal and Nenoatal Nursing* 37, no. 1 (2023), https://dx.doi.org/10.1097/JPN.0000000000000685.
367 Chalmers, and Levin.
368 E O Boundy et al., "Kangaroo Mother Care and Neonatal Outcomes: A Meta-Analysis," *Pediatrics* 137, no. 1 (2016), https://dx.doi.org/ DOI: 10.1542/peds.2015-2238, N Charpak, Z Figueroa, and J G Ruiz, "Kangaroo Mother Care," *Lancet* 351 (1998), N Charpak, J G Ruiz-Palaez, and Y Rey-Martinez, "Kangaroo Mother Program: An Alternate Way of Caring for Low Birth Weight Infants? One Year Mortality in a Two Cohort Study," *Pediatrics* 94 (1994).
369 D Murdock, "Handling during Neonatal Intensive Care," *Archives of Diseases in Children* 59 (1984).
370 J G Long, J F Lucey, and A G Philip, "Noise and Hypoxia in the Intensive Care Nursery," *Pediatrics* 65 (1980).
371 H Lagerkrantz et al., "Plasma Catecholamines Following Nursing Procedures in a Neonatal Ward," *Early Human Development* 14 (1986).
372 Chalmers, and Levin.
373 Sezgi Goksan et al., "fMRI Reveals Neural Activity Overlap between Adult and Infant Pain," *eLife* 4, no.:e06356 (2015), https://dx.doi.org/ http://dx.doi.org/10.7554/eLife.06356.

374 Bevilacqua et al.
375 Chalmers, and Levin.
376 Chalmers, and Levin.
377 H Als, "Program Guide: Newborn Individualized Developmental Care and Assessment Program. An Education and Training Program for Health Care Professionals," 2014, http://www.nidcap.org, H Als, " Individualized, Family-Focused Developmental Care for the Very-Low-Birthweight Preterm Infant in the NICU," in *The Psychological Development of Low-Birthweight Children*, ed. Sigman MD Friedman SL (Norwood, NJ: Ablex., 1992), H Als, and L Gilkerson, "The Role of Relationship-Based Developmentally Supportive Care in Strengthening Outcome of Preterm Infants," *Seminars in Perinatology* 21 (1997), H Als et al., "Individualized Perinatal Care for the Very-Low-Birth-Weight Preterm Infant," *Journal of the American Medical Association* 11 (1994), D M Buchler et al., "Effectiveness of Individualized Developmental Care for Low-Risk Preterm Infants: Behavioral and Electrophysiological Evidence," *Pediatrics* 96 (1995).
378 L Wallin, and M Eriksson, "Newborn Individual Development Care and Assessment Program (NIDCAP): A Systematic Review of the Literature," *Worldviews on Evidence-Based Nursing* 6, no. 54-69 (2009), B Westrup et al., "A Randomized Control Trial to Evaluate the Effects of the Newborn Individualized Developmental Care and Assessment Program in a Swedish Setting," *Pediatrics* 105 (2000), A J Symington, and J Pinelli, "Developmental Care for Promoting Development and Preventing Morbidity in Preterm Infants.," *Cochrane Library* (2009).
379 Chalmers, and Levin, A Levin, "The Mother-Infant Unit at Tallinn Children's Hospital, Estonia: A Truly Baby Friendly Unit," *Birth* 21, no. 1 (1994), A Levin, "Where Are You Going, Neonatal Medicine? Letter to Editor," *Intensive and critical care nursing* 11 (1995), A Levin, "Viewpoint: Humane Neonatal Care Initiative," *Acta Paediatrica* 88 (1999), Chalmers, and Levin, Chalmers, and Levin.
380 S Montero et al., "Experiences with Perinatal Loss from the Health Professionals' Perspective.," *Revista Latino-Americana de Enfermagem* 19, no. 6 (2011), D Nuzum, S Meaney, and K O'Donoghue, "The Impact of Stillbirth on Consultant Obstetrician Gynaecologists: A Qualitative Study," *BJOG* 121, no. 8 (2014).
381 K Schrøder et al., "Second Victims Need Emotional Support after Adverse Events: Even in a Just Safety Culture," *BJOG* 126, no. 4 (2018), https://dx.doi.org/DOI: 10.1111/1471-0528.15529.
382 Boundy et al, Chalmers, and Levin.
383 D Hall, and G Kirsten, "Kangaroo Mother Care - a Review," *Transfusion Medicine* 18 (2008), Moore et al, MJ Renfrew et al., "Breastfeeding

Promotion for Infants in Neonatal Units: A Systematic Review and Economic Analysis " *Health Technology Assessment* 13, no. 40 (2009).

384 Chalmers, and Levin, Levin, "Where Are You Going, Neonatal Medicine? Letter to Editor."

385 K D Bolton et al., "Black Mother's Experiences of a Neonatal Care Unit," *Journal of Reproductive and Infant Psychology* 11 (1993), K E Kahn, S Wayburne, and M Fouch, "Baragwanath Premature Unit: An Analysis of the Case Records of 1000 Consecutive Admissions," *South African Medical Journal* 28, no. 22 (1954), J Kennell, and M Klaus, "The Perinatal Paradigm: Is It Time for a Change?," *Clinical Perinatology* 15 (1988), N Tafari, and S M Ross, "On the Need for Organized Perinatal Care," *Ethiopian Medical Journal* 11 (1973).

386 J Kennell, "The Humane Neonatal Care Initiative," *Acta Paediatrica* 88 (1999).

387 K O'Brien et al., "Evaluation of the Family Integrated Care Model of Neonatal Intensive Care: A Cluster Randomized Controlled Trial in Canada and Australia.," *BMC Pediatrics* 15 (2015), https://dx.doi.org/*DOI: 10.1186/s12887-015-0527-0* , Karel O'Brien et al., "Evaluation of Family Integrated Care (FiCare): A Cluster Randomized Controlled Trail in Canada and Australia." (paper presented at the Pediatric Academic Societies Meeting, Baltimore, USA, April 30-May 3, 2016).

388 O'Brien et al.

389 Chalmers, and Levin.

390 S K Cone, S Short, and G Gutcher, "From "Baby Barn" to the "Single Family Room Designed NICU": A Report of Staff Perceptions One Year Post Occupancy.," *Newborn Infant Nursing Review* 10, no. 2 (2010), R Domanico et al., "Documenting the NICU Design Dilemma: Comparative Patient Progress in Open-Ward and Single Family Room Units," *Journal of Perinatology* 31, no. 4 (2011), L M Smithgall, "Perceptions of Maternal Stress and Neonatal Patient Outcomes in a Single Private Room Versus Open Room Neonatal Intensive Care Unit Environment." (East Tennessee State University, 2010), W F Walsh, K L McCullough, and R D White, "Room for Improvement: Nurses' Perceptions of Providing Care in a Single Room Newborn Intensive Care Setting.," *Advances in Neonatal Care* 6, no. 5 (2006), R D White, "Recommended Standards for Newborn ICU Design," Journal of Perinatology, 2006 2013, http://www.nature.com/jp/journal/v26/n3s/full/7211587a.html, R D White, "Single-Family Room Design in the Neonatal Intensive Care Unit - Challenges and Opportunities.," *Newborn Infant Nursing Review* 10, no. 2 (2010).

391 Westrup et al, J Muraskas, and K Parsi, "The Cost of Saving the Tiniest Lives: NICU's Versus Prevention," *Virtual Mentor* 10, no. 10 (2008).

392 W H Northway, "Bronchopulmonary Dysplasia: Twenty-Five Years Later," *Pediatrics* 89 (1992), CL Yeo, S Choo, and L Y Ho, "Chronic Lung Disease in Very Low Birthweight Infants: A 5 Year Review," *Journal of Pediatrics and Child Health* 33 (1997).

393 B Byland, T Cervin, and O Finnstrom, "Morbidity and Neurological Function of Very Low Birthweight Infants from the Newborn Period to 4 Years of Age: A Prospective Study from the South-East Region of Sweden," *Acta Pediatrica* 87 (1998), R W Cooke, "Factors Affecting Survival and Outcome at 3 Years in Extremely Preterm Infants," *Archives of Diseases in Children* 71 (1994), G J Escobar, B Littenberg, and D B Petitti, "Outcome among Surviving Very Low Birthweight Infants: A Meta-Analysis," *Archives of Diseases in Children* 66 (1991), Muraskas, and Parsi.

394 M Hack et al., "School-Age Outcomes in Children with Birthweights under 750g," *New England Journal of Medicine* 331 (1994), A Hall et al., "School Attainment, Cognitive Ability and Motor Function in a Total Scottish Very-Low-Birthweight Population at Eight Years: A Controlled Study," *Developmental* (1995), M Ornstein et al., "Neonatal Follow-up of Very Low Bithweight/Extremely Low Birthweight Infants to School Age: A Critical Review," *Acta Paediatrica* 80 (1991), E J Sell et al., "Early Identification of Learning Problems in Neonatal Intensive Care Graduates," *American Journal of Diseases of Childhood.* 139 (1985), K Stjernqvist, and W Svenningsen, "Ten Year Follow-up of Children Born before 29 Gestational Weeks: Health, Cognitive Development, Behaviour and School Achievement," *Acta Paediatrica* 88 (1999).

395 J E Grey, and D A Goldmann, "Medication Errors in the Neonatal Intensive Care Unit: Special Patients, Unique Issues," *Archives of Diseases of Children Fetal and Neonatal Edition.* 89 (2004), https://dx.doi.org/10.1136/adc.2003.046060.

396 Grey, and Goldmann.

397 Als et al, P T Berker et al., "Outcomes of Developmentally Supportive Care for Very Low Birthweight Infants," *Nursing Research* 40 (1991), L D Brown, and J A Heerman, "The Effect of Developmental Care on Preterm Infant Outcome," *Applied Nursing Research* 10 (1997), B E Fleischer, K VandenBerg, and et al, "Individualized Care for Very Low Birthweight Premature Infants Improves Medical and Developmental Outcome in the Neonatal Intensive Care Unit," *Clinical Pediatrics* 10 (1995), P Petryshen et al., "Comparing Nursing Costs for Preterm Infants Receiving Conventional Vs. Developmental Care," *Nursing Economics* 15 (1997), B Stevens et al., "Developmental Vs. Conventional Care: A Comparison of Clinical Outcomes for Very Low Birthweight Infants," *Canadian Journal of Nursing Research* 28 (1996).

398 Chalmers, and Levin.
399 Chalmers, and Levin.
400 Chalmers, and Levin.
401 Chalmers, and Levin.
402 B Chalmers, and D Meyers, "Babies with Abnormalities: Reactions of Mothers," *International Journal of Prenatal and Perinatal Studies* 1 (1990).
403 Chalmers, and Meyers.
404 Chalmers, and Meyers.
405 Chalmers, and Meyers.
406 Chalmers, and Meyers.
407 Chalmers, and Meyers.
408 The Lancet, "It Happened to Me: Responses to the Stillbirth Series," *The Lancet* 377, no. 9779 (2011).
409 Enkin et al.
410 Hodnett et al.
411 Enkin et al.
412 Hodnett et al.
413 Jennifer Worth, *Call the Midwife: A Memoir of Birth, Joy, and Hard Times* (London, UK: Penguin Books, 2002).
414 B Chalmers, and D Meyers, "What Men Say About Pregnancy, Birth and Parenthood.," *Journal of Psychosomatic Obstetrics and Gynaecology* 17 (1996).
415 Enkin et al.
416 Public Health Agency of Canada.
417 Hodnett et al, M H Klaus, and J H Kennell, "The Doula: An Essential Ingredient of Childbirth Rediscovered," *Acta Paediatrica* 86, no. 10 (1997).
418 Chalmers, and Levin.
419 Chalmers, and Levin.
420 N. Ko et al., "Can Patient Navigation Improve Receipt of Recommended Breast Cancer Care? Evidence from the National Patient Navigation Research Program," *Journal of Clinical Oncology* 32, no. 22 (2014), https://dx.doi.org/10.1200/JCO.2013.53.6037.
421 Chalmers, and Levin.
422 Chalmers, and Levin.
423 Chalmers, and Levin.
424 Chalmers, and Levin.
425 H Clinton, and B Obama, "Making Patient Safety the Centerpiece of Medical Liability Reform.," *New England Journal of Medicine* 354 (2006), S Kraman, and G Hamm, "Risk Management: Extreme Honesty May Be the Best Policy.," *Annals of Internal Medicine* 131

(1999), J Ogloff, and R Schuller, *Introduction to Psychology and Law: Canadian Perspectives* (Toronto: University of Toronto Press, 2001).

426 Canadian Medical Protective Association, "Apology Legislation in Canada: What It Means for Physicians," Canadian Medical Protective Association, last modified Originally published September 2008 / Revised April 2013, April 2013, accessed 17 April, 2015, https://www.cmpa-acpm.ca/-/apology-legislation-in-canada-what-it-means-for-physicians.

427 Laura MacGregor, "Unspoken Wounds: A Mother's Experience of Medical Error.," *CMAJ* 197, E815-6 (2025), https://dx.doi.org/doi: 10.1503/cmaj.25008.

428 MacGregor.

429 Kirsten Patrick, "The Importance of Saying Sorry When Things Go Wrong in Health Care," *CMAJ* 197, no. 27, E813-E814 (2025), https://dx.doi.org/https://doi.org/10.1503/cmaj.251210.

430 Public Health Agency of Canada.

431 Chalmers, and Omer-Hashi.

432 Kukura 787.

433 Chalmers, and Levin.

434 Chalmers, and Levin.

435 Public Health Agency of Canada.

436 Declercq, and Chalmers.

437 Wanda Barfield, "Transcript: One in 5 Women Reported Mistreatment While Receiving Maternity Care," Vital Signs Report CDC, 2023, accessed August 22, 2023, https://www.cdc.gov/media/releases/2023/t0822-vs-maternity-mistreatment.html#:~:text=This%20Vital%20Signs%20report%20found,and%2027%25%20were%20multiracial%20women.

438 Hazel Keedle et al., "What Women Want If They Were to Have Another Baby: The Australian Birth Experience Study (Best) Cross-Sectional National Survey," *BMJ* 13, no. 9 (2023), https://dx.doi.org/DOI: 10.1136/bmjopen-2023-071582.

439 Chalmers, "Childbirth across Cultures: Research and Practice."

440 M MacDorman, F Menacker, and E Declercq, "Trends and Characteristics of Home and Other out-of-Hospital Births in the United States 1990-2006," *National Vital Statistics Report* 58, no. 11 (2010).

441 CDC National Vital Statistics Reports, *Changes in Home Births by Race and Hispanic Origin and State of Residence of Mother: United States, 2018-20-19 and 2019 - 2020.*, by Elizabeth C.W. Gregory, Michelle J.K. Osterman, and Claudia P. Valenzuela. (USA: U S Deparment of Health and Social Sservices., 2021).

442 MacDorman, Menacker, and Declercq.

443 L Vogel, ""Do It Yourself" Births Prompt Alarm," *Canadian Medical Association Journal* 183, no. 6 (2011).

444 Sirin Kale, and Lucy Osborne, "Five Key Findings from Our Investigation into the Free Birth Society," *The Guardian* (UK), November 23 2025, https://www.theguardian.com/lifeandstyle/2025/nov/23five-key-findings-from-our-investigation-into-the-free-birth-society.

445 Kale, and Osborne.

446 Kale, and Osborne.

447 Sirin Kale, and Lucy Osborne, "Influencers Made Millions Pushing 'Wild' Births – Now the Free Birth Society Is Linked to Baby Deaths around the World," *The Guardian* (UK), 22 November, 2025, https://www.theguardian.com/world/ng-interactive/2025/nov/22/free-birth-society-linked-to-babies-deaths-investigation.

448 Beverley Chalmers, "Shame on Us!," *Birth* 38, no. 4 (2011).

449 Chalmers, "Shame on Us!."

450 Chalmers, and Dzakpasu.

451 Lauri van den Berg et al., "Childbirth Experiences in the United Kingdom Compared to the Netherlands: A Cross-Sectional Survey Study," *Birth* 0 (2025), https://dx.doi.org/doi.org/10.1111/birt.70006.

452 Karin Johnson et al., "Medical Interventions and Women's Perceptions of Respectful Intrapartum Care: A National Survey-Based Cohort Study," *BJOG* 0, no. 1-12 (2025), https://dx.doi.org/doi.org/10.1111/1471-0528.18329.

453 Public Health Agency of Canada.

454 H Keedle et al., "Women's Reasons for, and Experiences of, Choosing a Homebirth Following a Caesarean Section," *BMC Pregnancy and Childbirth* 15, no. 206 (2015), https://dx.doi.org/10.1186/s12884-015-0639-4, Keedle et al.

455 Society of Obstetricians and Gynaecologists of Canada, *Improving Sexual and Reproductive Health: Integrating Women's Empowerment and Reproductive Rights*, vol. July 16, 2011. http://iwhp.sogc.org/uploads/File/ISRH_booklet_web.pdf.

456 Society of Obstetricians and Gynaecologists of Canada, *Improving Sexual and Reproductive Health: Integrating Women's Empowerment and Reproductive Rights.*

457 E Declercq et al., "Is a Rising Cesarean Delivery Rate Inevitable? Trends in Industrialized Countries, 1987 to 2007," *Birth* 38, no. 2 (2011), M Keirse, "Commentary: The Freezing Aftermath of a Hot Randomized Controlled Trial.," *Birth* 38, no. 2 (2011), M Klein et al., "Attitudes of the New Generation of Canadian Obstetricians: How Do They Differ from Their Predecessors?," *Birth* 38, no. 2 (2011), A Kotaska, "Guideline-Centered Care: A Two-Edged Sword.," *Birth* 38, no. 2 (2011), A Kotaska,

"Commentary: Routine Cesarean Section for Breech: The Unmeasured Cost.," *Birth* 38, no. 2 (2011), G W Lawson, "Report of a Breech Cesarean Section Maternal Death.," *Birth* 38, no. 2 (2011), Declercq et al, Keirse, "Commentary: The Freezing Aftermath of a Hot Randomized Controlled Trial.", Klein et al, Kotaska, Kotaska, Lawson.

458 A Banaszek, "Medical Humanities Becoming Prerequisites in Many Medical Schools," *Canadian Medical Association Journal* 183, no. 8 (2011), Enkin et al.

459 Public Health Agency of Canada.

460 D Bowen et al., "Discussions after Death," *South African Medical Journal* 78 (1990), D Skibniewski-Woods, "A Review of Postnatal Debriefing of Mothers Following Traumatic Delivery.," *Community Practice.* 84, no. 12 (2011).

461 B E Chalmers, and B M Chalmers, "Post-Partum Depression: A Revised Perspective," *Journal of Psychosomatic Obstetrics and Gynaecology* 5 (1986), C Pesado et al., "Postpartum Depression and Culture: Maternal Child Nursing " *The American Journal of Maternal/Child Nursing* 35, no. 5 (2010).

462 F J Paulson, D Sharnail, and M S Bazemore, "Prenatal and Postpartum Depression in Fathers and Its Association with Maternal Depression a Meta-Analysis," *JAMA* 303, no. 19 (2010).

463 Public Health Agency of Canada.

464 M St-André, P N Reebye, and J-V Wittenberg, "Infant Mental Health in Canada: Initiatives from British Columbia, Québec and Ontario," *Journal of the Canadian Academy of Child and Adolescent Psychiatry* 19, no. 2 (2010).

465 Cindy-Lee Dennis, and Ellen Hodnett, "Psychosocial and Psychological Interventions for Treating Postpartum Depression.," *Cochrane Database of Systematic Reviews* 4 (2009).

466 B Chalmers, and D Meyers, "Adjustment to the Early Months of Parenthood.," *International Journal of Pre-natal and Perinatal Studies* 1 (1990), Skibniewski-Woods, Skibniewski-Woods, G W S Kong, T K H Chung, and I H Lok, "The Impact of Supportive Counselling on Women's Psychological Wellbeing after Miscarriage – a Randomised Controlled Trial.," *BJOG* 121, no. 10 (2014).

467 Public Health Agency of Canada.

468 A Maslow, *Motivation and Personality* (New York: Harper, 1943).

469 Beverley Chalmers, "How Often Must We Ask for Sensitive Care before We Get It?," *Birth* 29, no. 2 (2002).

470 Public Health Agency of Canada.

471 Public Health Agency of Canada.

472 Chalmers, and Levin, Penny Simkin, "Should ACOG Support Childbirth Education as Another Means to Improve Obstetric Outcomes? Response

to ACOG Committee Opinion # 687: Approaches to Limit Intervention during Labor and Birth," *Birth* 44, no. 4 (2017), https://dx.doi.org/doi.org/10.1111/birt.12306.

473 A J Gagnon, and J Sandall, "Individual or Group Antenatal Education for Childbirth or Parenthood, or Both.," *Cochrane Pregnancy and Childbirth Group* (2007), http://onlinelibrary.wiley.com/o/cochrane/clabout/articles/PREG/frame.html.

474 B Chalmers, and J McIntyre, "Do Antenatal Classes Have a Place in Modern Obstetric Care?," *International Journal of Psychosomatic Obstetrics and Gynaecology* 15 (1994).

475 B Chalmers, and G J Hofmeyr, "The Gestation of a Childbirth Education Diploma.," *Journal of Psychosomatic Obstetrics & Gynaecology* 10 (1989).

476 Chalmers, and Hofmeyr.

477 Public Health Agency of Canada.

478 Beverley Chalmers et al., "Use of Routine Interventions in Vaginal Labor and Birth: Findings from the Maternity Experiences Survey," *Birth* 36, no. 1 (2009).

479 L Gramling, K Hickman, and S Bennett, "What Makes a Good Family-Centered Partnership between Women and Their Practitioners? A Qualitative Study.," *Birth* 31, no. 1 (2004).

480 A M Romano, "Creating a Culture of Consumer Engagement in Maternity Care.," *Journal of Perinatal Education* 19, no. 2 (2010).

481 Public Health Agency of Canada.

482 Public Health Agency of Canada.

483 J Adams et al., "Attitudes and Referral Practices of Maternity Care Professionals with Regard to Complementary and Alternative Medicine: An Integrative Review," *Journal of Advanced Nursing* 67, no. 3 (2011).

484 Nikodem VC et al., "Do Cabbage Leaves Prevent Breast Engorgement? A Randomized, Controlled Study," *Birth* 20, no. 2 (1993).

485 Chalmers, and Levin.

486 Cristina Mattison et al., "Understanding the Conditions That Influence the Roles of Midwives in Ontario, Canada's Health System: An Embedded Single-Case Study.," *BMC Health Services Research* 20 (2020), https://dx.doi.org/https://doi.org/10.1186/s12913-020-5033-x.

487 Public Health Agency of Canada.

488 J Ratti et al., "Playing Nice: Improving the Professional Climate between Physicians and Midwives in the Calgary Area," *JOGC* 36, no. 7 (2014).

489 Harvey et al, Hueston, and Rudy.

490 Midwives Alliance North America, "What Is a Midwife?," 2015, accessed 24 June, 2015, http://mana.org/about-midwives/what-is-a-midwife, Canadian Association of Midwives, "Midwifery in Canada Is

Growing," *The Pinard: Newsletter of the Canadian Association of Midwives* 5, no. 1 (2015).
491 Chalmers, and Levin.
492 Chalmers, and Levin.
493 Beverley Chalmers, "The Case for Perinatal Psychologists," *Perinatology* 6, no. 6 (2004).
494 Evelyn Verbeke et al., "Cost-Effectiveness of Mental-Health Interventions during and after Pregnancy: A Systematic Review," *Birth* March (2022), https://dx.doi.org/https://doi.org/10.1111/birt.12623.
495 Beverley Chalmers, and Bernard Chalmers, "Post-Partum Depression: A Revised Perspective," *Journal of Psychosomatic Obsterics and Gynaecology* 5 (1986), Rieko Kishi Fukuzawa, and Chang Gi Park, "Role of Intrapartum Social Support in Preventing Postpartum Depression," *The Journal of Perinatal Education* 32, no. 2 (2023), https://dx.doi.org/10.1891/JPE-2022-0003, W-L Wolman et al., "Post-Partum Depression and Companionship in the Clinical Birth Environment: A Review and Randomized Controlled Study.," *American Journal of Obstetrics and Gynecology* 168 (1993).
496 Chalmers, and Levin.
497 Nicole Thompson, "Lessons on the Grief of Perinatal Loss as an Obstetric Provider," *JOGC* 47, no. 9 (2025), https://www.sciencedirect.com/science/article/pii/S1701216325003469?dgcid=author.
498 Chalmers, "The Case for Perinatal Psychologists."
499 Chalmers, "The Case for Perinatal Psychologists."
500 Chalmers, *Family-Centred Perinatal Care: Improving Pregnancy, Birth and Postpartum Care.*
501 Chalmers et al.
502 National Collaborating Centre for Womens and Childrens Health.
503 H C Brown, and H J Smith, "Giving Women Their Own Case Notes to Carry during Pregnancy," *Cochrane database of systematic reviews* (2):CD002856 (2004).
504 Brown, and Smith.
505 Beverley Chalmers, "Multicultural, Multidisciplinary, Psycho-Social Obstetric Care.," *Journal of Obstetrics and Gynaecology of Canada* 21 (1999), Ratti et al.
506 Chalmers, and Levin.
507 Banaszek.
508 Banaszek.
509 Chalmers, and McIntyre.
510 PHAC Public Health Agency of Canada, *Canadian Hospitals Maternity Policies and Practices Survey* (Ottawa, ON: Public Health Agency of Canada, 2012).

511 Public Health Agency of Canada, *Canadian Hospitals Maternity Policies and Practices Survey.*
512 Chalmers, and Levin.
513 Chalmers, and Levin, Beverley Chalmers, "Globalization and Perinatal Health Care.," *BJOG* 111, no. 9 (2004).
514 Chalmers, *African Birth: Childbirth in Cultural Transition.* , Chalmers, "Globalization and Perinatal Health Care."
515 Beverley Chalmers, "Cultural Issues in Perinatal Care.," *Birth* 40, no. 4 (2013).
516 Adams et al, Chalmers, *African Birth: Childbirth in Cultural Transition.* , Beverley Chalmers, "Western and African Conceptualizations of Birth.," *Psychology and Health* 12 (1996), Chalmers, "Multicultural, Multidisciplinary, Psycho-Social Obstetric Care.", Chalmers, Chalmers, "Childbirth across Cultures: Research and Practice.", Chalmers, "Cultural Issues in Perinatal Care.", Chalmers, and Jeckaite, Chalmers, and Omer-Hashi, Chalmers, and Qulieva, Chalmers et al., "Women's Experiences of Birth in St Petersburg, Russian Federation Following a Maternal-Child Health Intervention Program.", Chalmers et al., "What Women Say About Post-Partum Care and Breastfeeding in St Petersburg, Russian Federation.", Chalmers et al.
517 Chalmers, "Cultural Issues in Perinatal Care.", Chalmers, and Levin.
518 Jessica Gildersleeve, and Devaleena Das, *Birthing Stories: Silence, Trauma, and the Power of Narratives in Clinical Care.* (In Preparation, 2026).
519 Gildersleeve, and Das.
520 Chalmers, "Globalization and Perinatal Health Care."
521 Public Health Agency of Canada.
522 Chalmers, *African Birth: Childbirth in Cultural Transition.* .
523 Chalmers, "Psychosomatic Obstetrics and Gynaecology in the New Millenium: Some Thoughts and Observations.", Chalmers, and Omer-Hashi.
524 Chalmers, and Omer-Hashi.
525 Chalmers, and Omer-Hashi.
526 B Chalmers, and K Omer-Hashi., "What Somali Women Say About Birth in Canada.," *Journal of Reproductive and Infant Psychology* 20 (2002).
527 Chalmers, and Omer-Hashi.
528 Chalmers, and Omer-Hashi.
529 Chalmers, and Omer-Hashi.
530 Public Health Agency of Canada.
531 C Reading, and F Wein, *Health Inequalities and Social Determinants of Aboriginal Peoples' Health* (2009). http://www.nccah.ote

532 V K Douglas, "Childbirth among the Canadian Inuit: A Review of the Clinical and Cultural Literature " *International Journal of Circumpolar Health* 65, no. 2 (2006).
533 *In Plain Sight: Addressing Indigenous-Specific Racism and Discrimination in BC Health Care*, by B C Health Care (Vancouver: BC Government report, 2020).
534 *In Plain Sight.*
535 *In Plain Sight.*
536 Boyer, and Bartlett.
537 Yvonne Boyer, "Healing Racism in Canadian Health Care," *CMAJ* 189, no. 46 (2017), https://dx.doi.org/https://doi.org/10.1503/cmaj.171234.
538 Chalmers, and Levin, Chalmers, "Cultural Issues in Perinatal Care."
539 Chalmers, "Psychosomatic Obstetrics and Gynaecology in the New Millenium: Some Thoughts and Observations."
540 Chalmers, "Psychosomatic Obstetrics and Gynaecology in the New Millenium: Some Thoughts and Observations."
541 Gildersleeve, and Das.
542 Chalmers, "Cultural Issues in Perinatal Care.", Chalmers, and Levin.
543 Chalmers, "Cultural Issues in Perinatal Care.", Chalmers, and Levin.
544 Chalmers, "Cultural Issues in Perinatal Care.", Chalmers, and Levin.
545 Public Health Agency of Canada.
546 Chalmers, "Cultural Issues in Perinatal Care.", Chalmers, and Levin.
547 Chalmers, "Cultural Issues in Perinatal Care.", Chalmers, and Levin.
548 Chalmers, "Cultural Issues in Perinatal Care.", Chalmers, and Levin.
549 Chalmers, and Levin, Chalmers, "Cultural Issues in Perinatal Care."
550 Chalmers, "Cultural Issues in Perinatal Care.", Chalmers, and Levin.
551 K Sutton, and B Chalmers, "Contraception and Pregnancy Options," in *Human Sexuality*, ed. C Pukall (Toronto: Oxford University Press, 2014).
552 B Chalmers, "What Do International Health Consultants Need to Know?," *Journal of the Society of Obstetricians and Gynaecologists of Canada* 21 (1999).
553 Chalmers, "What Do International Health Consultants Need to Know? ."
554 WHO, "WHO Health for All Database," WHO 20212021, http://www.euro.who.int/en/data-and-evidence/databases/european-health-for-all-database-hfa-db.
555 Public Health Agency of Canada, *Perinatal Health Indicators for Canada 2011.*
556 Beck et al.
557 Declercq, Sakala, and Corry, Declercq, Sakala, and Corry.
558 BORN Ontario, "BORN: Better Outcomes Registry and Network," 2015, accessed 1 July 2015, https://www.bornontario.ca/en/about-born/.

559 Chelsea Gomez, and Tara Carman, "Canada Significantly Undercounts Maternal Deaths, and Doctors Are Sounding the Alarm," *CBC* (Canada), October 3, 2022, https://www.cbc.ca/news/canada/canada-maternal-deaths-undercount-1.6600905#:~:text=Canada%C2%B7CBC%20Investigates-,Canada%20significantly%20undercounts%20maternal%20deaths%2C%20and%20doctors%20are%20sounding%20the,maternal%20deaths%20and%20close%20calls.
560 Public Health Agency of Canada.
561 Declercq, Sakala, and Corry, Declercq, Sakala, and Corry.
562 Beck et al.
563 Green, Coupland, and Kitzinger, Green et al.
564 Brown, and Lumley, A Calder, and P Purton, *Maternity Care Matters: An Audit of Maternity Services in Scotland 1998. Scottish Program for Clinical Effectiveness in Reproductive Health* (Aberdeen: Douglas Baird Centre for Research on Women's Health, 1999), Chalmers, *African Birth: Childbirth in Cultural Transition.* , Chalmers, and Jeckaite, Chalmers et al, Chalmers, and Qulieva, Chalmers et al., "Women's Experiences of Birth in St Petersburg, Russian Federation Following a Maternal-Child Health Intervention Program.", Chalmers et al., "What Women Say About Post-Partum Care and Breastfeeding in St Petersburg, Russian Federation.", Chalmers et al, Declercq, Sakala, and Corry, Declercq, Sakala, and Corry, Heiberg et al, Stratulat et al.
565 Chalmers, and Jeckaite, Chalmers, and Meyers, "What Men Say About Pregnancy, Birth and Parenthood."
566 Public Health Agency of Canada.
567 Public Health Agency of Canada, *Canadian Hospitals Maternity Policies and Practices Survey.*
568 Public Health Agency of Canada.
569 Cavalli, and Copp.
570 Euiqui Cen et al., "Maternal Myo-Inositol Intake and Congenital Heart Defects in Offspring: A Population Based Case-Control Study," *BJOG* 0 (2025), https://dx.doi.org/doi.org/10.1111/1471-0528.70045.
571 Chalmers, and Meyers, "What Men Say About Pregnancy, Birth and Parenthood.", L Freedman, and M Kruk, "Disrespect and Abuse of Women in Childbirth: Challenging the Global Quality and Accountability Agendas," *The Lancet* Early Online Publication (23 June 2014), https://dx.doi.org/doi:10.1016/S0140-6736(14)60859-X, J O'Leary, and C Thorwick, "Father's Perspectives during Pregnancy, Postperinatal Loss," *Journal of Obstetrics, Gynecology, and Neonatal Nursing* 35, no. 1 (2006).
572 Chalmers, "Childbirth across Cultures: Research and Practice."
573 M E Hannah et al., "Planned Caesarean Section Versus Planned Vaginal Birth for Breech Presentation at Term: A Randomised Multicentre Trial.," *Lancet* 356, no. 1375-1383 (2000).

574 B Chalmers, “What Should International Health Consultants Know?,” *Bulletin of the World Health Organization* 77 (1999), Chalmers, “What Do International Health Consultants Need to Know?.”, Beverley Chalmers, “How Ethical Is International Perinatal Research? Challenges and Misconceptions,” *Birth* 34, no. 3 (2007).

575 Chalmers, “How Ethical Is International Perinatal Research? Challenges and Misconceptions.”

576 Chalmers, “How Ethical Is International Perinatal Research? Challenges and Misconceptions.”

577 Chalmers, “How Ethical Is International Perinatal Research? Challenges and Misconceptions.”

578 Kramer et al.

579 Chalmers, “How Ethical Is International Perinatal Research? Challenges and Misconceptions.”

580 Chalmers, “How Ethical Is International Perinatal Research? Challenges and Misconceptions.”

581 S Benatar, “Reflections and Recommendations on Research Ethics in Developing Countries.,” *Social Science and Medicine* 54 (2002), G Lindegger, and L M Richter, “HIV Vaccine Trials: Critical Issues in Informed Consent.,” *South African Journal of Science.* 96 (2000).

582 Simonovic.

583 Simonovic.

584 Simonovic.

585 Jill Arnold, ““Obstetric Violence” Introduced as a New Legal Term in Venezuela,” 2010, accessed 27 April, 2015, http://www.theunnecesarean.com/blog/2010/11/7/obstetric-violence-introduced-as-a-new-legal-term-in-venezue.html, Canada: Immigration and Refugee Board of Canada, *Venezuela: Implementation and Effectiveness of the 2007 Organic Law on the Right of Women to a Life Free of Violence*, 3 April 2008 ed., *Refworld* (Ottawa: Immigration and Refugee Board of Canada, 2008).

586 Arnold, Canada.

587 Arnold, Canada.

588 WHO, *The Prevention and Elimination of Disrespect and Abuse during Facility-Based Childbirth* (Geneva: World Health Organization, 2015).

589 WHO, *The Prevention and Elimination of Disrespect and Abuse during Facility-Based Childbirth.*

590 E Shakibazadeh et al., “Respectful Care during Childbirth in Health Facilities Globally: A Qualitative Evidence Synthesis,” *BJOG* 125, no. 8 (2018), https://dx.doi.org/https://doi.org/10.1111/1471-0528.15015.

591 Bowser, and Hill.

592 Rubino et al, Chalmers, and Omer-Hashi.

593 Bowser, and Hill, Freedman, and Kruk.

594 J P Vogel et al., “Promoting Respect and Preventing Mistreatment during Childbirth,” *BJOG* 123, no. 5 (2016).

Bibliography

Abalos, E, M Chamillard, V Diaz, O Tuncalp, and A M Gulmezoglu. "Antenatal Care for Healthy Pregnant Women: A Mapping of Interventions from Existing Guidelines to Inform the Development of New WHO Guidelines on Antenatal Care." *BJOG* (2015). Accessed 23 December 2015. https://dx.doi.org/DOI: 10.1111/1471-0528.13820.

Adams, J, C W Lui, D Sibbritt, A Broom, J Wardle, and C Homer. "Attitudes and Referral Practices of Maternity Care Professionals with Regard to Complementary and Alternative Medicine: An Integrative Review." *Journal of Advanced Nursing* 67, no. 3 (2011): 472-83.

Affonso, D, E Basque, V Wahlberg, and J Brady. "Reconciliation and Healing for Mothers through Skin-to-Skin Contact Provided in an American Tertiary Level Intensive Care Nursery." *Neonatal Network* 12 (1993): 25-32.

Alio, A P, H M Salihu, J L Kornosky, A M Richman, and P J Marty. "Feto-Infant Health and Survival: Does Paternal Involvement Matter?", *Maternal Child Health Journal* 14, no. 6 (2010): 931-37.

Alison Gemmill, Claire E. Margerison, Elizabeth A. Stuart, and Suzanne O. Bell. "Infant Deaths after Texas' 2021 Ban on Abortion in Early Pregnancy." *JAMA Paediatrics* 178, no. 8 (2024): 784-91. https://dx.doi.org/doi:10.1001/jamapediatrics.2024.0885.

Als, H. " Individualized, Family-Focused Developmental Care for the Very-Low-Birthweight Preterm Infant in the NICU." In *The Psychological Development of Low-Birthweight Children*. Edited by Sigman MD Friedman SL. Norwood, NJ: Ablex., 1992.

Als, H. "Program Guide: Newborn Individualized Developmental Care and Assessment Program. An Education and Training Program for Health Care Professionals." 2014. http://www.nidcap.org.

Als, H, and L Gilkerson. "The Role of Relationship-Based Developmentally Supportive Care in Strengthening Outcome of Preterm Infants." *Seminars in Perinatology* 21 (1997): 178-89.

Als, H, G Lawhon, F H Duffy, G B McAnulty, R Gibes-Grossman, and J G Blickman. "Individualized Perinatal Care for the Very-Low-Birth-Weight Preterm Infant." *Journal of the American Medical Association* 11 (1994): 853-58.

Althabe, F, C Sosa, J Belizán, L Gibbons, F Jacquerioz, and E Bergel. "Cesarean Section Rates and Maternal and Neonatal Mortality in Low-Middle- and High-Income Countries: An Ecological Study.", *Birth* 33, no. 4 (2006): 270-7.

Anderson, G C. "Current Knowledge About Skin-to-Skin (Kangaroo) Care for Preterm Infants." *Journal of Perinatology* 11 (1991): 216-26.

Anonymous. "Our Family Secrets." *Annuls of Internal Medicine* 163, no. 4 (2015): 321. https://dx.doi.org/10.7326/M14-2168.

Armstrong, Elizabeth Mitchell. "Making Sense of Advice About Drinking during Pregnancy: Does Evidence Even Matter?", *Journal of Perinatal Education* 26, no. 2 (2017): 65-9. https://dx.doi.org/10.1891/1058-1243.26.2.65.

Arnold, Jill. ""Obstetric Violence" Introduced as a New Legal Term in Venezuela." 2010. Accessed 27 April, 2015. http://www.theunnecesarean.com/blog/2010/11/7/obstetric-violence-introduced-as-a-new-legal-term-in-venezue.html.

Atkins, Bethany, Hannah Blencowe, Frances M. Boyle, Emma Sacks, Dell Horey, and Vicki Flenady. "Is Care of Stillborn Babies and Their Parents Respectful? Results from an International Online Survey." *BJOG: An International Journal of Obstetrics & Gynaecology* (2022). https://dx.doi.org/ https://doi.org/10.1111/1471-0528.17138.

Austin, M P, J Colton, S Priest, N Reilly, and D Hadzi-Pavlovic. "The Antenatal Risk Questionnaire: Acceptability and Use for Psychosocial Risk Assessment in the Maternity Setting.", *Women*

Birth 26, no. 1 (2013): 17-25. https://dx.doi.org/10.1016/j.wombi.2011.06.002.

Bahl, Rachna, Emily Hotton, Joanna Crofts, and Tim Draycott. "Assisted Vaginal Birth in 21st Century: Current Practice and New Innovations." *American Journal of Obstetrics and Gynecology*, no. March (2024): 917-31.

Banaszek, A. "Medical Humanities Becoming Prerequisites in Many Medical Schools." *Canadian Medical Association Journal* 183, no. 8 (2011): c441-c42.

Barfield, Wanda. "Transcript: One in 5 Women Reported Mistreatment While Receiving Maternity Care." Vital Signs Report CDC. 2023. Accessed August 22, 2023. https://www.cdc.gov/media/releases/2023/t0822-vs-maternity-mistreatment.html#:~:text=This%20Vital%20Signs%20report%20found,and%2027%25%20were%20multiracial%20women.

Batram-Zantvoort, Stephanie, Céline Miani, Ilaria Mariani, Emanuelle Pessa Valente, Mehreen Zaigham, Ingvild Hersoug Nedberg, Magdalena Kurbanović, Elizabete Pumpure, Anja Bohinec, Antigone Sarantaki, Barbara Baranowska, Aessia Abderhalden-Zellweger, Elise de La Rochebrochard, Raquel Costa, Marina Ruxandra Otelea, Alina Liepinaitienė, Jelena Radetic, Amira Ćerimagić, Maryse Arendt, Martina König-Bachmann, Stefano Delle Vedove, Karolina Linden, Sigrun Kongslien, Daniela Drandić, Darta Kreslina, Zalka Drglin, Dimitra Metallinou, Urszula Tataj-Puzyna, Michael Gemperle, Virginie Rozée, Heloísa Dias, Marija Mizgaitienė, Jovana Ruzicic, Imola Simon, Simona Fumagalli, Helen Elden, Eline Skirnisdottir Vik, Barbara Mihevc Ponikvar, Aikaterini Lykeridou, Beata Szlendak, Claire de Labrusse, Tiago Miguel Pinto, Simona Jazdauskienė, Christoph Zenzmaier, Ilana Chertok, Emma Sacks, Marzia Lazzerini, and on behalf of IMAgiNE EURO Study group. "The Association between Women's Perception of Birth during the Pandemic, Companion of Choice and Support from Health Professionals: A Cross-Sectional Study in 20 Countries in the WHO European Region." *Birth* 52 (2025): 677-89. https://dx.doi.org/doi.org/10.1111/birt.12915.

Beck, L F, C H Johnson, B Morrow, and et al. *PRAMS 1999 Surveillance Report*. Atlanta, GA: Division of Reproductive Health, National

Center for Chronic Disease Prevention and Health Promotion, Centers for Disease Control and Prevention, 2003.

Bell, Susan. "Quebec Indigenous Groups Collecting Stories of Forced Sterilization." (Canada)2021, https://www.cbc.ca/news/canada/north/indigenous-forced-sterilization-quebec-study-cree-1.6186212.

Bellafante, Ginia. "JD Vance and the Age-Old Trope of 'Childless Cat Ladies'." *The New York Times* (New York)2024, https://www.nytimes.com/2024/07/25/nyregion/jd-vance-kamala-harris-cat-lady.html.

Benatar, S. "Reflections and Recommendations on Research Ethics in Developing Countries.", *Social Science and Medicine* 54 (2002): 1131-41.

Berg, Lauri van den, Jens Henrichs, Jeroesnvan Dillen, Soo Downe, and Corine Verhoeven. "Childbirth Experiences in the United Kingdom Compared to the Netherlands: A Cross-Sectional Survey Study." *Birth* 0 (2025): 1-10. https://dx.doi.org/doi.org/10.1111/birt.70006.

Berghella, V, E Buchanan, L Pereira, and J K Baxter. "Preconception Care.", *Obstetrical & Gynecological Survey* 65, no. 2 (2010): 119-31.

Berker, P T, P C Grunwald, J Moorman, and S Stuhr. "Outcomes of Developmentally Supportive Care for Very Low Birthweight Infants." *Nursing Research* 40 (1991): 150-55.

Betran, A P, M R Torloni, J Zhang, A M Gülmezoglu, and and the WHO Working Group on Caesarean Section. "WHO Statement on Caesarean Section Rates.", *BJOG* 123, no. 5 (2016): 667-70. https://dx.doi.org/10.1111/1471-0528.13526.

Bevilacqua, G, M Corradi, G P Donzelli, V Fanos, D Gianotti, C Magnani, M Orzalesi, S Parmigiani, D Pedrotti, and G PSalvioli. "The Parma Charter of the Rights of the Newborn." Accessed 13 February, 2016. http://www.uenps.com/media/Parma%20Charter%20Rights%20of%20the%20newborn.pdf.

Boffey, Daniel. "Netherlands Fertility Doctor Used Own Sperm to Father 21 Children " *The Guardian* (Brussels)2022, https://www.theguardian.com/world/2022/feb/02/netherlands-fertility-doctor-jos-beek-father-21-children.

Bohren, Meghan, Joshua P Vogel, Erin C Hunter, Otha Lutsiv, Suprita K Makh, Joao Paulo Souza, Carolina Agular, Fernando Sariava Coneglian, Alex Luiz Araujo Diniz, Ozge Tuncalp, Dena Javadi, Olufemi T Oladapo, Rajat Khosia, Michelle J Hindin, and A Metin Gulmezoglu. "The Mistreatment of Women during Childbirth in Health Facilities Globally: A Mixed-Methods Systematic Review." *PLOS Medicine* 12, no. 6 (2015). https://dx.doi.org/10.1371/journal.pmed.1001847.

Bolton, K D, B Chalmers, P Cooper, and E Wainer. "Black Mother's Experiences of a Neonatal Care Unit." *Journal of Reproductive and Infant Psychology* 11 (1993): 229-34.

BORN Ontario. "BORN: Better Outcomes Registry and Network." 2015. Accessed 1 July 2015. https://www.bornontario.ca/en/about-born/.

Boundy, E O, R Dastjerdi, D Spiegelman, W W Fawzi, S A Missmer, E Lieberman, S Kajeepeta, S Wall, and G J Chan. "Kangaroo Mother Care and Neonatal Outcomes: A Meta-Analysis." *Pediatrics* 137, no. 1 (2016): 1-16. https://dx.doi.org/ DOI: 10.1542/peds.2015-2238.

Bowen, D, C Van Gelderen, B Chalmers, and A Hamilton. "Discussions after Death." *South African Medical Journal* 78 (1990): 760.

Bowser, D, and K Hill. *Exploring Evidence for Disrespect and Abuse in Facility-Based Childbirth: Report of a Landscape Analysis* Washington, DC: USAID-TRAction Project. Harvard School of Public Health and University Research Co, 2010.

Boyer, Yvonne. "Healing Racism in Canadian Health Care." *CMAJ* 189, no. 46 (2017): E1408-E09. https://dx.doi.org/https://doi.org/10.1503/cmaj.171234.

Boyer, Yvonne, and Judith Bartlett. External Review: Tubal Ligation in the Saskatoon Health Region: The Lived Experience of Aboriginal Women. Health Region Saskatoon. Canada. https://www.saskatoonhealthregion.ca/DocumentsInternal/Tubal_Ligation_intheSaskatoonHealthRegion_the_Lived_Experience_of_Aboriginal_Women_BoyerandBartlett_July_22_2017.pdf.

Bragg, F, D A Cromwell, L C Edozien, I Gurol-Urganci, T A Mahmood, and A Templeton. "Variation in Rates of Caesarean Section among English NHS Trusts after Accounting for Maternal and Clinical

Risk: Cross Sectional Study." *British Medical Journal* 341 (2010): c5065.

Brown, H C, and H J Smith. "Giving Women Their Own Case Notes to Carry during Pregnancy." *Cochrane database of systematic reviews* (2):CD002856 (2004).

Brown, L D, and J A Heerman. "The Effect of Developmental Care on Preterm Infant Outcome." *Applied Nursing Research* 10 (1997): 190-97.

Brown, S, and J Lumley. "Satisfaction with Care in Labour and Birth: A Survey of 790 Australian Women." *Birth* 21 (1994): 4-13.

Buchler, D M, H Als, F M Duffy, G B McAnulty, and J Leiderman. "Effectiveness of Individualized Developmental Care for Low-Risk Preterm Infants: Behavioral and Electrophysiological Evidence." *Pediatrics* 96 (1995): 923-32.

Byland, B, T Cervin, and O Finnstrom. "Morbidity and Neurological Function of Very Low Birthweight Infants from the Newborn Period to 4 Years of Age: A Prospective Study from the South-East Region of Sweden." *Acta Pediatrica* 87 (1998): 758-63.

Cai, Derek. "Japan Sterilisation Law Victims Included Nine-Year-Olds." BBC. 2023. Accessed 20 June, 2023. https://www.bbc.com/news/world-asia-65958119.

Calder, A, and P Purton. *Maternity Care Matters: An Audit of Maternity Services in Scotland 1998. Scottish Program for Clinical Effectiveness in Reproductive Health.* Aberdeen: Douglas Baird Centre for Research on Women's Health, 1999.

Canada, Canada: Immigration and Refugee Board of. *Venezuela: Implementation and Effectiveness of the 2007 Organic Law on the Right of Women to a Life Free of Violence.* 3 April 2008 ed. Refworld. Ottawa: Immigration and Refugee Board of Canada, 2008.

Canada, Obesity. "Overcoming Weight Bias: Do You Have It in You." Obesity Canada. 2024. Accessed 19 February, 2024. https://obesitycanada.ca/wp-content/uploads/2022/07/Overcoming-Weight-Bias-11x17-May-2018-Eng-Fr4-4.pdf.

Canadian Medical Protective Association. "Apology Legislation in Canada: What It Means for Physicians." Canadian Medical Protective Association. Last modified Originally published September 2008 / Revised April 2013, April 2013. Accessed

17April,2015.https://www.cmpa-acpm.ca/-/apology-legislation-in-canada-what-it-means-for-physicians.

In Plain Sight: Addressing Indigenous-Specific Racism and Discrimination in BC Health Care, by Care, B C Health. Vancouver, 2020.

Cavalli, P, and A J Copp. "Inositol and Resistant Neural Tube Defects." *Journal of Medical Genetics* 39, no. e5 (2002). https://dx.doi.org/DOI 10. 1136/jmg.39.2.e5.

Cedergren, M I. "Maternal Morbid Obesity and the Risk of Adverse Pregnancy Outcomes." *Obstetrics and Gynaecology* 103, no. 2 (2004): 219-24.

Cen, Euiqui, I L Joseph Su, Jun Ying, Mohammed S Orloff, Elijah H Bolin, Xiangyang Lou, Lynn Almli, Lorenzo D Botto, Marilyn L Browne, Tichard H Finell, Mary M Jenkins, Eirini Nestoridi, Andrew Olshan, Paul Romitti, Gary M Shaw, Wendy Nembhard, and the National Birth Defects Study. "Maternal Myo-Inositol Intake and Congenital Heart Defects in Offspring: A Population Based Case-Control Study." *BJOG* 0 (2025): 1-12. https://dx.doi.org/doi.org/10.1111/1471-0528.70045.

US Center for Reproductive Rights Declarations, by Center for Reproductive Rights. 1992-2013.

Chalmers, B. *African Birth: Childbirth in Cultural Transition.* Sandton, South Africa: Berev Publications, 1990.

Chalmers, B. *Birth, Sex and Abuse: Women's Voices under Nazi Rule*. UK: Grosvenor House Publishing, 2015

Chalmers, B. "Maternity Care in the Former Soviet Union." *British Journal of Obstetrics and Gynaecology* 112 (2005): 495-99.

Chalmers, B. "What Do International Health Consultants Need to Know?." *Journal of the Society of Obstetricians and Gynaecologists of Canada* 21 (1999): 556-63.

Chalmers, B. "What Should International Health Consultants Know? ." *Bulletin of the World Health Organization* 77 (1999): 97.

Chalmers, B, and S Dzakpasu. "Interventions in Labour and Birth and Satisfaction with Care: The Canadian Maternity Experiences Survey Findings." *Journal of Reproductive and Infant Psychology* 33, no. 4 (2015): 374-87.

Chalmers, B, S Dzakpasu, M Heaman, J Kaczorowski, and for the Maternity Experiences Study Group. "The Maternity Experiences Survey: An Overview of Findings." *Journal of Obstetrics and Gynaecology of Canada* 30 (2008): 217-28.

Chalmers, B E, and B M Chalmers. "Post-Partum Depression: A Revised Perspective." *Journal of Psychosomatic Obstetrics and Gynaecology* 5 (1986): 93-105.

Chalmers, B, and G J Hofmeyr. "The Gestation of a Childbirth Education Diploma.", *Journal of Psychosomatic Obstetrics & Gynaecology* 10 (1989): 179-87.

Chalmers, B, and D Jeckaite. "Giving Birth in Two Maternity Hospitals in Lithuania.", *Birth* 37, no. 2 (2010): 116-23.

Chalmers, B, J Kaczorowski, E Darling, M Heaman, D Fell, B O'Brien, and L Lee. "Cesarean and Vaginal Birth in Canadian Women: A Comparison of Experiences." *Birth* 37, no. 1 (2010): 44-49.

Chalmers, B, J Kaczorowski, B O'Brien, and C Royle. "Rates of Interventions in Labor and Birth across Canada: Findings of the Canadian Maternity Experiences Survey.", *Birth* 39, no. 3 (2012): 203-10.

Chalmers, B, and A Levin. *Humane Perinatal Care*. Tallinn, Estonia: TEA Publishers, 2001.

Chalmers, B, C Levitt, M Heaman, B O'Brien, R Sauve, J Kaczorowski, and and the Maternity Experiences Study Group of the Canadian Perinatal Surveillance System. "Breastfeeding Rates and Hospital Breastfeeding Practices in Canada: A National Survey of Women.", *Birth* 36, no. 2 (2009): 122-23.

Chalmers, B, and V Mangiaterra. "Appropriate Perinatal Technology: A WHO Perspective." *Journal of the Society of Obstetricians and Gynaecologists of Canada* 23 (2001): 574-75.

Chalmers, B, V Mangiaterra, and R Porter. "WHO Principles of Perinatal Care: The Essential Antenatal, Perinatal and Postpartum Care Course." *Birth.* 28 (2001): 202-07.

Chalmers, B, and J McIntyre. "Do Antenatal Classes Have a Place in Modern Obstetric Care?", *International Journal of Psychosomatic Obstetrics and Gynaecology* 15 (1994): 119-23.

Chalmers, B, and J McIntyre. "Integrating Psychology and Obstetrics for Medical Students: Shared Labour Ward Teaching." *Medical Teacher* 15, no. 1 (1993): 35-40.

Chalmers, B, J McIntyre, and D Meyers. "South African Obstetricians' Views on Caesarean Section." *South African Medical Journal* 82 (1991): 161-64.

Chalmers, B, and D Meyers. "Adjustment to the Early Months of Parenthood.", *International Journal of Pre-natal and Perinatal Studies* 1 (1990): 229-40.

Chalmers, B, and D Meyers. "Babies with Abnormalities: Reactions of Mothers." *International Journal of Prenatal and Perinatal Studies* 1 (1990): 13-29.

Chalmers, B, and D Meyers. "What Men Say About Pregnancy, Birth and Parenthood.", *Journal of Psychosomatic Obstetrics and Gynaecology* 17 (1996): 47-52.

Chalmers, B, H Muggah, M Samarskaya, and E Tkatchenko. "What Women Say About Antenatal Care in St Petersburg, Russian Federation." *Journal of Psychosomatic Obstetrics and Gynaecology* 20 (1999): 1-10.

Chalmers, B, and K Omer-Hashi. *Female Genital Mutilation and Obstetric Care*. Vancouver, BC, Canada: Trafford Publishers, 2003.

Chalmers, B, and K Omer-Hashi. "What Somali Women Say About Birth in Canada.", *Journal of Reproductive and Infant Psychology* 20 (2002): 267-82.

Chalmers, B, and R Porter. "Assessing Management of Normal Labour: The Bologna Score." *Birth* 28, no. 2 (2001): 79-83.

Chalmers, B, R Porter, D Sheratt, A Peat, and C Tucker. *Essential Antenatal, Perinatal and Post-Partum Care Course*. Copenhagen: World Health Organization Regional Office for Europe, 1999.

Chalmers, B, and D Qulieva. "A Report of Women's Birth Experiences in Baku, Azerbaijan." *Journal of Psychosomatic Obstetrics and Gynaecology* 25 (2004): 3-14.

Chalmers, B, M Samarskaya, E Tkatchenko, and H Muggah. "What Women Say About Post-Partum Care and Breastfeeding in St Petersburg, Russian Federation." *Journal of the Society of Obstetricians and Gynaecologists of Canada* 21 (1999): 127-37.

Chalmers, B, M Samarskaya, E Tkatchenko, and H Muggah. "Women's Experiences of Birth in St Petersburg, Russian Federation Following a Maternal-Child Health Intervention Program." *Birth* 25, no. 107-116 (1998).

Chalmers, B, M Sand, H Muggah, L Oblivanova, N Almazova, and E Tkatchenko. "Contraceptive Knowledge, Attitudes and Use among Women Attending Health Clinics in St Petersburg, Russian Federation." *Canadian Journal of Human Sexuality* 7 (1998): 129.

Chalmers, B., and D. Meyers. "A Cross-Cultural View of the Psychosocial Management of Miscarriage." *Journal of Psychosomatic Obstetrics & Gynecology* 13, no. 3 (1992): 163-76. https://dx.doi.org/10.3109/01674829209019573.

Chalmers, Beverley. "The Baby Friendly Hospital Initiative: Where Next?", *British Journal of Obstetrics and Gynaecology* 111, no. 3 (2004): 198-9.

Chalmers, Beverley. *Birth, Sex and Abuse: Women's Voices under Nazi Rule*. UK: Grosvenor House Publishers, 2015.

Chalmers, Beverley. "Breastfeeding Unfriendly in Canada?", *Canadian Medical Association Journal* 185, no. 5 (2013): 375-6. https://dx.doi.org/10.1503/cmaj.121309.

Chalmers, Beverley. "The Case for Perinatal Psychologists." *Perinatology* 6, no. 6 (2004): 320-25.

Chalmers, Beverley. *Child Sex Abuse: Power, Profit, Perversion*. UK: Grosvenor House Publishers 2022.

Chalmers, Beverley. "Childbirth across Cultures: Research and Practice." *Birth* 39, no. 4 (2012): 276-80.

Chalmers, Beverley. "Cultural Issues in Perinatal Care.", *Birth* 40, no. 4 (2013): 217-19.

Chalmers, Beverley. *Early Parenthood: Heaven or Hell*. South Africa: Juta and Co., 1984.

Chalmers, Beverley. *Family-Centred Perinatal Care: Improving Pregnancy, Birth and Postpartum Care*. Cambridge: Cambridge University Press, 2017.

Chalmers, Beverley. "Family-Centred, Evidence-Based, Psycho-Socially Sensitive, and Culturally Respectful Perinatal Care." In *Birthing Techno-Sapiens;: Human Technology Co-Evolution and *the Future of Reproduction*. Edited by Robbie Davis-Floyd. USA: Routledge, 2021.

Chalmers, Beverley. "Globalization and Perinatal Health Care." *BJOG* 111, no. 9 (2004): 889-91.

Chalmers, Beverley. "How Ethical Is International Perinatal Research? Challenges and Misconceptions." *Birth* 34, no. 3 (2007): 191-3.

Chalmers, Beverley. "How Often Must We Ask for Sensitive Care before We Get It?", *Birth* 29, no. 2 (2002): 79-82.

Chalmers, Beverley. "Implementing the Baby Friendly Hospital Initiative.", *Journal of the Society of Obstetricians and Gynaecologists of Canada* 20 (1997): 271-79.

Chalmers, Beverley. "Multicultural, Multidisciplinary, Psycho-Social Obstetric Care.", *Journal of Obstetrics and Gynaecology of Canada* 21 (1999): 975-79.

Chalmers, Beverley. "Over-Reliance on a Medical Approach to Care: Some Thoughts for Consideration." *Journal of the Society of Obstetricians and Gynaecologists of Canada* 21, no. 11 (1999): 1081-86.

Chalmers, Beverley. *Pregnancy and Parenthood: Heaven or Hell*. Sandton, South Africa: Berev Publications, 1990.

Chalmers, Beverley. "Psychosocial Factors and Obstetric Complications", *Psychology and Medicine* 13 (1983): 333-39.

Chalmers, Beverley. "Psychosomatic Obstetrics and Gynaecology in the New Millenium: Some Thoughts and Observations." *Journal of Psychosomatic Obstetrics and Gynaecology* 19 (1998): 62-69.

Chalmers, Beverley. "Shame on Us!", *Birth* 38, no. 4 (2011): 279-81.

Chalmers, Beverley. "Terminology Used in Early Pregnancy Loss." *British Jourrnal of Obstetrics and Gynaecology* 99 (1992): 357-58.

Chalmers, Beverley. "Types of Life Events and Factors Influencing Their Seriousness Ratings." *Journal of Social Psychology* 121 (1983): 283-95.

Chalmers, Beverley. "Western and African Conceptualizations of Birth." *Psychology and Health* 12 (1996): 1-10.

Chalmers, Beverley. "WHO Appropriate Technology for Birth Revisited." *British Journal of Obstetrics and Gynaecology* 99 (1992): 709-10.

Chalmers, Beverley, and Bernard Chalmers. "Post-Partum Depression: A Revised Perspective." *Journal of Psychosomatic Obsterics and Gynaecology* 5 (1986): 93-105.

Chalmers, Beverley, and Robbie Davis-Floyd. "Birthing Techno-Sapiens in Disruptive Times." In *Birthing Techno-Sapiens: Human Technology Co-Evolution and the Future of Reproduction*. Edited by Robbie Davis-Floyd. USA: Routledge, 2021.

Chalmers, Beverley, and Justus Hofmeyr. *Miscarriage: A Crisis Discarded*. 1989.

Chalmers, Beverley, Janusz Kaczorowski, Cheryl Levitt, Susie Dzakpasu, Beverley O'Brien, Lily Lee, Madeline Boscoe, and David Young. "Use of Routine Interventions in Vaginal Labor and Birth: Findings from the Maternity Experiences Survey." *Birth* 36, no. 1 (2009): 13-25.

Chalmers, Beverley, and Dana Solomon. "Actually Empowering Women during Childbirth." *The Lancet* 406 (2025): 1470-1.

Chalmers, I, M Enkin, and M Keirse. *Effective Care in Pregnancy and Childbirth* Oxford: Oxford University Press, 1989.

Charpak, N, Z Figueroa, and J G Ruiz. "Kangaroo Mother Care." *Lancet* 351 (1998): 914.

Charpak, N, J G Ruiz-Palaez, and Y Rey-Martinez. "Kangaroo Mother Program: An Alternate Way of Caring for Low Birth Weight Infants? One Year Mortality in a Two Cohort Study." *Pediatrics* 94 (1994): 804-10.

Chazan, David. "Dutch Fertility Doctor Used Own Sperm to Artificially Inseminate Patients." *Daily Telegraph* (London, England)2019, https://www.telegraph.co.uk/news/2019/04/14/dutch-fertility-doctor-used-sperm-inseminate-patients/.

Chedda S, Tullius Z, Tejeda K, and Leiner M. "Virtual Visitation in a Neonatal Intensive Care Unit: Insights from 5 Years Using a PDSA Model to Improve Family-Centred Care." *The Journal of Perinatal and Nenoatal Nursing* 37, no. 1 (2023): 50-60. https://dx.doi.org/10.1097/JPN.0000000000000685.

Childbirth Connection. *The Rights of Childbearing Women.* USA: Childbirth Connection, 2012.

Clark-Coates, Zoe, and Samantha Collinge. .*The Independent Pregnancy Loss Review - Care and Support When Baby Loss Occurs before 24 Weeks Gestation.* Edited by Secretary of State for Health and Social Care. UK, 2023.

Clinton, H, and B Obama. "Making Patient Safety the Centerpiece of Medical Liability Reform.", *New England Journal of Medicine* 354 (2006): 2205-8.

Cochrane Library. "The Cochrane Database of Systematic Reviews." John Wiley and Sons. 2015. Accessed 17 April 2015. http://www.cochranelibrary.com/cochrane-database-of-systematic-reviews/index.html.

Cone, S K, S Short, and G Gutcher. "From "Baby Barn" to the "Single Family Room Designed NICU": A Report of Staff Perceptions One Year Post Occupancy.", *Newborn Infant Nursing Review* 10, no. 2 (2010): 97-103.

Cooke, R W. "Factors Affecting Survival and Outcome at 3 Years in Extremely Preterm Infants." *Archives of Diseases in Children* 71 (1994): F28-F31.

Cooney, Christy. "Greenland Women Seek Compensation over Involuntary Birth Control." BBC News. 2023. Accessed 3 October 2023. https://www.bbc.com/news/world-europe-66990670.

Csosz, Sylvia. "The Psychological and Physiological Effects of Social Support during Childbirth in African Women." 1992.

Daalen, Kim Robin van, Jeenan Kaiser, Samuel Kebede, Gabriela Cipriano, Hassan Maimouni, Ekiomoado Olumese, Anthea Chu, Isla Kuhn, and Clare Oliver-Williams. "Racial Discrimination and Adverse Pregnancy Outcomes: A Systematic Review and Meta-Analysis." *BMJ Global Health* 7, no. e009227 (2022). https://dx.doi.org/10.1136/bmjgh-2022-009227.

Davis-Floyd, Robbie, ed., *Birthing Techno-Sapiens: Human Technology Co-Evolution and the Future of Reproduction*. First ed. USA: Routledge, 2020.

Declercq, E, and B Chalmers. "Mothers' Reports of Their Maternity Experiences in the USA and Canada." *Journal of Reproductive and Infant Psychology* 26, no. 4 (2008): 295-308.

Declercq, E R, C Sakala, and M P Corry. *Listening to Mothers: Report of the First National U.S. Survey of Women's Childbearing Experiences* New York: Maternity Center Association: Maternity Center Association, 2002.

Declercq, E, C Sakala, and M Corry. *Listening to Mothers II: Report of the Second National US Survey of Women's Childbearing Experiences*. New York: Childbirth Connections, 2006.

Declercq, E, R Young, H Cabral, and J Ecker. "Is a Rising Cesarean Delivery Rate Inevitable? Trends in Industrialized Countries, 1987 to 2007." *Birth* 38, no. 2 (2011): 99-104.

Dennis, Cindy-Lee, and Ellen Hodnett. "Psychosocial and Psychological Interventions for Treating Postpartum Depression.", *Cochrane Database of Systematic Reviews* 4 (2009).

Department of Health. *Breastfeeding Mothers' Bill of Rights* by Department of Health, New York State. State of New York, 2010.

DeRegil, M L, G Fernandez, A C. Dowswell, T. Rosas, and P Juan. "Effects and Safety of Periconceptional Folate Supplementation for Preventing Birth Defects." *Cochrane database of systematic reviews* 10 (2010).

Dobson, Juliet. "Ignoring Women's Experiences Led to the NHS's Biggest Maternity Scandal." *BMJ* 377, no. 0899 (2022). https://dx.doi.org/https://doi.org/10.1136/bmj.o899.

Domanico, R, D K Davis, F Coleman, and B O Davis. "Documenting the NICU Design Dilemma: Comparative Patient Progress in Open-Ward and Single Family Room Units." *Journal of Perinatology* 31, no. 4 (2011): 281-88.

Douglas, V K. "Childbirth among the Canadian Inuit: A Review of the Clinical and Cultural Literature ", *International Journal of Circumpolar Health* 65, no. 2 (2006): 117-32.

Downe, S, K Finlayson, O Tuncalp, and A Metin Gulmezoglu. "What Matters to Women: A Systematic Scoping Review to Identify the Processes and Outcomes of Antenatal Care Provision That Are Important to Healthy Pregnant Women.", *BJOG* (2015). https://dx.doi.org/10:1111/1471-0528.13819.

Editorial. "Cancer Care : Beoynd Survival." *The Lancet* 399, no. 10334 (2022): 1441. https://dx.doi.org/https://doi.org/10.1016/S0140-6736(22)00698-5.

Enkin, M, M Keirse, and I Chalmers. *A Guide to Effective Care in Pregnancy and Childbirth*. Oxford: Oxford University Press, 1989.

Enkin, M, M Keirse, M Renfrew, and J Neilson. *A Guide to Effective Care in Pregnancy and Childbirth*. 3rd ed. Oxford: Oxford University Press, 2000.

Enkin, Murray, Marc Keirse, James Neilson, Caroline Crowther, Lelia Dudley., Ellen Hodnett, and Justus Hofmeyr, eds., *A Guide to Effective Care in Pregnancy and Childbirth*. Oxford: Oxford University Press, 2000.

Enkin, Murray, Marc Keirse, Mary Renfrew, and James Neilson. *A Guide to Effective Care in Pregnancy and Childbirth*. 2nd ed. Oxford: Oxford University Press, 1995.

Escobar, G J, B Littenberg, and D B Petitti. "Outcome among Surviving Very Low Birthweight Infants: A Meta-Analysis." *Archives of Diseases in Children* 66 (1991): 204-11.

Evans, Meredith, Lesley Tarasoff, Yona Lunsky, Kate Welsh, Laurie Prouls, Susan Havercamp, Sisan Parish, and Hilary Brown. "Disability Justice and Collective Access to Labour and Delivery Care: A Qualitative Study." *MBC Pregnancy and Childbirth* 24, no. 832 (2024). Https://bmcpregnancychildbirth.biomedcentral.com/articles/10.1186/s12884-024-07036-3.

Family Care International. *Action for the 21st Century: Reproductive Health and Rights for All*. New York: Family Care International, 1994.

Fleischer, B E, K VandenBerg, and et al. "Individualized Care for Very Low Birthweight Premature Infants Improves Medical and Developmental Outcome in the Neonatal Intensive Care Unit." *Clinical Pediatrics* 10 (1995): 523-29.

Fornah, Frances. "The Childbirth Experiences and Perceptions of Sierra Leonean Women Relating to Basic Maternal Rights." Walden University, Minneapolis, 2022.

Fournier, Sylvie. "Black, Indigenous Mothers Say They Were Sterilized without Full Consent at Quebec Hospitals." CBC. 2021. Accessed 30 September, 2021. https://www.cbc.ca/news/canada/montreal/quebec-hospital-sterilization-1.6188269.

Fox, Rebekah, Sara McMullen, and Mary Newburn. "UK Women's Experiences of Breastfeeding and Additional Breastfeeding Support: A Qualitative Study of Baby Cafe Services.", *BMC Pregnancy & Childbirth* 15 (2015): 147. https://dx.doi.org/10.1186/s12884-015-0581-5.

Freedman, L, and M Kruk. "Disrespect and Abuse of Women in Childbirth: Challenging the Global Quality and Accountability Agendas." *The Lancet* Early Online Publication (23 June 2014). https://dx.doi.org/doi:10.1016/S0140-6736(14)60859-X.

Frieson, Phoebe, Wan-Li Sun, and Sarah Towle. "Consent and Educational Sensitive Exams on Anaesthetized Patients: Experiences of Medical Students across Canada." *Education* 46, no. 11 (2024).

Fukuzawa, Rieko Kishi, and Chang Gi Park. "Role of Intrapartum Social Support in Preventing Postpartum Depression." *The Journal of Perinatal Education* 32, no. 2 (2023). https://dx.doi.org/10.1891/JPE-2022-0003.

Gadeski, Emma. "Dozens More Women Say Provo Ob-Gyn Sexually Assaulted Them." *The Daily Universe* (Utah). March 24 2022, https://universe.byu.edu/2022/03/24/dozens-more-women-say-provo-ob-gyn-sexually-assaulted-them/.

Gagnon, A J, and J Sandall. "Individual or Group Antenatal Education for Childbirth or Parenthood, or Both.", *Cochrane Pregnancy and Childbirth Group* (2007). http://onlinelibrary.wiley.com/o/cochrane/clabout/articles/PREG/frame.html.

Gallagher, James, Natalie Truswell, and Jonathan Sumberg. "Female Surgeons Sexually Assaulted While Operating." BBC News. 2023. Accessed 12 September, 2023. https://www.bbc.com/news/health-66775015.

Garcia, J, M Redshaw, B Fitzsimons, and et al. *First Class Delivery: A National Survey of Women's Views of Maternity Care*. London: Audit Commission, 1998.

The Global Numbers and Costs of Additionally Needed and Unnecessary Caesarean Sections Performed Per Year: Overuse as a Barrier to Universal Coverage, by Gibbons, L, J M. Belizán, J A Lauer, A P Betrán, M Merialdi, and F Althabe. Geneva 2010.

Gildersleeve, Jessica, and Devaleena Das. *Birthing Stories: Silence, Trauma, and the Power of Narratives in Clinical Care.*: In Preparation, 2026.

Goer, H, and A Romano. *Optimal Care in Childbirth: The Case for a Physiologic Approach* USA: Classic Day Publishing, 2012.

Goksan, Sezgi, Caroline Hartley, Faith Emery, Naomi Cockrill, Ravi Poorun, Fiona Moultrie, Richard Rogers, Jon Campbell, Michael Sanders, Eleri Adams, Stuart Clare, Mark Jenkinson, Irene Tracey, and Rebeccah Slater. "fMRI Reveals Neural Activity Overlap between Adult and Infant Pain." *eLife* 4, no.:e06356 (2015). https://dx.doi.org/http://dx.doi.org/10.7554/eLife.06356.

Gomez, Chelsea, and Tara Carman. "Canada Significantly Undercounts Maternal Deaths, and Doctors Are Sounding the Alarm." *CBC* (Canada). October 3, 2022, https://www.cbc.ca/news/canada/canada-maternal-deaths-undercount-1.6600905#:~:text=Canada%C2%B7CBC%20Investigates-,Canada%20significantly%20undercounts%20maternal%20deaths%2C%20and%20doctors%20are%20sounding%20the,maternal%20deaths%20and%20close%20calls.

Gramling, L, K Hickman, and S Bennett. "What Makes a Good Family-Centered Partnership between Women and Their Practitioners? A Qualitative Study.", *Birth* 31, no. 1 (2004): 43-48.

Green, J, V Coupland, and J Kitzinger. "Expectations, Experiences and Psychological Outcomes of Childbirth: A Prospective Study of 825 Women." *Birth* 17 (1990): 15-24.

Green, J M, H A Baston, S C Easton, and F McCormick. *Greater Expectations: The Inter- Relationship between Women's Expectations and Experiences of Decision Making, Continuity, Choice and Control in Labour, and Psychological Outcomes. Summary Report*. Leeds: Mother & Infant Research Unit, University of Leeds, 2003.

Green, J M, V A Coupland, and J V Kitzinger. *Great Expectations: A Prospective Study of Women's Expectations and Experiences of Childbirth*. 2nd ed. UK Books for Midwives Press, 1998.

CDC National Vital Statistics Reports. *Changes in Home Births by Race and Hispanic Origin and State of Residence of Mother: United States, 2018-20-19 and 2019 - 2020.*, by Gregory,

Elizabeth C.W., Michelle J.K. Osterman, and Claudia P. Valenzuela. USA, 2021.

Grey, J E, and D A Goldmann. "Medication Errors in the Neonatal Intensive Care Unit: Special Patients, Unique Issues." *Archives of Diseases of Children Fetal and Neonatal Edition.* 89 (2004): F472-F73. https://dx.doi.org/10.1136/adc.2003.046060.

Guzikevits, Mika, Tom Gordon-Hecker, David Rekhtman, Shaden Salameh, Salomon Israel, Moses Shayo, David Gozal, Anat Perry, Alex Gileles-Hillel, and Shoham Choshen-Hillel. "Sex Bias in Pain Management Decisions." *Proceedings of the National Academy of Sciences* 121, no. e2401331121., 33 (2024).

Gynecologists, American College of Obstetricians and. "Sexual Misconduct: ACOG Committee Opinion 796." *Obstetics and Gynaecology* 135, no. 1 (2020): e43-e50. https://www.acog.org/en/clinical/clinical-guidance/committee-opinion/articles/2020/01/sexual-misconduct.

Habeka, Dubravko, Anis Cerovac, Ana Luetić, Ingrid Marton, Matija Prka, Tomislav Kulaš, and Boris Ujevića. "Modified Stark's (Misgav Ladach) Caesarean Section: 15 – Year Experience of the Own Techniques of Caesarean Section." *European Journal of Obstetrics and Gynecology and Reproductive Biology* 247 (2020): 90-3.

Hack, M, H G Taylor, N Klein, R Eiben, C Schatschneider, and N Mercuri-Minich. "School-Age Outcomes in Children with Birthweights under 750g." *New England Journal of Medicine* 331 (1994): 753-59.

Hall, A, A MacCloed, C Counsell, L Thomson, and L Mutch. "School Attainment, Cognitive Ability and Motor Function in a Total Scottish Very-Low-Birthweight Population at Eight Years: A Controlled Study." *Developmental* (1995).

Hall, D, and G Kirsten. "Kangaroo Mother Care - a Review." *Transfusion Medicine* 18 (2008): 77-82.

Hannah, M E, W J Hannah, S A Hewson, and et al. "Planned Caesarean Section Versus Planned Vaginal Birth for Breech Presentation at Term: A Randomised Multicentre Trial.", *Lancet* 356, no. 1375-1383 (2000).

Harvey, S, J Jarell, R Brant, C Stainton, and D Rach. "A Randomized Control Trial of Nurse-Midwifery Care.", *Birth* 23 (1996): 128-35.

Hatem, M, J Sandall, D Devane, H Soltani, and S Gates. "Midwife-Led Versus Other Models of Care for Childbearing Women. ." *Cochrane Database of Systematic Reviews.* (4):CD004667. (2008).

Heiberg, E, S Skurtveit, E Helsing, and B Chalmers. "Women's Experiences of Giving Birth in Northwest Russia in 2000 and 2002 and in Northern Norway 2000." *Acta Obstetrica et Gynecologica Scandinavica* 86, no. 3 (2007): 373-5.

Hellerstein, S, S Feldman, and T Duan. "China's 50% Caesarean Delivery Rate: Is It Too High?", *BJOG* (2014). https://dx.doi.org/10.1111/1471-0528.12971.

Hensing, Gunnel, Erik Eriksson, Ida Gremyr, and Anke Samulowitz. ""Brave Men" and "Emotional Women": A Theory-Guided Literature Review on Gender Bias in Health Care and Gendered Norms Towards Patients with Chronic Pain." *Pain Research & Management* 2018 (2018): 1-14.

Hodnett, E D, S Gates, G J Hofmeyr, and C Sakala. "Continuous Support for Women during Childbirth.", *Cochrane database of systematic reviews* 10:CD003766 (2012).

Hodnett, E, S Gates, J Hofmeyr, and C Sakala. "Continuous Support for Women in Childbirth.", *Cochrane Database of Systematic Reviews* 3 (2007): Art No: DOI: 10.1002/14651858.CD003766.pub2.

Hodson, Nathan, and Susan Bewley. "Abuse in Assisted Reproductive Technology: A Systematic Qualitative Review and Typology." *European journal of obstetrics & gynecology and reproductive biology* 238 (2019): 170-77. https://dx.doi.org/10.1016/j.ejogrb.2019.05.027.

Hofmeyr, G J. "50 Years of 'Active Management of Labour' Is Enough.", *BJOG* (2023). https://dx.doi.org/10.1111/1471-9528.17377.

Hofmeyr, G J, C Nikodem, Wolman W-L, Chalmers B, and Kramer T. "Companionship to Modify the Clinical Birth Environment: Effects on Progress and Perception of Labour and Breastfeeding." *British Journal of Obstetrics and Gynaecology* 98 (1991): 756-64.

Hofmeyr, GJ, S Bernitz, M Bonet, M Bucagu, B Dao, S Downe, H Galadanci, CSE Homer, V Hundley, T Lavender, B Levy,

D Lissauer, P Lumbiganon, FE Conville, R Pattison, Z Quershi, JP Souze, ME Stanton, P ten_Hoope-Bender, V Vannevel, JPO Vogel, and OT Oladapo. "WHO Next-Generation Partograph: Revolutionary Steps Towards Individualised Labour Care." *BJOG* 128, no. 10 (2002): 1658-62. https://dx.doi.org/htttps://doi.org/10.1111/1471-0528.16694.

Holmgren, Gunna, MLennart Sjoholm, and Michael Stark. "The Misgav Ladach Method or Cesarean Section, Method Description." *Acta Obstetrica et Gynecologia Scandinavica* 78, no. 7 (1999): 615-21.

Hong, Y R, and J S Park. "Impact of Attachment, Temperament and Parenting on Human Development.", *Korean Journal of Pediatrics* 55, no. 12 (2012): 449-54.

Horta, B L, R Bahl, J C Martinés, and C G Victora. "Evidence on the Long-Term Effects of Breastfeeding.", *World Health Organization* (2007). http://www.who.int/maternal_child_adolescent/documents/9241595230/en/index.html.

Hueston, W, and M Rudy. "A Comparison of Labour and Delivery Management between Nurse-Midwives and Family Physicians." *The Journal of Family Practice* 37 (1993): 449-54.

Hutting, Charlotte. "What Is a Kraamverzorgster and Where Can I Find One?" Amsterdam Mamas. Accessed 30 May, 2023. https://amsterdam-mamas.nl/articles/what-is-a-kraamverzorgster-and-where-can-i-find-one/.

Isobel, Sophie. "Trauma and the Perinatal Period: A Review of the Theory and Practice of Trauma□Sensitive Interactions for Nurses and Midwives." *Nursing Open* 10, no. 12 (2023): 7585–95. https://dx.doi.org/doi: 10.1002/nop2.2017

Johnson, Karin, Charlotte Elvander, Karl Johansson, Sissel Saltvedt, and Malin Edqvist. "Medical Interventions and Women's Perceptions of Respectful Intrapartum Care: A National Survey-Based Cohort Study." *BJOG* 0, no. 1-12 (2025). https://dx.doi.org/doi.org/10.1111/1471-0528.18329.

Joy, S B De, and K Bittner. "Obesity Stigma as a Determinant of Poor Birth Outcomes in Women with High BMI: A Conceptual Framework." *Maternal Child Health Journal* 19, no. 693-9 (2015). https://dx.doi.org/10.1007/s10995-014-1577-x.

Jung, Elaine. "Doctors Fitted a Contraceptive Coil without My Consent." *BBCNews* (UK) 2022, www.bbc.com/news/world-europe-63863088.

Kahn, K E, S Wayburne, and M Fouch. "Baragwanath Premature Unit: An Analysis of the Case Records of 1000 Consecutive Admissions." *South African Medical Journal* 28, no. 22 (1954): 453-56.

Kale, Sirin, and Lucy Osborne. "Five Key Findings from Our Investigation into the Free Birth Society." *The Guardian* (UK). November 23 2025, https://www.theguardian.com/lifeandstyle/2025/nov/23/five-key-findings-from-our-investigation-into-the-free-birth-society.

Kale, Sirin, and Lucy Osborne. "Influencers Made Millions Pushing 'Wild' Births – Now the Free Birth Society Is Linked to Baby Deaths around the World." *The Guardian* (UK). 22 November, 2025, https://www.theguardian.com/world/ng-interactive/2025/nov/22/free-birth-society-linked-to-babies-deaths-investigation.

Keedle, H, V Schmied, E Burns, and H Dahlen. "Women's Reasons for, and Experiences of, Choosing a Homebirth Following a Caesarean Section." *BMC Pregnancy and Childbirth* 15, no. 206 (2015). https://dx.doi.org/10.1186/s12884-015-0639-4.

Keedle, Hazel, Risharda Lockwood, Warren Keedle, Daniella Susic, and Hannah G Dahlen. "What Women Want If They Were to Have Another Baby: The Australian Birth Experience Study (Best) Cross-Sectional National Survey." *BMJ* 13, no. 9 (2023). https://dx.doi.org/DOI: 10.1136/bmjopen-2023-071582.

Keilar, Brianna, Isabelle Khurshudyan, and Haley Britzky. "Exclusive: What Led the Army to Investigate Gynecologist Described in Lawsuit as a 'Predator in Uniform'." *CNN* (USA)2025, https://www.cnn.com/2025/11/21/politics/army-investigation-gynecologist-sexual-misconduct.

Keirse, M. "Commentary: The Freezing Aftermath of a Hot Randomized Controlled Trial.", *Birth* 38, no. 2 (2011): 165-67.

Keirse, M. "Just Roar-Rely on Acronym Rhetoric. Roundtable Discussion on the Language of Birth." *Birth* 39, no. 2 (2012): 163-64.

Kennell, J. "The Humane Neonatal Care Initiative." *Acta Paediatrica* 88 (1999): 367-70.

Kennell, J, and M Klaus. "The Perinatal Paradigm: Is It Time for a Change?", *Clinical Perinatology* 15 (1988): 801-03.

Kirubarajan, Abirami, Jackie Tsang, Susan Dong, Jeanette Hui, Padmaja Sreeram, Zuhal Mohmand, Shannon Leung, Alessandra Ceccacci, and Mara Sobel. "Pregnancy and Childbirth during Incarceration: A Qualitative Systematic Review of Lived Experiences." *BJOG* 129, no. 9 (2022): 1460-72. https://dx.doi.org/ https://doi.org/10.1111/1471-0528.17137.

Klaus, M H, and J H Kennell. "The Doula: An Essential Ingredient of Childbirth Rediscovered." *Acta Paediatrica* 86, no. 10 (1997): 1034-36.

Klaus, M, J Kennell, S Robertson, and R Sosa. "Effects of Social Support during Parturition on Maternal and Infant Morbidity." *British Medical Journal* 293 (1986): 585-7.

Klein, M, R Liston, W Fraser, and and the Maternity Research Group et al. "Attitudes of the New Generation of Canadian Obstetricians: How Do They Differ from Their Predecessors?", *Birth* 38, no. 2 (2011): 129-39.

Klein MC, Gryzybowski S, Harris S, Liston R, Spence A, Le G, Brummendorf D, Kim S, and Kaczorowski J. "Epidural Analgesia Use as a Marker for Physician Approach to Birth: Implications for Maternal and Newborn Outcomes.", *Birth* 28, no. 4 (2001): 243-8.

Ko, N., J Darnell, E Calhoun, K Freund, K Wells, C Shapiro, D Dudley, S Patierno, K Fiscella, P Raich, and T Battaglia. "Can Patient Navigation Improve Receipt of Recommended Breast Cancer Care? Evidence from the National Patient Navigation Research Program." *Journal of Clinical Oncology* 32, no. 22 (2014): DOI 10.1200/JCO.2013.53.6037. https://dx.doi.org/10.1200/JCO.2013.53.6037.

Kong, G W S, T K H Chung, and I H Lok. "The Impact of Supportive Counselling on Women's Psychological Wellbeing after Miscarriage – a Randomised Controlled Trial.", *BJOG* 121, no. 10 (2014): 1253–62, .

Kotaska, A. "Commentary: Routine Cesarean Section for Breech: The Unmeasured Cost.", *Birth* 38, no. 2 (2011): 162-64.

Kotaska, A. "Guideline-Centered Care: A Two-Edged Sword.", *Birth* 38, no. 2 (2011): 97-98.

Kraman, S, and G Hamm. "Risk Management: Extreme Honesty May Be the Best Policy.", *Annals of Internal Medicine* 131 (1999): 963-7.

Kramer, M, F Aboud, E Mironova, I Vanilovich, PW Platt, L Matush, S Igunov, E Fombonne, N Bogdanovich, T Ducruet, J-P Collet, B Chalmers, E Hodnet, S Davidovsky, O Skugarevsky, O Trofimovic, L Shapiro, and for the Promotion of Breastfeeding Intervention Trial (PROBIT) Study Group. "Breastfeeding and Child Cognitive Development: New Evidence from a Large Randomized Trial. ." *Archives of General Psychiatry* 65, no. 5 (2008): 578-84.

Kramer, M, B Chalmers, E Hodnett, Z Sevkovskaya, I Dzikovitch, S Shapiro, J-P Collett, I Vanilovich, I Mezen, T Ducruet, G Shishko, V Zubovish, D Miknuik, E Gluchanina, V Dombrowsky, A Ustinovich, T Kot, N Bogdanovich, L Ovchinikova, E Helsing, and for the PROBIT study group. "Promotion of Breastfeeding Intervention Trial (Probit): A Cluster-Randomized Trial in the Republic of Belarus. ." *Journal of the American Medical Academy,* 285 (2001): 413-20.

Kramer, M S, and R Kakuma. "Optimal Duration of Exclusive Breastfeeding.", *Cochrane Database of Systematic Reviews* 8 (2012).

Kukura, Elizabeth. "Obstetric Violence." *The Georgetown Law Journal* 106 (2018): 721-801.

Lagerkrantz, H, E Nilsson, I Redham, and P Hjelmdahl. "Plasma Catecholamines Following Nursing Procedures in a Neonatal Ward." *Early Human Development* 14 (1986): 61-65.

Lamont, Ronald, Laura Fraser, Carmen Amezcua-Prieto, and Jan Jorgensen. "Obstetric Trauma Due to Abuse and Preventable Events: A Commentary on Definition, Classification and Qualitative Research." *BJOG An International Journal of Obstetrics & Gynaecology* 132 (2025): 1951-5. https://dx.doi.org/doi.org/10.1111/1471-0528.18316.

Lawrence, R A, and R M Lawrence. *Breastfeeding: A Guide for the Medical Profession*. 7th ed. USA: Elsevier, Mosby, 2011.

Lawson, G W. "Report of a Breech Cesarean Section Maternal Death.", *Birth* 38, no. 2 (2011): 159-61.

Leisher, Susannah H. "Respectful Stillbirth Care Is a Human Right." *BJOG* 22 March (2022). https://dx.doi.org/https://doi.org/10.1111/1471-0528.17157.

Levin, A. "The Mother-Infant Unit at Tallinn Children's Hospital, Estonia: A Truly Baby Friendly Unit." *Birth* 21, no. 1 (1994): 39-44.

Levin, A. "Viewpoint: Humane Neonatal Care Initiative." *Acta Paediatrica* 88 (1999): 353-55.

Levin, A. "Where Are You Going, Neonatal Medicine? Letter to Editor." *Intensive and critical care nursing* 11 (1995): 49-52.

Lindegger, G, and L M Richter. "HIV Vaccine Trials: Critical Issues in Informed Consent.", *South African Journal of Science.* 96 (2000): 313-7.

Long, J G, J F Lucey, and A G Philip. "Noise and Hypoxia in the Intensive Care Nursery." *Pediatrics* 65 (1980): 143-45.

Lu, M C. "Recommendations for Preconception Care.", *American Family Physician* 76, no. 3 (2007): 397-400.

Ludington, S M. "Energy Conservation during Skin-to-Skin Contact between Premature Infants and Their Mothers." *Heart and Lung* 19 (1990): 445-51.

Ma, K. " Attachment Theory in Adult Psychiatry. Part 1: Conceptualisations, Measurement and Clinical Research Findings.", *Advances in Psychiatric Treatment* 12 (2006): 440-49.

MacDorman, M, F Menacker, and E Declercq. "Trends and Characteristics of Home and Other out-of-Hospital Births in the United States 1990-2006." *National Vital Statistics Report* 58, no. 11 (2010): 1-7.

MacGregor, Laura. "Unspoken Wounds: A Mother's Experience of Medical Error.", *CMAJ* 197, E815-6 (2025). https://dx.doi.org/doi: 10.1503/cmaj.25008.

Mackinnon, Amy. "What Actually Happens When a Country Bans Abortion?" *Foreign Policy* (USA). May 16 2019, https://foreign-policy.com/2019/05/16/what-actually-happens-when-a-country-bans-abortion-romania-alabama/.

Magee, S R., C Battle, J Morton, and M Nothnagle. "Promotion of Family-Centered Birth with Gentle Cesarean Delivery." *Journal of the American Board of Family Medicine* 27, no. 5 (2014): 690-93.

Marr, Mollie C., Jessica Beeghly, Katherine Au, and Katherine Jorda. "Creating a Trauma-Informed Multidisciplinary Clinic." (2025). https://dx.doi.org/doi.org/10.1111/birt.70032.

Maslow, A. *Motivation and Personality*. New York: Harper, 1943.

Mattison, Cristina, John Lavis, Eileen Hutton, Michelle Dion, and Michael Wilson. "Understanding the Conditions That Influence the Roles of Midwives in Ontario, Canada's Health System: An Embedded Single-Case Study.", *BMC Health Services Research* 20 (2020): 197. https://dx.doi.org/https://doi.org/10.1186/s12913-020-5033-x.

McClellan, M S, and W A Cabianca. "Effects of Early Mother-Infant Contact Following Cesarean Birth.", *Obstetrics and Gynecology* 56 (1980): 52-5.

McNiven, P, Klein M C, Baradaran N, Tomkinson, Hearps S J C, and Saxell L. "Midwives' Belief in Normal Birth: The Canadian Survey of Maternity Care Provider's Attitudes toward Labour and Birth." *The Canadian Journal of Midwifery Research and Practice* 10, 2 (2011): 11-21.

Melzer, K, Y Schutz, N Soehnchen, and et al. "Effects of Recommended Levels of Physical Activity on Pregnancy Outcomes.", *American Journal of Obstetrics and Gynecology* 202, no. 266 (2010): e1-6.

Mercer, J S, D A Erickson-Owens, B Graves, and M M Haley. "Evidence-Based Practices for the Fetal to Newborn Transition.", *Journal of Midwifery & Women's Health* 52, no. 3 (2007): 262-72, 312-3.

Midmer, D, A Biringer, J Caroll, A Reid, L Wilson, D Stewart, M Tate, and B Chalmers. *The ALPHA Form - Antenatal Psychosocial Health Assessment Form*. 2nd edition ed. Toronto: University of Toronto, Faculty of Medicine, Department of Family and Community Medicine, 1966.

Midwives Alliance North America. "What Is a Midwife?", 2015. Accessed 24 June, 2015. http://mana.org/about-midwives/what-is-a-midwife.

Midwives, Canadian Association of. "Midwifery in Canada Is Growing." *The Pinard: Newsletter of the Canadian Association of Midwives* 5, no. 1 (2015): 5-6.

Mitra, Monika, Michael McKee, Ilhom Akobirshoev, Jianying Zhang, Kimberly McKee, and Lisa Iezzoni. "Pregnancy, Birth, and Infant Outcomes among Women Who Are Deaf or Hard of Hearing." *American Journal of Preventive Medicine* 58, no. 3 (2020): 418-26. https://www.ajpmonline.org/article/S0749-3797(19)30477-5/abstract.

Montero, S, J Sanchez, C Montoro, M Crespo, A Jaén, and M Tirado. "Experiences with Perinatal Loss from the Health Professionals' Perspective.", *Revista Latino-Americana de Enfermagem* 19, no. 6 (2011): 1405-12.

Moore, E R, G C Anderson, N Bergman, and T Dowswell. "Early Skin-to-Skin Contact for Mothers and Their Healthy Newborn Infants.", *Cochrane database of systematic reviews* 5 (2012).

Morris, T, K McNamara, and C Morton. "Hospital-Ownership Status and Cesareans in the United States: The Effect of for-Profit Hospitals." 44 (2017): 325-30. https://dx.doi.org/10.1111/birt.12299.

Morton, H, and P Simkin. "Can Respectful Maternity Care Save and Improve Lives?", *Birth* 46, no. 3 (2019): 391-5. https://dx.doi.org/DOI: 10.1111/birt.12444.

Moxon, Sarah, Wendy Graham, Veronique Filippi, Hannah Blencowe, Tanya Doherty, Tamar Kabakian-Khasholian, Meghan Kumar, Dorothy Olouch, and Lisa Hinton. "Nothing About Us without Us: Consolidating Experiences of Maternity Care to Advance Equity." *BJOG* 0 (2025): 1-6. https://dx.doi.org/doi.org/10.1111/1471-0528.18300.

Mundasad, Smitha, and Tulip Mazumdar. "Baby Loss in Pregnancy: Pledge to Store Remains in Dignified Way." *BBC News* (UK)2023, https://www.bbc.com/news/health-66259223.

Muraskas, J, and K Parsi. "The Cost of Saving the Tiniest Lives: NICU's Versus Prevention." *Virtual Mentor* 10, no. 10 (2008): 655-8.

Murdock, D. "Handling during Neonatal Intensive Care." *Archives of Diseases in Children* 59 (1984): 957-61.

Murray, Heather, Christopher Gillies, and Armand Aalamain. "Physician Incivility in the Health Care Workplace." *CMAJ* 196, no. 9 (2024). https://dx.doi.org/doi.org/10.1503/cmaj.231377.

Nagpal, J, A Sachdeva, R Sengupta Dhar, VL Bhargava, and A Bhartia. "Widespread Non-Adherence to Evidence-Based Maternity Care Guidelines: A Population-Based Cluster Randomised Household Survey." *BJOG* (2014). https://dx.doi.org/10.1111/1471-0528.13054 (http://dx.doi.org/10.1111/1471-0528.13054).

Nagpal, Taniya S, Harry Prapavessis, Christina G. Campbell, Barbra de Vrijer, Isabelle Giroux, and Michelle F. Mottola. "Are Pre-Pregnancy Weight Fluctuations and Adherence to Prenatal Nutrition and Exercise Recommendations Related to Excessive Gestational Weight Gain?", *Journal of Behavioral Medicine* 43, no. 6 (2022): 1047-55.

National Collaborating Centre for Womens and Childrens Health., UK. "Antenatal Care. Routine Care for the Healthy Pregnant Woman." (2008). www.nice.org.uk/nicemedia/live/11947/40145/40145.pdf.

National Health Services. "Pelvic Pain in Pregnancy." UK Government. 2014. Accessed 24 April, 2015. http://www.nhs.uk/conditions/pregnancy-and-baby/pages/pelvic-pain-pregnant-spd.aspx.

National Institute for Health and Care Excellence, NICE. "Intrapartum Care: Care of Healthy Women and Their Babies during Childbirth." (2014). www.nice.org.uk/guidance/cg190.

National Institute for Health and Care Excellence, UK. "Weight Management before, during and after Pregnancy. Quick Reference Guide." (2010). www.nice.org.uk/nicemedia/live/13056/49929/49929.pdf.

National Institute for Health and Clinical Excellence, UK. *NICE Guideline: Routine Care for the Healthy Pregnant Woman* Vol. PMID: 21370514. CG 62 update, Reprint. London: RCOG Press, March 2008.

Nikodem VC, Danziger D, Gebka N, A M Gulmezoglu AM, and Hofmeyr GJ. "Do Cabbage Leaves Prevent Breast Engorgement? A Randomized, Controlled Study." *Birth* 20, no. 2 (1993): 61-4.

Northway, W H. "Bronchopulmonary Dysplasia: Twenty-Five Years Later." *Pediatrics* 89 (1992): 969-73.

Novick, G. "Women's Experience of Prenatal Care: An Integrative Review." *Journal of Midwifery and Womens Health* 54, no. 3 (2009): 226-7.

Nuzum, D, S Meaney, and K O'Donoghue. "The Impact of Stillbirth on Consultant Obstetrician Gynaecologists: A Qualitative Study." *BJOG* 121, no. 8 (2014): 1020-8.

O'Brien, Elizabeth, and Miriam Rich. "Obstetric Violence in Historical Perspective." *The Lancet* 399, no. June (2022): 2183-5.

O'Brien, Karel, Marianne Bracht, Kate Robson, Xiang Y Ye, Lucia Maria, Melinda Cruz, Eugene Ng, Luis Monterrosa, Amuchou Soraisham, Ruben Alvaro, Michael Narvey, Orlando Da Silva, Kei Lui, William Tarnow-Mordi, and Shoo Lee. "Evaluation of Family Integrated Care (FiCare): A Cluster Randomized Controlled Trail in Canada and Australia." Paper presented at the Pediatric Academic Societies Meeting, Baltimore, USA, April 30-May 3, 2016.

O'Leary, C M, L Heuzenroeder, E J Elliott, and C Bower. "A Review of Policies on Alcohol Use during Pregnancy in Australia and Other English-Speaking Countries.", *Medical Journal of Australia* 186, no. 9 (2007): 466-71.

O'Brien, K, M Bracht, M Robson, X Ye, L Mirea, M Cruz M, E Ng, L Monterrosa, A Soraisham, R Alvaro, M Narvey, O Da Silva, L Kei, W Tarnow-Mordi, and S Lee. "Evaluation of the Family Integrated Care Model of Neonatal Intensive Care: A Cluster Randomized Controlled Trial in Canada and Australia.", *BMC Pediatrics* 15 (2015): 210. https://dx.doi.org/*DOI: 10.1186/s12887-015-0527-0*

O'Leary, J, and C Thorwick. "Father's Perspectives during Pregnancy, Postperinatal Loss." *Journal of Obstetrics, Gynecology, and Neonatal Nursing* 35, no. 1 (2006): 78-86.

Oakley, D, T Murland, F Mayes, R Hayashi, B Petersen, C Rorie, and F Anderson. "Comparisons of Certified Nurse-Midwives and Obstetricians." *Journal of Nurse-Midwifery* 40 (1995): 399-409.

Ogloff, J, and R Schuller. *Introduction to Psychology and Law: Canadian Perspectives*. Toronto: University of Toronto Press, 2001.

Open Society Foundation. "Against Her Will: Forced and Coerced Sterilization of Women Worldwide." Open Society Foundation. 2011. Accessed 20 June, 2023. https://www.opensociety

foundations.org/publications/against-her-will-forced-and-coerced-sterilization-women-worldwide#:~:text=Women%20world-wide%20have%20been%20forced,Africa%2C%20Asia%2C%20and%20Europe.

Ornstein, M, A Ohlsson, J Edmonds, and E Asztalos. "Neonatal Follow-up of Very Low Bithweight/Extremely Low Birthweight Infants to School Age: A Critical Review." *Acta Paediatrica* 80 (1991): 741-48.

Osterman, M J.K., and J A. Martin. "Primary Cesarean Delivery Rates, by State: Results from the Revised Birth Certificate, 2006–2012.", *National Vital Statistics Report* 63, no. 1 (2014). http://www.cdc.gov/nchs/fastats/delivery.htm.

Patel, Kripalini, Liz Newnham, Katherine Gillltt, and Allison Cummins. "A Simultaneous Concept Analysis to Provide Clarity between Obstetric Violence and Birth Trauma." *Birth* 0 (2025): 1-13.

Patrick, Kirsten. "The Importance of Saying Sorry When Things Go Wrong in Health Care." *CMAJ* 197, no. 27, E813-E814 (2025). https://dx.doi.org/https://doi.org/10.1503/cmaj.251210.

Paulson, F J, D Sharnail, and M S Bazemore. "Prenatal and Postpartum Depression in Fathers and Its Association with Maternal Depression a Meta-Analysis." *JAMA* 303, no. 19 (2010): 1961-69.

Pesado, C, R L. Beckstrand, L Clark Callister, and C Corbett. "Postpartum Depression and Culture: Maternal Child Nursing ", *The American Journal of Maternal/Child Nursing* 35, no. 5 (2010): 254-61.

Petryshen, P, B Stevens, J Hawkins, and M Stewart. "Comparing Nursing Costs for Preterm Infants Receiving Conventional Vs. Developmental Care." *Nursing Economics* 15 (1997): 138-45.

Phelan, S M, D J Burgess, M W Yeazel, W L Hellerstedt, J M Griffen, and M van Ryn. "Impact of Weight Bias and Stigma on Quality of Care and Outcomes for Patients with Obesity." *Obesity Reviews* 16 (2015): 319-26.

Physiotherapy, Pelvic Obstetric and Gynaecological. "Pregnancy-Related Pelvic Girdle Pain - for Health Professionals Formerly Known as Symphysis Pubis Dysfunction", 2015. Accessed

24 April, 2015. http://pogp.csp.org.uk/publications/pregnancy-related-pelvic-girdle-pain-pgp-health-professionals.

Pijl, Marit S. G. van der, Corine J. M. Verhoeven, Rachel Verweij, Tineke van der Linden, Elselijn Kingma, Martine H. Hollander, and Ank de Jonge. "Disrespect and Abuse during Labour and Birth Amongst 12,239 Women in the Netherlands: A National Survey." *Reproductive Health Matters* 19, no. 160 (2022). https://dx.doi.org/https://doi.org/10.1186/s12978-022-01460-4.

Posner, S F, D L Broussard, W M Sappenfield, N Streeter, L B Zapata, and M G Peck. "Where Are the Data to Drive Policy Changes for Preconception Health and Health Care?", *Womens Health Issues* 18, no. 6 (2008): S81-6.

Price, M, and J Broomberg. "The Impact of Fee-for-Service Reimbursement System on the Utlization of Health Services: Part III. A Comparison of Caesarean Section Rates in White Nulliparous Women in Private and Public Sectors." *South African Medical Journal* 78 (1990): 136-38.

Public Health Agency of Canada. *Family-Centred Maternity and Newborn Care Guidelines* Ottawa, Ontario: Government of Canada, 2021.

Public Health Agency of Canada, PHAC. *Canadian Hospitals Maternity Policies and Practices Survey*. Ottawa, ON: Public Health Agency of Canada, 2012.

Public Health Agency of Canada, PHAC. *Perinatal Health Indicators for Canada 2011*. Ottawa, ON: Public Health Agency of Canada, 2012. http://www.phac-aspc.gc.ca/rhs-ssg/phi-isp-2011-eng.php.

Public Health Agency of Canada, PHAC. *What Mothers Say: The Maternity Experiences Survey* Ottawa, ON: Public Health Agency of Canada, 2009.

Puhl, R, and K D Brownell. "Bias, Discrimination, and Obesity." *Obesity Research* 9, no. 12 (2001): 788-805.

Pukall, Caroline. *Human Sexuality: A Contemporary Introduction*. Third ed. Canada: Oxford University Press, 2020.

Radtke, Laura, Ricarda Dukatz, Carolin Biele, Alexander Paping, Khaled Sameez, Christine Klapp, Wolfgang Henrich, and Anna M

Dückelmann. "Charité Caesarean Birth Improves Birth Experience in Planned and Unplanned Caesarean Sections While Maintaining Maternal and Neonatal Safety: A Prospective Cohort Study." *CEOG* 49, no. 6 (2022-06-28 2022). https://dx.doi.org/10.31083/j.ceog4906124.

Rajani, Pilli, and Manjula Pathri. "A Comparative Evaluation of the Paperless Partograph and the Modified WHO Partograph in Labor Management." *Journal of Contemporary Clinical Practice* 11, no. 7 (2025): 112-7. https://dx.doi.org/doi:10.61336/jccp/25-07-15.

Ratakonda, Sanjana, Tiffany L. Panko, Sasha Alber, Lauren D. Smith, Margarita M. Cooley, Monika Mitra, and Michael McKee. "Wait, What? What's Going On?— Pregnancy Experiences of Deaf and Hard of Hearing Mothers Who Do Not Sign." *Birth* 52, no. 2 (2024): 261-68. https://dx.doi.org/doi.org/10.1111/birt.12881.

Ratti, J, S Ross, K Stephanson, and T Williamson. "Playing Nice: Improving the Professional Climate between Physicians and Midwives in the Calgary Area." *JOGC* 36, no. 7 (2014): 590-97.

Reading, C, and F Wein. *Health Inequalities and Social Determinants of Aboriginal Peoples' Health* 2009. http://www.nccah.

Redshaw, M, R Rowe, C Hockley, and P Brocklehurst. *Recorded Delivery: A National Survey of Women's Experience of Maternity Care* Oxford: National Perinatal Epidemiology Unit, University of Oxford, 2007

Renfrew, MJ, D Craig, L Dyson, F McCormick, S Rice, and SE King. "Breastfeeding Promotion for Infants in Neonatal Units: A Systematic Review and Economic Analysis ", *Health Technology Assessment* 13, no. 40 (2009): 1-146.

Rivelli, Elizabeth. "How Much Does It Cost to Have a Baby?" Forbes. 2025. Accessed 4 May, 2025. https://www.forbes.com/advisor/health-insurance/how-much-does-it-cost-to-have-a-baby/.

Roach, Jason O'Neale, and Gavin Yamey. "Witnessing Unethical Conduct: The Effects." *Student BMJ* 322, no. 011022 (2201). www.studentbmj,com/current_issue/editorials/2.html.

Rodrigues, V A D S, Abreu Y R, and Santos C A G et al. "Nonpharmacological Labor Pain Management Methods and Risk of Cesarean Birth: A Retrospective Cohort Study." *Birth* (2022): 1-10. https://dx.doi.org/doi:10.1111/birt.12617.

Roehling, Mark V, Patricia V. Roehling, and Shaun Pichler. "The Relationship between Body Weight and Perceived Weight-Related Employment Discrimination: The Role of Sex and Race.", *Journal of Vocational Behavior* (2007).

Rollins, N, N Bhandari, N Hajeebhoy, S Horton, C Lutter, J Martines, WE Plwoz, L Richter, C Victora, and on behalf of The Lancet Breastfeeding Series Group. "Why Invest, and What Will It Take to Improve Breastfeeding Practices?", *The Lancet* 387, no. 10017 (2016): 491-504.

Romano, A M. "Creating a Culture of Consumer Engagement in Maternity Care.", *Journal of Perinatal Education* 19, no. 2 (2010): 50-4.

Romano, A M, and J A Lothian. "Promoting, Protecting and Supporting Normal Birth: A Look at the Evidence." *Journal of Obstetric, Gynecology and Neonatal Nursing* 37 (2008): 94-105.

Roudebush, J R, J Kaufman, B H Johnson, M R Abraham, and S P Clayton. "Patient- and Family-Centered Perinatal Care: Partnerships with Childbearing Women and Families ", *Journal of Perinatal & Neonatal Nursing* 20, no. 3 (2006): 201-9.

Royal College of Obstetricians and Gynaecologists, Royal College of Midwives, and National Childbirth Trust. *Making Normal Birth a Reality: Consensus Statement from the Maternity Care Working Party* London: Maternity Care Working Party 2007. http://www.rcog.org.uk/womens-health/clinical-guidance/making-normal-birth-reality.%20Accessed%206%20March%202013.

Rubino, Francesco, Rebecca M. Puhl, David E. Cummings, Robert H. Eckel, Donna H. Ryan, Jeffrey I. Mechanick, Joe Nadglowski, Ximena Ramos Salas, Phillip R. Schauer, Douglas Twenefour, Caroline M. Apovian, Louis J. Aronne, Rachel L. Batterham, Hans-Rudolph Berthoud, Camilo Boza, Luca Busetto, Dror Dicker, Mary De Groot, Daniel Eisenberg, Stuart W. Flint, Terry T. Huang, Lee M. Kaplan, John P. Kirwan, Judith Korner, Ted K. Kyle, Blandine Laferrère, Carel W. le Roux, LaShawn McIver, Geltrude Mingrone, Patricia Nece, Tirissa J. Reid, Ann M. Rogers,

Michael Rosenbaum, Randy J. Seeley, Antonio J. Torres, and John B. Dixon. "Joint International Consensus Statement for Ending Stigma of Obesity." *Nature medicine* (2020). https://dx.doi.org/https://doi.org/10.1038/s41591-020-0803-x.

Rubinoa, Francesco, David E Cummings, Robert H Eckel, Ricardo V Cohen, John P H Wilding, and Wendy A Brown. "Definition and Diagnostic Criteria of Clinical Obesity." *The Lancet Diabetes and Endocrinology* 13, no. 3 (2025): 221-62.

Rush, J. "A Randomized Control Trial of the Effects of the Bath in Labour." PhD, University of Toronto, 1999.

Schachter, C L O, C A Stalker, E Teram, G C Lasiuk, and A Danilkewich. *Handbook on Sensitive Practice for Health Care Practitioners: Lessons from Adult Survivors of Childhood Sexual Abuse.* Ottawa Public Health Agency of Canada., 2008.

Schrøder, K, R F Lamont, J S Jørgensen, and N C Hvidt. "Second Victims Need Emotional Support after Adverse Events: Even in a Just Safety Culture." *BJOG* 126, no. 4 (2018): 440-2. https://dx.doi.org/DOI: 10.1111/1471-0528.15529.

Scott, J. "Folic Acid Consumption Throughout Pregnancy: Differentiation between Trimesters." *Annals of Nutrition & Metabolism* 59, no. 1 (2011): 46-9.

Scottish Programme for Clinical Effectiveness in Reproductive Health. *Maternity Care Matters: An Audit of Maternity Services in Scotland 1998* Aberdeen: Douglas Baird Centre for Research on Women's Health, 1999.

Sell, E J, J A Gaines, C Gluckman, and E Williams. "Early Identification of Learning Problems in Neonatal Intensive Care Graduates." *American Journal of Diseases of Childhood.* 139 (1985): 460-63.

Sellers, P. *Midwifery* Vol. 1 and 2. Cape Town: Juta & Co, 1993.

Shah, Neel. "A Nice Delivery- the Cross-Atlantic Divide over Treatment Intensity in Childbirth." *The New Englsnd Journal of Medicine* 372, no. 23 (2015). https://dx.doi.org/DOI: 10.1056/NEJMp1501461.

Shakibazadeh, E, M Namadian, M A Bohren, J P Voge, A Rashidian, V Nogueira Pileggi, S Madeira, S Leathersich, Ö Tunçalp, O T Oladapo, J P Souza, and A M Gülmezoglu. "Respectful Care during Childbirth in Health Facilities Globally: A Qualitative Evidence Synthesis." *BJOG* 125, no. 8 (2018): 932-42. https://dx.doi.org/https://doi.org/10.1111/1471-0528.15015.

Shearer, B. "Failure to Progress or Failure to Wait? In Roundtable Discussion on the Language of Birth.", *Birth* 39, no. 2 (2011): 158-9.

Shenouda, Caroline, Aloka Wijesooriya, Amanda Toufeili, Michael R. Miller, Debbie Penava, and Barbra de Vrijer. "Labour Progression in Obese Women: Are Women with Increased Body Mass Index Having Unnecessary Cesarean Sections?", *Journal of Obstetrics and Gynaecology of Canada* 42 no. 3 (2020): 293-300. https://dx.doi.org/DOI:https://doi.org/10.1016/j.jogc.2019.04.014.

Simkin, P. "Non-Pharmacological Methods of Pain Relief during Labour." In *Effectiveness and Satisfaction in Pregnancy and Childbirth.* Edited by M Enkin I Chalmers, M Keirse. Oxford: Oxford Medical Publications, 1989.

Simkin, P, M Stewart, B Shearer, J C Glantz, J Rooks, A Lyerly, B Chalmers, and M Keirse. "Roundtable Discussion on the Language of Birth." *Birth* 39, no. 2 (2012): 156-64.

Simkin, Penny. "Should ACOG Support Childbirth Education as Another Means to Improve Obstetric Outcomes? Response to ACOG Committee Opinion # 687: Approaches to Limit Intervention during Labor and Birth." *Birth* 44, no. 4 (2017): 293-7. https://dx.doi.org/doi.org/10.1111/birt.12306.

Simonovic, Dybravka. *A Human Rights-Based Approach to Mistreatment and Violence against Women in Reproductive Health Services with a Focus on Childbirth and Obstetric Violence*, edited by UN Human Rights Council. New York: United Nations General Assembly, 2019. https://digitallibrary.un.org/record/3823698?ln=en.

Singh, Priya Fielding, and Amelia Dmowska. "Obstetric Gaslighting and the Denial of Mothers' Realities.", *Social Science and Medicine* 301, no. 114938 (2022): 1-8.

Singh, S, and G Posner. "Doctors Behaving Badly and the Tyranny of Peer Pressure." *Journal of Obsterics and Gynaecology of Canada* 37, no. 12 (2015): 1113-15.

Singla, Daisy R., Richard K. Silver, Simone N. Vigod, Nour Schoueri-Mychasiw, J. Jo Kim, Laura M. La Porte, Paula Ravitz, Crystal E. Schiller, Andrea S. Lawson, Alex Kiss, Steven D. Hollon, Cindy-Lee Dennis, Tara S. Berenbaum, Holly A. Krohn, Jamie E. Gibori, Jaime Charlebois, David M. Clark, Ariel K. Dalfen, Wendy Davis, Bradley N. Gaynes, Molyn Leszc, Sarah Rachel Katz, Kellie E. Murphy, John A. Naslund, and Samantha Meltzer-Brody. "Task-Sharing and Telemedicine Delivery of Psychotherapy to Treat Perinatal Depression: A Pragmatic, Noninferiority Randomized Trial." *Nature Medicine* 31 (2025): 1214-24. https://dx.doi.org/doi.org/10.1038/s41591-024-03482-w.

Skibniewski-Woods, D. "A Review of Postnatal Debriefing of Mothers Following Traumatic Delivery.", *Community Practice.* 84, no. 12 (2011): 29-32.

Smith, J, F Plaat, and N Fisk. "The Natural Caesarean: A Woman-Centred Technique." *BJOG: An International Journal of Obstetrics and Gynaecology* 115, no. 1037-42 (2008). http://www.ncbi.nlm.nih.gov/pmc/articles/PMC2613254/.

Smithgall, L M. "Perceptions of Maternal Stress and Neonatal Patient Outcomes in a Single Private Room Versus Open Room Neonatal Intensive Care Unit Environment." East Tennessee State University, 2010.

Society of Obstetricians and Gynaecologists of Canada. *Improving Sexual and Reproductive Health: Integrating Women's Empowerment and Reproductive Rights*, vol. July 16, 2011. http://iwhp.sogc.org/uploads/File/ISRH_booklet_web.pdf.

Society of Obstetricians and Gynaecologists of Canada. *International Women's Health Program. Sexual and Reproductive Rights and Health* vol. 2013 Mar 12. Ottawa, ON: SOGC, 2009. http://iwhp.sogc.org/index.php?page=sexual-reproductive-rights&hl=en_US.

Society of Obstetricians and Gynaecologists of Canada. "Joint Policy Statement on Normal Birth.", *Journal of Obstetrics and Gynaecology of Canada* 30, no. 12 (2008): 1163-65.

Solomon, Magan, Jack Moncado, Mouna Latouf, Mayaluna Bierlich, Gabe Polidori, Lois Chen, and Diane Sautter. "A Health Care System Divided: How Apartheid's Lingering Effects Harm South

African Maternal Health." *McGill Journal of Global Health* 9 (2020). https://mghjournal.com/2020/09/24/vol-ix-a-health-care-system-divided-how-apartheids-lingering-effects-harm-south-african-maternal-health/.

Somasundaram, Praveena. "Hospitals to Pay Nearly 150 Patients Who Say Gynecologist Abused Them." *Washington Post* (Washington). October 8 2022, https://www.washingtonpost.com/nation/2022/10/08/columbia-university-doctor-sexual-abuse/.

Sroufe, L A. "Attachment and Development: A Prospective, Longitudinal Study from Birth to Adulthood.", *Attachment and Human Development* 7, no. 349-367 (2005).

St-André, M, P N Reebye, and J-V Wittenberg. "Infant Mental Health in Canada: Initiatives from British Columbia, Québec and Ontario." *Journal of the Canadian Academy of Child and Adolescent Psychiatry* 19, no. 2 (2010): 116-19.

Starrs, A. "A Lancet Commission on Sexual and Reproductive Health and Rights: Going Beyond the Sustainable Development Goals." *The Lancet* 386, no. 9999 (2015): 1111-2.

Statistics Canada. *Overwhelming Majority of Canadian Women Start Breastfeeding Soon after Giving Birth, and More Than Half Stop within Six Months*, by StatCan. 2022, 2022.

Stephenson, P, M Wagner, M Badea, and F Serbanescu. "Commentary: The Public Health Consequences of Restricted Induced Abortion--Lessons from Romania.", *American Journal of Public Health* 82, no. 10 (1992): 1328-31. https://dx.doi.org/doi: 10.2105/ajph.82.10.1328.

Stevens, B, P Petryshen, J Hawkins, B Smith, and P Taylor. "Developmental Vs. Conventional Care: A Comparison of Clinical Outcomes for Very Low Birthweight Infants." *Canadian Journal of Nursing Research* 28 (1996): 97-113.

Stewart, M. "Talking to, and About, Women in Labour. In Roundtable Discussion on the Language of Birth.", *Birth* 39, no. 2 (2011): 157-8.

Stjernqvist, K, and W Svenningsen. "Ten Year Follow-up of Children Born before 29 Gestational Weeks: Health, Cognitive Development, Behaviour and School Achievement." *Acta Paediatrica* 88 (1999): 557-62.

Stratulat, P, O Bivol, M Stratila, and et al. "Evaluarea Rezultatelor Implementarii Technologiilor Programului National De Ameliorare a Asistentei Medicale Perinatale in Republica Moldova." *Buletin de Perinatologie* 3 (2002): 3-41.

Suozzo, Andrea, Sophie Chou, and Lizzie Presser. "Texas Won't Study How Its Abortion Ban Impacts Women, So We Did." Propublica. Propublica. 2025. Accessed 7 November 2025. https://www.propublica.org/article/texas-maternal-mortality-analysis-methodology.

Sutton, K, and B Chalmers. "Contraception and Pregnancy Options." In *Human Sexuality*. Edited by C Pukall. Toronto: Oxford University Press, 2014.

Swenson, Karli, Sydney Comstock, and Darah Briley. "Reducing Stigma among Providers Caring for Pregnant People with Substance Abuse Disorders: A Systematic Review of Interventions.", *Birth* (2025): 1-8. https://dx.doi.org/doi.org/10.1111/birt.70027.

Symington, A J, and J Pinelli. "Developmental Care for Promoting Development and Preventing Morbidity in Preterm Infants.", *Cochrane Library* (2009).

Tafari, N, and S M Ross. "On the Need for Organized Perinatal Care." *Ethiopian Medical Journal* 11 (1973): 93-100.

Tarasoff, Lesley, Gul Saeed, Yona Lunsky, Kate Welsh, Laurie Proulx, Susan Havercamp, Susan Parish, and Hilary Brown. "Prenatal Care Experiences of Childbearing People with Disabilities in Ontario, Canada." *Journal of Obstetrics, Gyanaecology, and Neonatal Nursing* 52 (2023): 235-47. https://dx.doi.org/doi.org/10.1016/j.jogn.2023.02.001.

The Associated Press. "China Forces Birth Control on Uighurs to Suppress Population." *The Associated Press* (Canada). 29 June, 2020, https://www.voanews.com/a/east-asia-pacific_china-forces-birth-control-uighurs-suppress-population/6191919.html#:~:text=The%20Chinese%20government%20is%20taking,majority%20to%20have%20more%20children.

The Lancet. "Empowering Women during Childbirth.", *The Lancet,* 406, no. 10498 (2025): 1.

The Lancet. "It Happened to Me: Responses to the Stillbirth Series." *The Lancet* 377, no. 9779 (2011): 1720.

The Transforming Maternity Care Vision Team. "2020 Vision for a High-Quality, High-Value Maternity Care System." *Women's Health Issues* 20, no. 1 (2010). http://transform.childbirthconnection.org/vision/high-quality-high-value/.

Thompson, Nicole. "Lessons on the Grief of Perinatal Loss as an Obstetric Provider." *JOGC* 47, no. 9 (2025). https://www.sciencedirect.com/science/article/pii/S1701216325003469?dgcid=author.

Tikkanen, Roosa, Munira Z. Gunja, Molly FitzGerald, and Laurie C. Zephyrin. "Maternal Mortality and Maternity Care in the United States Compared to 10 Other Developed Countries." The Commonwealth Fund. 2020. Accessed 14 September, 2023. https://www.commonwealthfund.org/publications/issue-briefs/2020/nov/maternal-mortality-maternity-care-us-compared-10-countries.

Tilden, Ellen, Rebecca Jungbauer, Erica Hart, and Amy Cantor. "One Hundred Yeas of Seeking Respectfiul Maternity Care: History and Evolution." *Birth* (2024). https://dx.doi.org/Httpe://doi.org/10.1111/birt.12876.

Tucker, Sarah Yahr. "A Growing Number of Women Allege Doctors Abused Them during Childbirth." *Vice* (Canada). October 16 2019.

UNICEF. *The State of the World's Children*, 2014. http://www.unicef.org/sowc/.

United Nations. *LGBTQ+ People*. Geneva: United Nations, 2024. www.un.org/lgbtiq-people.

United Nations. *Reproductive Rights* 2014. http://www.un.org/en/development/desa/population/theme/rights/index.shtml.

The United Nations Convention on the Rights of the Child, by United Nations. 1989.

Draft Outcome Document of the United Nations Summit for the Adoption of the Post-2015 Development Agenda, by United Nations General Assembly. A/69/L.85. New York, 2015.

Vedeler, Carina, Anne Britt Vika Nilsen, Ellen Blix, Soo Downe, and Tine S. Eri. "What Women Emphasise as Important Aspects of

Care in Childbirth - an Online Survey." *BJOG* Preprint (2021). https://dx.doi.org/https://doi.org/10.1111/1471-0528.16926.

Verbeke, Evelyn, Annick Bogaerts, Tinne Nuyts, Neeltje Cromberg, and Jeroen Luyten. "Cost-Effectiveness of Mental-Health Interventions during and after Pregnancy: A Systematic Review." *Birth* March (2022). https://dx.doi.org/https://doi.org/10.1111/birt.12623.

Victora, C, R Bahl, A Barros, G Franca, S Horton, J Krasevic, S Murch, M Sankar, N Walker, N Rollins, and for The Lancet Breastfeeding Series Group. "Breastfeeding in the 21st Century: Epidemiology, Mechanisms and Lifelong Effect." *The Lancet* 387, no. 10017 (2016): 475-90.

Villar, J, E Valladares, D Wojdyla, N Zavaleta, A Shah, L Campodónico, and et al. " Caesarean Delivery Rates and Pregnancy Outcomes: The 2005 WHO Global Survey on Maternal and Perinatal Health in Latin America ", *Lancet* 367, no. 9525 (2006): 1819-29.

Vogel, J P, M A Bohren, Ö Tuncalp, O T Oladapo, and A M Gülmezoglu. "Promoting Respect and Preventing Mistreatment during Childbirth." *BJOG* 123, no. 5 (2016): 671-74.

Vogel, L. ""Do It Yourself" Births Prompt Alarm." *Canadian Medical Association Journal* 183, no. 6 (2011): 648-50.

Wagner, M. *Pursuing the Birth Machine: The Search for Appropriate Birth Technology*. Australia: ACE Graphica, 1994.

Waldenstrom, U, I Hildingsson, C Rubertsson, and I Radestad. "A Negative Birth Experience: Relevance and Risk Factors in a National Sample." *Birth* 31 (2004): 17-27.

Wallin, L, and M Eriksson. "Newborn Individual Development Care and Assessment Program (NIDCAP): A Systematic Review of the Literature." *Worldviews on Evidence-Based Nursing* 6, no. 54-69 (2009).

Walsh, W F, K L McCullough, and R D White. "Room for Improvement: Nurses' Perceptions of Providing Care in a Single Room Newborn Intensive Care Setting.", *Advances in Neonatal Care* 6, no. 5 (2006): 261-70.

Warren, SL, L Huston, B Egeland, and LA Sroufe. "Child and Adolescent Anxiety Disorders and Early Attachment ", *Journal of the American Academy of Child and Adolescent Psychiatry* 36 (1997): 637-44.

Weisenthal, Simon. *Justice Not Vengeance*. London: Weidenfeld and Nicolson, 1989.

Westrup, B, A Kleberg, K von Eichwald, K Stjernqvist, and H Lagerkrantz. "A Randomized Control Trial to Evaluate the Effects of the Newborn Individualized Developmental Care and Assessment Program in a Swedish Setting." *Pediatrics* 105 (2000): 66-72.

White, R D. "Recommended Standards for Newborn ICU Design." Journal of Perinatology. 2006 2013. http://www.nature.com/jp/journal/v26/n3s/full/7211587a.html.

White, R D. "Single-Family Room Design in the Neonatal Intensive Care Unit - Challenges and Opportunities.", *Newborn Infant Nursing Review* 10, no. 2 (2010): 83-86.

The Respectful Maternity Care Charter: The Universal Rights of Childbearing Women by White Ribbon Alliance. 2011.

Whitworth, M, and T Dowswell. "Routine Pre-Pregnancy Health Promotion for Improving Pregnancy Outcomes." *Cochrane database of systematic reviews* 4 (2009).

WHO. "Appropriate Technology for Birth.", *Lancet* 8452 (1985): 436-7.

WHO. *Code of Marketing of Breastmilk Substitutes*. Geneva: World Health Organization, 1981.

WHO. *Essential Antenatal, Perinatal and Postpartum Care Course*. Copenhagen: WHO Regional Office for Europe 2002.

WHO. *Global and Regional Estimates of Violence against Women: Prevalence and Health Effects of Intimate Partner Violence and Non-Partner Sexual Violence*. Geneva: World Health Organization, 2013.

WHO. *Having a Baby in Europe*. Copenhagen: World Health Organization, 1985.

WHO. *The Prevention and Elimination of Disrespect and Abuse during Facility-Based Childbirth.* Geneva: World Health Organization, 2015.

WHO. "Safe Motherhood: Mother-Baby Package: Implementing Safe Motherhood in Countries " World Health Organization, Maternal Health and Safe Motherhood Programme. 19962013 http://whqlibdoc.who.int/hq/1994/WHO_FHE_MSM_94.11_Rev.1.pdf.

Second Meeting of Focal Points of Reproductive Health/Health of Women and Children in the European Region by WHO. Copenhagen, 1998.

WHO. *Ten Steps to Successful Breastfeeding*. Geneva: WHO, 2020. https://www.who.int/activities/promoting-baby-friendly-hospitals/ten-steps-to-successful-breastfeeding.

WHO. "WHO Health for All Database." WHO 20212021. http://www.euro.who.int/en/data-and-evidence/databases/european-health-for-all-database-hfa-db.

WHO. *WHO Recommendations: Intrapartum Care for a Positive Childbirth Experience* Geneva: World Health Organization, 2018.

WHO Statement on Caesarean Section Rates, by WHO. WHO/RHR/15.02. Geneva, 2015.

WHO. *Workshop on Perinatal Care Proceedings: Venice* Copenhagen: World Health Organization, 1998.

Department of Reproductive Health and Research. *Managing Complications in Pregnancy and Childbirth: A Guide for Midwives and Doctors*, by WHO, UNFPA, UNICEF, and World Bank. WHO/RHR/oo.7. Geneva, 2000.

WHO/UNICEF. *Global Strategy for Infant and Young Child Feeding*. Geneva: World Health Organization; United Nations Children's Fund, 2003.

WHO/UNICEF. *Protecting, Promoting and Supporting Breastfeeding: The Special Role of Maternity Services* Geneva: World Health Organization and UNICEF, 1989.

Winberg, J. "Mother and Newborn Baby: Mutual Regulation of Physiology and Behavior— a Selective Review." *Developmental Psychobiology* 47 (2005): 217-29.

Witt, W P, K Litzelman, E R Cheng, F Wakeel, and E S Barker. "Measuring Stress before and during Pregnancy: A Review of Population-Based Studies of Obstetric Outcomes." *Maternal Child Health Journal* 18, no. 1 (2014): 52-63. https://dx.doi.org/10.1007/s10995-013-1233-x.

Wolman, W-L, B Chalmers, G J Hofmeyr, C Nikodem, and T Kramer. "Post-Partum Depression and Companionship in the Clinical Birth Environment: A Review and Randomized Controlled Study.",

American Journal of Obstetrics and Gynecology 168 (1993): 1388-93.

Worth, Jennifer. *Call the Midwife: A Memoir of Birth, Joy, and Hard Times*. London, UK: Penguin Books, 2002.

Yeo, CL, S Choo, and L Y Ho. “Chronic Lung Disease in Very Low Birthweight Infants: A 5 Year Review.” *Journal of Pediatrics and Child Health* 33 (1997): 102-06.

Yoo, H I, B N Kim, M S Shin, S C Cho, and K E Hong. “Parental Attachment and Its Impact on the Development of Psychiatric Manifestations in School-Aged Children.” *Psychopathology* 39 (2006): 165-74.

Zanardo, V, G Svegliado, F Cavallin, A Giustardi, E Cosmi, P Litta, and D Trevisanuto. “Elective Cesarean Delivery: Does It Have a Negative Effect on Breastfeeding? .” *Birth* 37, no. 4 (2010): 275-9.

Zonshine, Idan. “Gynecologist Gets 18 Months in Prison after Sexually Assaulting Patients.” *Jerusalem Post* (Israel). Aprtil 21, 2021, https://www.jpost.com/israel-news/gynecologist-gets-18-months-in-prison-after-sexually-assaulting-patients-665887.

Zwelling, E, and C R Phillips. “Family-Centered Maternity Care in the New Millennium: Is It Real or Is It Imagined?”, *Journal of Perinatal and Neonatal Nursing* 15, no. 3 (2001): 1-12.

Index

N

O

P

R

S

T

V

W

www.ingramcontent.com/pod-product-compliance
Ingram Content Group UK Ltd.
Pitfield, Milton Keynes, MK11 3LW, UK
UKHW040228290926
15471UKWH00001B/67

9 781836 156345